The Muscle and Bone Palpation Manual

with Trigger Points, Referral Patterns, and Stretching

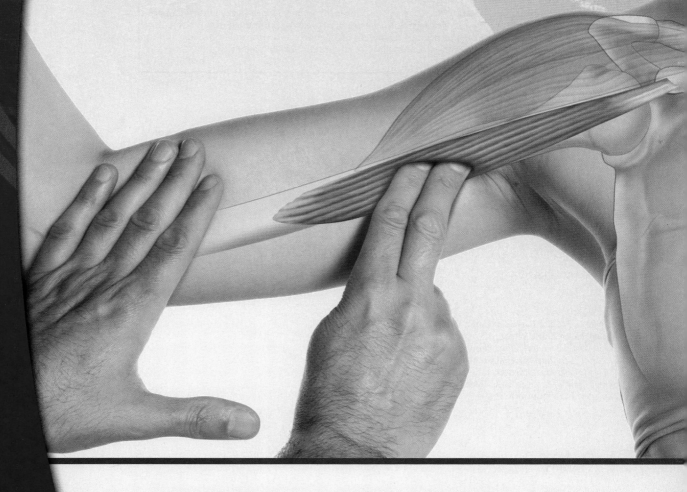

JOSEPH E. MUSCOLINO, DC

Instructor, Connecticut Center for Massage Therapy
Westport, Connecticut
Owner, The Art and Science of Kinesiology
Redding, Connecticut

MOSBY

ELSEVIER

MOSBY
ELSEVIER

11830 Westline Industrial Drive
St. Louis, Missouri 63146

THE MUSCLE AND BONE PALPATION MANUAL
WITH TRIGGER POINTS, REFERRAL PATTERNS,
AND STRETCHING   ISBN: 978-0-323-05171-2
Copyright © 2009 by Mosby, Inc., an affiliate of Elsevier Inc.

Notice

Neither the Publisher nor the Author assume any responsibility for any loss or injury and/or damage to persons or property arising out of or related to any use of the material contained in this book. It is the responsibility of the treating practitioner, relying on independent expertise and knowledge of the patient, to determine the best treatment and method of application for the patient.

The Publisher

Library of Congress Cataloging-in-Publication Data

Muscolino, Joseph E.
  The muscle and bone palpation manual with trigger points, referral patterns, and stretching / Joseph E. Muscolino. -- 1st ed.
      p. ; cm.
  Includes index.
  ISBN 978-0-323-05171-2 (pbk. : alk. paper) 1. Palpation. 2. Massage therapy. I. Title.
  [DNLM: 1. Palpation. 2. Muscle Stretching Exercises. 3. Musculoskeletal System--physiology. WB 275
M985m 2009]
  RC76.5.M87 2009
  615.8'22--dc22
                                                                        2008042526

ISBN 978-0-323-05171-2

Vice President and Publisher: Linda Duncan
Senior Editor: Kellie White
Senior Developmental Editor: Jennifer Watrous
Editorial Assistant: April Falast
Publishing Services Manager: Julie Eddy
Senior Project Manager: Laura Loveall
Designer: Julia Dummitt

Printed in China

Last digit is the print number: 9 8 7 6 5 4 3 2

DEDICATION

This book is dedicated to all of my students, past, present, and future. I have always felt that the classroom and life are about learning and growing. It was a gift to be a part of your lives as we meandered through the intricacies as well as the bigger picture of anatomy, physiology, kinesiology, palpation, and treatment. So much of my learning took place in the classroom along with you.

Thank you.

SPECIAL DEDICATION

This book is lovingly dedicated to Diane C. Schwartz. Her courage, spirit, and passion for life, learning, and love have always been and always will be an inspiration to me, and everyone's life she touched.

Sandra K. Anderson, BA, NCTMB

Sandra has a BA in biology from Ithaca College in Ithaca, New York, and has been a professional bodyworker since 1992, with certification in massage therapy, shiatsu, and Thai massage. She taught at Cortiva-Desert Institute of the Healing Arts in Tucson, Arizona, for twelve years, in subjects ranging from anatomy and physiology to shiatsu, and was Director of Education for one year. Sandra is co-owner of Tucson Touch Therapies, a massage and bodywork treatment center located in Tucson. She maintains a private clientele and also presents workshops on Asian bodywork techniques. Additionally, she is author of *The Practice of Shiatsu* (Mosby, 2008).

Leon Chaitow, ND, DO

Leon Chaitow is a graduate of the British College of Osteopathic Medicine. Since 1983, he has been a visiting lecturer at numerous chiropractic, physiotherapy, osteopathic, naturopathic schools in Europe, the United States, Canada, and Australia. In 1993, Leon was the first naturopath/osteopath who was appointed as a consultant by the UK government. He is the author/editor of over 70 books, and he is the Founder/Editor-in-Chief of the peer-reviewed *Journal of Bodywork and Movement Therapies* (Elsevier). After 11 years as Senior Lecturer/Module Leader in Therapeutic Bodywork and Naturopathy, Leon retired from the University of Westminster in 2004. In November of 2005, he was awarded the Honorary Fellowship by the University in recognition of "services to Complementary and Osteopathic medicine." Leon lives and works in London and Corfu, Greece. He is happily married to Alkmini since 1972!

Judith DeLany, LMT

Judith DeLany has spent over two decades developing neuromuscular therapy techniques in continuing education format for manual therapy practitioners and for massage school curriculum. In addition to instructing NMT seminars internationally, she serves as director of NMT Center in St. Petersburg, Florida.

Ms. DeLany served for over a decade as associate editor for the *Journal of Bodywork and Movement Therapies* (a multidisciplinary Elsevier journal) and con-

tinues on *JBMT's* advisory board. She has co-authored three NMT textbooks and has written numerous articles on chronic pain management for both magazines and journals. Her professional focus aims to advance education in all health care professions to include myofascial therapies in the treatment of patients with acute and chronic pain.

Neal Delaporta, NCTMB, Chair-Elect for National Certification Board for Therapeutic Massage & Bodywork

An honors graduate of the National Holistic Institute in California, Neal passed the NCE in 2000 and established a private practice that includes sports, rehabilitative and spa modalities, and traditional healing practices such as aromatherapy and ear candling.

He has served as a faculty member at the Connecticut Center for Massage Therapy and is a member of the American Massage Therapy Association—Connecticut Chapter.

Neal is a prominent speaker, author, and workshop/seminar facilitator, as well as the creator of Top (Therapeutic Optimal Performance) Massage: A Sports-Based Protocol Designed For All Active People.

Mike Dixon, RMT

Mike is a twenty-two year veteran of Massage Therapy. He is an educator, a published author, and an international presenter in massage therapy continuing education (Arthrokinetic Therapy). He is the senior practical advisor for the West Coast College of Massage Therapy (WCCMT).

He has developed specialty courses in continuing education for massage therapist and naturopaths in the field of orthopedics and rehabilitation therapy called "Arthrokinetic Therapy."

His latest achievement is the release of his new text book *Joint Play the Right Way for the Axial Skeleton* (2006), which involves a multidimensional approach to treating the spine and pelvis.

He has been teaching at WCCMT since 1993 and has taught most courses in the practical department. His specialty is in orthopedics assessment and treatments. Mike also teaches at the Boucher Institute of Naturopathic Medicine.

Mike has trained over 2000 massage therapist and naturopathic doctors.

Sandy Fritz, MS, NCTMB

Sandy is the Owner, Director, and Head Educator of the Health Enrichment Center, which provides education for over 75 massage students per year. Part of her private practice includes working with mental health, in conjunction with a psychologist who provides support care and education for attention deficit/hyperactivity disorder, anxiety, depression, fatigue and pain management. She also provides massage for those dealing with everything from stress management massage to rehabilitative care upon physician referral. Additionally, Sandy has developed and supervises a student massage clinic with the Detroit Lions professional football team. She also provides professional sports massage and rehabilitation for individual professional football players and basketball players. As a worldwide public speaker and stress management educator, Sandy provides programs for the public in the corporate arena.

Beverley Giroud, LMT, NCTMB

Beverley Giroud is a massage therapist and personal trainer with a private practice in Tucson, Arizona. She is a graduate of the Desert Institute of the Healing Arts and holds additional certifications in orthopedic massage through OMERI and Exercise Coaching through the Chek Institute. She has been a massage therapy instructor for eight years. She also teaches business and ethics classes. Her private practice specializes in injury assessment, management and rehabilitation, as well as corrective exercise for injury and postural dysfunction. Prior to becoming a massage therapist, Beverley earned a Bachelor of Science degree in civil engineering at the University of Delaware.

Gil Hedley, PhD

Gil Hedley has taught his 6-Day Intensive Hands-On Human Dissection Workshops to professionals from virtually all health and fitness modalities internationally since 1995. Documenting his unique approach to human anatomy, his Integral Anatomy Series on DVD has now been sold into 27 countries. A presenter at the First International Fascia Congress in 2007, Gil is also a regular contributor of feature articles for *Spirituality & Health Magazine,* among others, and his second book is due out in 2009.

Glenn M. Hymel, EdD, LMT

Glenn M. Hymel is Professor and Chair of the Department of Psychology at Loyola University New Orleans. His principal areas of specialization include educational psychology, research and statistics, and the psychology of personal adjustment. Dr. Hymel is a graduate of the Blue Cliff School of Therapeutic Massage in Metairie, Louisiana, and maintains a practice in the Greater New Orleans Area. Glenn is the author of the textbook, *Research Methods for Massage and Holistic Therapies* (Mosby, 2006) and the tertiary author (along with Sandy Fritz and Leon Chaitow) of *Clinical Massage in the Healthcare Setting* (Mosby, 2008).

Bob King, LMT, NCTMB

Bob King has authored manuals, books, videos, curricula and numerous clinical articles in a massage therapy career spanning more than three decades. He is a Cortiva Educational Consultant and conducts advanced myofascial trainings throughout the country. He is the founder and past president of the Chicago School of Massage Therapy, served two terms as AMTA National President, and is widely regarded as a successful innovator, activist, and educator within the profession. Bob serves on the Editorial Advisory Board of the *Journal of Bodywork and Movement Therapies.* In 2004, he received the Distinguished Service Award for the Massage Therapy Foundation for visionary leadership.

George Kousaleos, BA, LMT, NCTMB

George Peter Kousaleos is the founder and President of the CORE Institute School of Massage Therapy and Structural Bodywork in Tallahassee, Florida. A graduate of Harvard University, George has taught Structural Integration, Myofascial Therapy, and Sports and Performance Bodywork workshops and certification seminars throughout the United States, Canada, and Europe. During his career he has volunteered for leadership positions on the National Certification Board, the Florida Licensure Board, and the Massage Therapy Foundation. His involvement in Olympic Sports Massage included serving as General Manager of the 1996 British Olympic Preparation Camp Sports Massage Team and Co-Director of the 2004 Athens Olympic International Sports Massage Team.

Whitney Lowe, LMT

Whitney Lowe is a recognized authority on pain and injury treatment with massage therapy. He is the author of the books, *Orthopedic Assessment in Massage Therapy* (David Scott, 2006), and *Orthopedic Massage: Theory and Technique* (Mosby, 2003). In 1994 he founded the Orthopedic Massage Education & Research Institute (OMERI) to provide massage therapists the advanced education they would need for treating orthopedic soft-tissue disorders. He is currently a member of the editorial advisory board of the *Journal of Bodywork & Movement Therapies* and has been a regular featured author in publications such as *Massage Magazine, Massage Today* and *The Journal of Soft-Tissue Manipulation*.

Bob McAtee, NCTMB, CSCS, CPT

Bob McAtee is a veteran sports massage therapist, author, educator, and inventor. He maintains an active, international sports massage practice in Colorado Springs, Colorado, and regularly presents workshops on facilitated stretching, massage, and soft-tissue injury care nationally and internationally.

Bob is nationally certified in Therapeutic Massage and Bodywork (1992), is a Certified Strength and Conditioning Specialist (NSCA, 1998), and a certified personal trainer (ACE, 2006).

He is also the author of the book, *Facilitated Stretching* (Human Kinetics Publishers, 2007), from which the stretches demonstrated in the video are taken.

Thomas Myers, LMT, NCTMB, ARP

Thomas Myers is the author of *Anatomy Trains: Myofascial Meridians for Manual and Movement Therapists* (Churchill Livingstone, 2001), as well as numerous articles. Tom directs Kinesis, Inc., which offers professional certification trainings and continuing education worldwide. Tom studied with Drs. Ida Rolf, Moshe Feldenkrais, and Buckminster Fuller, and has practiced integrative bodywork for over 30 years in a variety of clinical and cultural settings.

Fiona Rattray, RMT

A registered massage therapist since 1983, Fiona is co-author of *Clinical Massage Therapy: Understanding, Assessing and Treating Over 70 Conditions* (Talus, 2001). She has 11 years experience teaching the treatment of injuries and postural dysfunction in the professional 2200-hour program in Ontario, Canada, and an additional 15 years experience in leading post-graduate workshops.

Monica J. Reno, LMT, NCTMB

Monica Reno has been an LMT since 1984. She is licensed in both New York and Florida. She is co-owner of the Tuscany Day Spa & Salon, in The Villages, Florida. Prior to that, she operated Allied Therapeutic Protocols in Winter Park, Florida, specializing in the treatment of endurance athletes. Monica was Director of Education for the Central Florida School of Massage Therapy for 8 years. She practiced Massage for 12 years in New York where she was part of the treatment team for the New York Jets, and she worked with George Rizos, DC. Currently, Monica is a member of the Board of Directors for NCBTMB.

Susan G. Salvo, BEd, LMT, NCTMB

Susan Salvo graduated from the New Mexico School of Natural Therapeutics in 1982. Ms. Salvo is a nationally known author, having written *Massage Therapy: Principles and Practice* (Saunders, 2007) and *Mosby's Guide to Pathology for the Massage Therapist* (Mosby, 2008). She has written the chapter "Teaching to Students with Learning Challenges" for *Teaching Massage* (Lippincott Williams & Wilkins, 2008). She has also contributed "Geriatric Massage" for *Modalities for Massage and Bodywork* (Mosby, 2008). Ms. Salvo is one of the featured experts interviewed in the documentary film, "History of Massage Therapy in the United States" released in 2007. She holds a baccalaureate degree in education and is currently working on her Masters of Science in Educational Leadership and Instructional Technology. Ms. Salvo is the director of the Louisiana Institute of Massage Therapy.

Diana L. Thompson, LMP

Diana L. Thompson, a licensed massage therapist for 25 years, has a private practice in Seattle, Washington, treating acute and chronic neuromusculo-skeletal and lymphatic disorders. She authored *Hands Heal: Communication, Documentation and Insurance Billing for Manual Therapists,* Third Edition (Lippincott Williams & Wilkins, 2005). Diana lectures at massage, acupuncture, midwifery, chiropractic, physician and physical therapy conferences internationally, and is a consultant for massage therapy research with The Center for Health Studies in Seattle. She is the President of the Massage Therapy Foundation, a philanthropic non-profit organization whose mission is to advance the knowledge and practice of massage therapy by supporting scientific research, education, and community service.

Benny Vaughn, LMT, ATC, CSCS, NCTMB

Benny has 35 years experience treating athletes and active adults; he is an expert in the assessment, treatment, and care of athletic related soft-tissue dysfunction using manual techniques. Mr. Vaughn is a graduate of the University of Florida, College of Health and Human Performance. He is a Certified Athletic Trainer (NATA), a Certified Strength and Conditioning Specialist (NSCA), and is Nationally Certified in Therapeutic Massage and Bodywork (NCTMB). He also holds a Florida Massage Therapy License. Benny has been on medical staff of the USA Olympic and World Championship Track & Field.

Tracy Walton, MS, LMT

Tracy Walton consults, writes, does research and teaches in massage therapy. She has also practiced since 1990. She teaches "Caring for Clients with Cancer," a CE course for massage therapists, and she has taught oncology massage nationally since 1998. Tracy has researched massage therapy and cancer for several projects, including one with Harvard Medical School's Osher Institute. She helped develop "Touch, Caring and Cancer," a DVD of massage instruction for caregivers. She was the 2003 AMTA Teacher of the Year. Tracy is the author of *Medical Conditions in Massage Therapy* (Lippincott Williams & Wilkins, 2009), a textbook for massage therapy students, professionals, and clinics.

Ruth Werner, LMP, NCTMB

Ruth Werner is a massage therapist, writer, and award-winning educator with a passionate interest in the role of bodywork for people who struggle with health. Her book, *A Massage Therapist's Guide to Pathology* (Lippincott Williams & Wilkins, 2008), is in its 4th edition and is used in massage schools worldwide. She writes columns for *Massage Today* and *Massage and Bodywork* magazine, and she teaches continuing education workshops all over the country. She is also the Education Chair for the Massage Therapy Foundation, an organization dedicated to advancing the knowledge and practice of massage therapy by supporting scientific research, education, and community service.

ABOUT THE AUTHOR

Dr. Joe Muscolino has been teaching musculoskeletal and visceral anatomy and physiology, kinesiology, neurology, and pathology courses at the Connecticut Center For Massage Therapy (CCMT) for over 22 years. He has also been instrumental in course manual development and assisted with curriculum development at CCMT He has published *The Muscular System Manual, Musculoskeletal Anatomy Coloring Book, Musculoskeletal Anatomy Flashcards, Kinesiology: The Skeletal System and Muscle Function,* and *Flashcards for Bones, Joints, and Actions of the Human Body,* as well as articles in the *Massage Therapy Journal* and the *Journal of Bodywork and Movement Therapies. Flashcards for Palpation, Trigger Points, and Referral Patterns* and *Mosby's Trigger Point Flip Chart with Referral Patterns and Stretching* will both publish in December of 2008. Dr. Muscolino runs continuing education workshops on such topics as anatomy and physiology, kinesiology, deep tissue massage, joint mobilization, as well as cadaver workshops. He is an NCBTMB approved provider of continuing education and CEUs are available for Massage Therapists toward certification renewal. In 2002, Dr. Muscolino participated on the NCBTMB Job Analysis Survey Task Force as well as the Test Specification Meeting as a Subject Matter Expert in Anatomy, Physiology and Kinesiology. He is also a member of the NCBTMB Exam Committee and has served on the NCBTMB Continuing Education Committee. Dr. Muscolino is also a member of the Educational Review Operational Committee (EROC) of the *Massage Therapy Journal.*

Dr. Muscolino holds a Bachelor of Arts degree in Biology from the State University of New York at Binghamton, Harpur College. He attained his Doctor of Chiropractic Degree from Western States Chiropractic College in Portland, Oregon, and is licensed in Connecticut, New York, and California. Dr. Joe Muscolino has been in private practice in Connecticut for over 23 years and incorporates soft tissue work into his chiropractic practice for all his patients.

If you would like further information regarding Dr. Muscolino's publications listed above, or if you are an instructor and would like information regarding the many supportive materials such as Power Point slides, test banks of questions, or TEACH Instructor Resources, please visit http://www.us.elsevierhealth.com. If you would like to contact Dr. Muscolino directly, please contact him at his website: www.learnmuscles.com.

FOREWORD

As a massage therapy educator and writer well into my third decade in this field, I know a few things about communicating with students and practicing therapists. I know that students and practitioners of massage and bodywork have remarkable diversity in age, ethnicity, and basic skill levels—and educators have to find a way to reach everyone regardless of these differences. People in this field often don't connect well with dry or abstract material; educators have to find a way to make information come alive. And massage therapists get especially excited when they find that what they are learning has a direct application to the work they want to do. The goal for educators is always to find ways to make their topics pertinent to the choices their students make in the session room.

Many massage therapy students approach the project of learning muscle anatomy with a certain degree of apprehension. They look at those long lists of muscles with attachments and functions, and feel utterly overwhelmed. The topic seems abstract, the language is unfamiliar, and the goal of truly "getting it" seems out of reach. Gifted educators find ways to make this information jump off the page, but the process is nonetheless daunting. What a gift to have a text that illustrates these concepts with thoroughness, clarity, and beauty.

Learning the muscles is a critical milestone in the education of every massage therapist, but those of us who have been in this business for a while know that it is only the first step. Putting that information to use—whether we're helping someone get a good night's sleep, recover from an injury, or train for a marathon—requires an ability to use facts about muscles in ways that can be hard to predict. This work requires a solid foundation in the basics, along with imagination and the ability to analyze subtle bits of information that only comes with experience. It helps, though, to have a text that instills this kind of thinking.

One of the features that truly distinguishes *The Muscle and Bone Palpation Manual with Trigger Points, Referral Patterns,* *and Stretching* is its emphasis on how muscles don't act independently, but interact seamlessly in an integrated whole. This awareness helps users of the book to understand how weakness or restriction in one area can create pain and dysfunction in another. The critical thinking skills associated with this level of understanding are necessary for every outstanding massage therapist.

The Muscle and Bone Palpation Manual identifies the needs of massage practitioners and students, and consistently meets them with accessible language, beautiful art that represents a wide range of bodies, and a sharp focus on how this knowledge can inform the way every massage therapist touches another human being. Meticulous attention to detail and obvious care about accuracy is visible on every page. This book can provide tools for massage therapists and students not only to become soft tissue experts, but to communicate professionally with other health care providers in order to obtain the best outcomes for their clients.

I have always worked hard to raise the bar for massage education. In my writing, my work in the classroom, in continuing education workshops, and with the Massage Therapy Foundation I have looked for opportunities to make it clear that the potential for massage to impact lives is greater than we can imagine. *The Muscle and Bone Palpation Manual* is a tool that can help to launch new generations of therapists in that ambitious direction, and I am delighted to see it enter the marketplace. It, and texts like it, will continue to set the best possible standards in massage education: a goal that supports us all.

Ruth Werner, LMP, NCTMB
Layton, Utah
August 2008

PREFACE

ORGANIZATION

The Muscle and Bone Palpation Manual is organized into three parts and contains a set of 2 DVDs.

Part I covers assessment and treatment techniques. Two chapters are provided that explain the art and science of how to palpate. These chapters simply and clearly explain the guidelines that will help you become an effective and confident palpator. There is also a chapter that explains how to reason out stretches for the muscles of the body, and explains how to perform advanced stretching techniques, such as contract relax (CR) stretching (also known as proprioceptive neuromuscular facilitation [PNF] stretching), and agonist contract (AC) stretching. Another chapter explains what trigger points are and how they are formed, along with what is likely a treatment method superior to ischemic/sustained compression. Given the crucial importance of body mechanics to the student and therapist, there is also a chapter that offers 10 guidelines that will appreciably improve the efficiency with which you work. Another chapter rounds out logistics of treatment by providing an atlas of massage strokes and draping methods for massage.

Part II is composed of three chapters that cover palpation of the bones, bony landmarks, and joints of the body, as well as covering the ligaments of the body. Effective palpation of the bones and bony landmarks of the body is a crucial first step before muscle palpation can be tackled. Effective palpation of the joints is also a necessary skill for assessment of clients. Each chapter in Part II also contains a thorough set of anterior, posterior, and lateral illustrations, depicting the ligaments of the body.

Part III is the masterpiece of the book. It contains 11 chapters that cover palpation of the skeletal muscles of the body. Each chapter presents a tour of the muscles of a region of the body. For each muscle, a step by step palpation is presented, with the reasoning given for the steps so that the palpation can be understood and easily remembered, instead of being memorized. The illustrations are superbly done with the bones and muscles drawn over photographs of real people, offering the most accurate and clear renderings of the muscles and muscle palpations possible. In addition, a unique muscle stretch illustration is given for each and every muscle covered, as well as trigger point and trigger point referral zone information and illustrations for all the muscles.

ANCILLARIES FOR THE INSTRUCTOR

In addition to the clear and simple, yet thorough, approach to the content of this book, the entire book is available in 50-minute Power Point presentations complimentary for any school that adopts this book into their curriculum. The Power Point presentations are accompanied by complete lesson plans along with learning objectives, critical reasoning questions, classroom activities, and more. An image bank containing every illustration in the book, as well as a 1,000 question test bank, are also available complimentary to schools that adopt this book.

ELECTRONIC RESOURCES

To enhance muscle palpation illustrations and text in Part III of this book, a set of 2 DVDs (included free in the book) contains over 4 hours of video demonstrating the muscle palpations of the book. This DVD set also contains cameo presentations by some of the most prestigious names in the world of massage therapy education, including Tom Myers, Leon Chaitow, Whitney Lowe, Bob King, Gil Hedley, and many more. Additional free online resources are included on the companion Evolve website, including technique videos for the intrinsic muscles of the hands and feet, interactive review exercises, a massage research PowerPoint presentation, and joint motion information.

OTHER RESOURCES

Also available for the student and practitioner is a companion set of full color flashcards covering all of the muscle and bone palpations, as well as the majority of muscle trigger point and referral zone illustrations. These flashcards provide an excellent study aid for the student and therapist alike to help learn the palpation protocols and trigger points. A full color practitioner flip chart containing the trigger point and referral zone illustrations and stretching illustrations is also available. This flip chart is an invaluable addition to every practice, offering a quick review at a glance of the trigger points and their referral zones as well as the stretches for your clients. It also serves as an excellent client education tool when explaining to clients how tight spots in their muscles can refer pain to other parts of the body, as well as visually showing your clients stretches that you recommend for them.

FINAL NOTE

No other book offers as much to you as *The Muscle and Bone Palpation Manual*. It contains the most thorough and clear palpation methods accompanied by the highest quality illustrations possible, and it includes a 2-DVD set demonstrating the palpations, too! Further, it offers a complete set of stretches and trigger point illustrations for the skeletal muscles of the body. With chapters on how to palpate, how to stretch, and understanding trigger points, a complete coverage of the ligaments, a compendium of all major massage strokes and draping methods, and a thorough chapter on body mechanics, *The Muscle and Bone Palpation Manual* will easily take the place of three or four books needed in your library.

Joseph E. Muscolino
August 2008

DISTINCTIVE FEATURES OF THIS BOOK

General muscle information, including attachments, actions, and a drawing of the individual muscle.

An Alternate Palpation Position is given when appropriate, often with an accompanying illustration.

Full-color musculoskeletal drawings depict muscles and bones exactly as they appear when palpated to help locate tissues and landmarks with confidence, explained by detailed palpation steps and supplemented with a photo of the starting position.

Trigger points, referral patterns, and a stretch included for each muscle provide convenient access to guidelines for additional client assessment and treatment.

Palpation Notes and Palpation Key for each muscle palpation provide more in-depth information to enhance palpation knowledge, and provide interesting notes to trigger memory recall.

Included throughout the chapters are Detours to individual muscles that are not featured in a full spread, briefly discussing palpation and trigger point aspects of those muscles.

Chapters 7, 8, and 9 contain comprehensive coverage of bones and how to palpate bones and their landmarks. These chapters feature four-color line drawings of bone palpation showing the therapist palpating the client's bone, with the bone visible beneath the skin.

Each chapter begins with a chapter overview, outline, objectives, and key terms.

Two companion DVDs demonstrate and reinforce correct palpation of the muscles of the body. Cameo footage features industry-leading experts presenting unique presentations of individual muscles. Presenters include Tom Myers, Leon Chaitow, Whitney Lowe, Bob King, Gil Hedley, and many more! Refer to DVD icons throughout the book directing you to DVD 1 or DVD 2 for this content.

ACKNOWLEDGMENTS

The longer I have been writing, the more I have come to realize that a book of this scope does not come to fruition without enormous contributions from many, many people. I am so thankful that this Acknowledgements page offers me the chance to publicly thank everyone who helped create this book.

First, I am indebted to all of my students, both at the Connecticut Center for Massage Therapy (CCMT), and in the continuing education classes that I teach throughout the United States. Few people may realize it, but teaching in front of a group of sharp, motivated students is the best way to learn a subject! Each and every time a student questioned my presentation of content, it helped me to hone how to best say and present it the next time. This has helped me immeasurably as a teacher and as an author!

A number of students specifically helped me by either modeling for photos that were the basis for the artwork in Chapters 7 through 9, or modeling for the photos used in Chapters 4 and 6. Thank you so very much. As always, I reserve a special thank you for William Courtland, the student who first sparked my interest in writing books. His statement, "You should write a book," nine years ago placed me on my current path as an author.

I would also like to thank the entire staff, administration, and faculty at CCMT. I have always appreciated the role they have given me, not only in the classroom, but also in helping to shape curriculum content and delivery. My 22 years at CCMT have been a pleasure. A special thanks to Kathy Watt, the Dean of Students at the Westport campus, for her extraordinary support and encouragement!

Many years ago, a professor of mine once said that we all stand on the shoulders of those who have come before us. This is so true. I would like to thank the authors of past and present books on musculoskeletal anatomy, physiology, kinesiology, palpation, assessment, and treatment. We all learn from each other and then offer our best to the students and therapists who buy our books.

One of the highlights of this book is the artwork. Indeed, much of the time, my writing is more of an addendum to the artwork than the other way around. I am indebted to Jeanne Robertson for her sharp, clean, and clear figures in Parts I and II of this book. I am also indebted to Ken Vanderstoep of LaserWords out of Canada who provided the wonderful trigger point and stretching illustrations in Part III. For the muscle and bone artwork superimposed over photographs of models (also found in Part III), I cannot thank Frank Forney and Dave Carlson of Colorado and Giovanni Rimasti of LaserWords enough. Their stunning artwork makes this book shine. A big thank you also goes out to Jodie Bernard of LaserWords, who was fabulous to work with. She was super competent, always available by phone, and fun to work with; a great combination of traits! And a fond thank you to my son, JC, for the illustration that accompanies the Special Dedication on the Dedication page.

For the beautiful photographs that were the basis of most of the artwork for Part III, as well as the other photographs throughout this book, I thank Yanik Chauvin, another great Canadian, once again. Yanik is a wonderful photographer and a pleasure to work with.

At Elsevier, thank you to my entire editorial, design, and production team. Specifically, Laura Loveall, Ellen Kunkelmann, and Linda McKinley in production; Julia Dummitt in design; and April Falast and Linda Duncan in editorial. A tremendously big thank you goes to Kellie White, my acquisitions editor, who created the means for this project to be as wonderful as it has turned out to be. And I cannot begin to thank my developmental editor, Jennifer Watrous, who has been my partner throughout this entire project. No author could ask for a better editor!

A special thank you to Sandy Fritz and Susan Salvo for writing the principal body of the chapter on massage strokes and draping. This book also contains a great number of cameo presentations, both in the DVDs and on the Evolve website. Thank you to the extraordinary assemblage of massage therapy educators who donated their time to be a part of this project. I am humbled and honored by your participation. I am also honored to have my good friend, Ruth Werner, write the foreword to this book.

Thank you also to all the models for the artwork in the book and DVDs that accompany the book. A special thank you goes to Betsyann Baron for her invaluable assistance in finding many of the models! Thank you to Chuck and his video team at Visionary Production for making the video shoot efficient and fun. Thank you to Steve and Lois at Top Graphics, for their fast and excellent work. And a blanket "thank you!" to all the people who worked on this project who I do not know personally. You all share in the success of this book.

Finally, a huge thank you to my entire family, especially my wife and angel, Simona Cipriani. Thank you for your patience, understanding, and support during all the hours that I have spent away from you to create this book. I love you all and look forward to spending more time with you now that this project is finally completed!

And thank you Diane, for all the love and support that you gave me; and the inspiration that you continue to give me every day of my life!

TABLE OF CONTENTS

Part III:
Muscle Palpation

Chapter 1

Introduction to Palpation

Overview

This chapter is an introduction to the general principles of palpation. The two major objectives of palpation, location and assessment of the target structure, are discussed first. General principles that explain how to palpate are then presented. The importance of palpating not only during a client examination but also during treatment is emphasized. The chapter concludes with an exercise that can help develop palpation skills and a recommendation to incorporate the practice of palpatory skills whenever our hands are on a client.

Note: The introductory palpation information covered in this chapter is sufficient to allow the reader to successfully palpate the bones and bony landmarks of the skeleton presented in Chapters 7 to 9. Palpating skeletal landmarks is relatively easy because they are hard tissue surrounded by the many soft tissues of the body; therefore their many features, such as tubercles, shafts, fossas, and condyles, stand out amongst the surrounding tissues. However, muscle palpation can be more nuanced and challenging. For this reason, it is strongly recommended that Chapter 2, The Art and Science of Muscle Palpation, is read before attempting the muscle palpations covered in Chapters 10 to 20. Chapter 2 explores palpation in much greater depth and offers more subtle and sophisticated methods and guidelines that are directly applicable to muscle palpation.

Chapter Outline

Chapter Objectives

After completing this chapter, the student should be able to perform the following:

1. Define the key terms of this chapter.
2. Discuss how palpation with mindful touch incorporates both the therapist's hands and mind.
3. State and discuss the importance of the two major objectives of palpation.
4. Describe the importance of moving slowly when palpating.
5. Discuss the importance of using appropriate pressure when palpating.
6. Discuss the importance of tissue barrier and how it relates to palpation.
7. Discuss the importance of the quality of palpation.
8. Discuss the importance of palpating not only during the examination of the client, but also when treating the client.
9. Describe one exercise that can be used to improve palpatory skills.
10. Explain the importance of constantly practicing palpation skills.

Key Terms

appropriate pressure
mindful intent
mindful touch

palpation
palpatory literacy
target muscle

target structure
tissue barrier

What Is Palpation?

Palpation may be defined in many ways. The word *palpation* itself derives from the Latin *palpatio*, meaning "to touch." However, defining palpation as simply touching is too simplistic because there is more involved. Inherent in the term *palpation* is not just touching, but also the act of sensing or perceiving what is being touched. In this sense, palpation involves more than just the fingers and hands. Palpation also involves the mind. Successful palpation requires us to feel with our brains as well as our fingers. When palpating, the therapist should be focused with a mindful intent; in other words, the therapist must *be* in his/her hands. All of the therapist's correlated knowledge of anatomy must be integrated into the sensations that the therapist's fingers are picking up from the client's body and sending to the brain. The therapist's mind must be open to the sensations that are coming in from the client, yet at the same time interpret these sensations with an informed mind (Figure 1-1). Incorporating mindful intent into examination and treatment sessions creates mindful touch.

> ### BOX 1-1
>
> A therapist may touch and palpate the client with more than just the fingers or hands. Sometimes the forearm, elbow, or even the feet are employed to contact the client. As a rule, this text will refer to fingers or hands when referring to the therapist's contact upon the client.

Figure 1-1 Palpation is as much an act of the mind as it is of the palpating fingers. Sensory stimuli entering through the therapist's hands must be correlated with a knowledge base of anatomy.

Objectives of Palpation: Location and Assessment

There are two main objectives when palpating. Step one is locating the target structure. Step two is assessing the target structure.

> ### BOX 1-2
>
> The term target structure is often used to name the particular structure of the body that the therapist is targeting to palpate. If the target structure is a muscle or muscle group, it is often called the target muscle.

The first objective, and indeed perhaps the major objective of the novice bodyworker, is to locate the target structure being palpated. This is no easy feat to achieve. It is one thing to simply touch the tissues of the client. It is an entirely different matter to be able to touch the tissues and discern the target structure from all the adjacent tissues. This requires the therapist to be able to locate all borders of the structure, superiorly, inferiorly, medially, laterally, and even superficially and deep. If the structure is immediately superficial to the skin, this may not be very difficult. Indeed, the olecranon process of the ulna or a well-developed deltoid muscle may be visually obvious and located without even touching the client's body. However, if the target structure is deeper in the client's body, locating the structure may present a great challenge.

> ### BOX 1-3
>
> As a rule, it is always best to first visually inspect the region that is to be palpated before placing your hands on the client. Once palpating hands are placed on the client, they will block any visual information that might be present. See Chapter 2, The Art and Science of Muscle Palpation, for more on this idea.

As basic as palpation for the purpose of determining location seems, it is a supremely important first step because it follows that if a structure cannot be accurately located, it cannot be accurately assessed. Once the target structure is located, then the process of assessment can begin. Assessment requires interpretation of the sensations that the palpating fingers pick up from the target structure. It involves becoming aware of the qualities of the target structure; its size, shape, and other characteristics. Is it soft? Is it swollen? Is it tense or hard? All of these factors must be considered when assessing the health of the target structure.

It is worthy of note that as high-tech diagnostic and assessment equipment continues to be developed in Western medicine, palpating hands remain the primary assessment tool of a bodyworker. Indeed, for a bodyworker, palpation, the act of gathering information through touch, lies at the very heart of assessment. Armed with both an accurate location and an accurate assessment of the health of the target structure through careful palpation, the bodyworker can develop an effective treatment plan that can be confidently carried out.

How to Palpate

Move Slowly

Given that palpation is a cooperative effort between the hands and the mind, it is important that the therapist's mind has sufficient time to interpret and make sense of the sensory stimuli that are coming in through the palpating fingers. This requires that palpation is performed slowly. Moving too quickly or frenetically jumping around the client's body does not allow for effective and mindful palpation.

Use Appropriate Pressure

The next question that arises when exploring how to palpate is how much pressure do we use? In other words, what is appropriate pressure? Because palpation is an exercise in sensation, it is imperative that the therapist's fingers are sensitive to the client's tissues that underlie them. However, quantifying palpation pressure is difficult. Recommendations for the degree of palpation pressure vary from 5 grams to 4 kilograms of pressure; there is an 800-fold difference between these two figures! One method recommended to gauge light pressure is to press on your eyelids; whatever pressure is comfortable there would then be considered appropriate pressure when palpating lightly. How much pressure is too much when palpating with deep pressure? A good measure of this is to look for blanching of the fingernails of the palpating fingers. If they are blanched, sensitivity is most likely lost.

Generally, most new therapists use too little pressure, probably because they are afraid of hurting the client. Being unfamiliar with exactly what tissues and structures are under the client's skin, they fear damaging tissue and hurting the client. With a stronger knowledge base of the underlying anatomy and more hands-on experience, this fear usually recedes. Conversely, there are those therapists who are heavy handed, using too much pressure and being oblivious to the comfort of the client. If a client tightens the target musculature because your palpation pressure is causing pain, then an accurate assessment of the tone of the muscle is not possible. This pressure would be considered to be too much.

The optimal pressure to use is whatever pressure is appropriate to the circumstance. Some clients are not comfortable with strong pressure because it hurts them; others prefer it. Some clients are not comfortable with very light pressure because it tickles their skin and/or it feels like a tease because the subcutaneous tissues are not being engaged; others prefer light pressure. The same client may even prefer light pressure in one region of the body, but deeper pressure in another.

Although the health and comfort of the client must be kept foremost in mind, the therapist should remember that the primary purpose of palpation is to locate and assess the structures of the client's body. When pressing into the client's tissues, palpating fingers usually sink in until a tissue barrier is felt. A tissue barrier is felt when the client's tissues offer an increased resistance to the pressure of the therapist's fingers. The tissue that is providing the barrier is often the tissue that is important to locate and assess. It is important to not blindly push past this tissue barrier, but rather to match the resistance of this tissue and explore it more fully. Therefore appropriate pressure employed to palpate a client's tissues is usually whatever pressure is necessary to reach and explore the tissue that is providing the tissue barrier.

If a structure is located three layers down, then it may be impossible to palpate it unless deeper pressure is employed. For example, accessing the psoas major muscle within the abdominopelvic cavity requires a good amount of pressure. This does not mean that the therapist should be rough, but if enough pressure is not used, the muscle cannot be reached and therefore cannot be palpated, located, and assessed. When we are working clinically, if we do not accurately assess the health of a client's structure because it requires deeper pressure that might temporarily be slightly uncomfortable for the client, then we will never be able to assess the client's condition; without an accurate assessment, we cannot treat the client to help them improve and feel better. Having said that, whenever lighter pressure can be used, it should. For example, if the medial or lateral epicondyle of the humerus is being palpated, there is simply no reason to press with anything more than light pressure, because these structures are located superficially (Figure 1-2). The same may be said for a thin superficial muscle of the body.

Quality of Palpation Touch

There is another aspect of palpation that must be addressed, which is the quality of the palpation touch. The quality of the palpation touch should be comfortable to the client. Generally, palpation is best achieved by the therapist using their fingers. When palpating with fingers, finger pads should ide-

A   B

Figure 1-2 This figure illustrates the idea of using pressure that is appropriate to the structure being palpated. When the medial and lateral epicondyles of the humerus are being palpated, only light pressure is needed **(A)**. However, when the psoas major muscle is palpated, deeper pressure is required **(B)**.

ally be used, not fingertips. Fingertip palpation tends to feel to the client as though he or she is being poked, not palpated. From the point of view of the therapist, finger pad palpation is also more desirable because the pads of the fingers are much more sensitive than the fingertips and better able to pick up subtle palpatory clues in the client's body.

When Do We Palpate?

Always. Whenever we are contacting the client, we should be palpating. This is true not only during the assessment phase of the session, but also during the treatment phase. Too many therapists view palpation and treatment as separate entities that are compartmentalized within a session. A therapist often spends the first part of the session palpating and gathering sensory input for the sake of assessment and evaluation. Using the information gathered during this palpation assessment stage, a treatment plan is determined and the therapist then spends the rest of the session implementing the treatment plan by outputting pressure into the client's tissues. Rigidly seen in this manner, palpation and treatment might each be viewed as a one-way street: palpation is *sensory information in* from the client, and treatment is *motor pressure out* to the client. The problem with this view is that we can also glean valuable assessment information while we are treating.

Treatment should be a two-way street that involves not just motor pressure out to the tissues of the client, but also continued sensory information in from the tissues of the client's body (Figure 1-3). While we are exerting pressure on the client's tissue, we are also sensing the quality of the tissue and its response to our pressure. This new information might guide us to alter or fine-tune our treatment for the client. Thus while we work, we continue to assess, gathering information that guides the pace, depth, or direction of the next strokes. Ideally, no stroke should be carried out in a cookbook manner, performed as if on autopilot. Treatment is a dynamic process. How the middle and end of each stroke are performed should be determined from the response of the client to that stroke as we perform it. This is the essence of mindful touch, having a fluid interplay between assessment and treatment; assessment

Figure 1-3 This figure illustrates the idea that palpation should be done whenever the therapist contacts the client, even when administering treatment strokes. At the same time that motor pressure is being applied to the client's tissues, the hands should be picking up all palpatory sensory signals that help with assessment. In other words, treatment is a two-way street: motor signals go out; and sensory signals come in, informing the treatment as it is administered.

informs treatment and treatment informs assessment, creating optimal therapeutic care for the client.

How to Learn Palpation

A long-standing exercise to learn palpation is to take a hair and place it under a page of a textbook without seeing where you placed it. With your eyes closed, palpate for the hair until you find it and can trace its shape under the page. Once found, now replace the hair, this time under two pages, and palpate to locate and trace it. Continue to increase the number of pages placed over the hair until you cannot find it. If this exercise is repeated, the number of pages under which you can locate and trace the hair will gradually increase, and your sensitivity will improve.

Even more important than performing palpation exercises with textbooks, it is imperative that palpation is applied directly to the client. When your hands are on your fellow students in school, or on your clients if you are in professional practice, constantly try to feel for the structures about which you have learned in your anatomy, physiology, and kinesiology classes. As your hands are moving on the client's skin, close your eyes so that you block out extraneous sensory stimuli and try to picture all the subcutaneous structures over which your hands are passing. The better you can picture an underlying structure, the better you will be able to feel it, with your palpating hands and your mind. Once felt, you can focus on locating its precise location and assessing its tissue quality.

Given that the foundation of all manual skills rests upon our palpatory ability to read the clues and signs that a client's body offers, the better we hone this skill, the greater palpatory literacy we gain. Perfecting our palpatory literacy is a work in progress, an endless journey. The greater we polish and perfect this skill, the greater our therapeutic potential becomes, bringing greater benefit to our clients. However, written chapters can only provide guidelines and a framework for how to palpate. Ultimately, palpation is a kinesthetic skill, and as such can only be learned by kinesthetic means. In other words, "palpation cannot be learned by reading or listening; it can only be learned by palpation."[1]

Reference

1. Frymann VM: Palpation, its study in the workshop, *AAO Yearbook*:16-31, 1963.

Chapter 2

The Art and Science of Muscle Palpation

Overview

This chapter expands on the principles of palpation covered in Chapter 1, specifically discussing palpation as it applies to the skeletal muscles of the body. Twenty guidelines are discussed that comprise the art and science of muscle palpation. The two most basic guidelines, described as the *science of muscle palpation*, are knowing the attachments and actions of the target muscle. The additional 18 guidelines describe how to begin and perfect the *art of muscle palpation*. In all, these guidelines can help increase palpatory literacy of the muscles of the body. The chapter concludes with a summary list of all 20 guidelines.

Chapter Outline

Chapter Objectives

After completing this chapter, the student should be able to perform the following:

1. Define the key terms of this chapter.
2. Explain why and demonstrate how knowing the attachments of a muscle is useful for its palpation.
3. Explain why and demonstrate how knowing the actions of a muscle is useful for its palpation.
4. Discuss and give an example of the importance of choosing the best action of a target muscle to isolate its contraction.
5. Discuss and give an example of the idea of using critical reasoning to figure out how to palpate a muscle instead of memorizing its palpation procedure.
6. Discuss the value of and be able to demonstrate how to add resistance to the client's contraction of the target muscle.
7. Explain and give an example of why another joint should not be crossed when adding resistance to the client's contraction of the target muscle.
8. Explain why it is best to look for a target muscle before placing the palpating hand on the client.
9. Explain why it is best to first locate a target muscle in the easiest place possible.
10. Discuss the value of and demonstrate strumming perpendicularly across the belly or tendon of a target muscle.
11. Explain the value of and be able to use baby steps when palpating a muscle.
12. Discuss the importance of alternately contracting and relaxing the target muscle.
13. Explain, give an example of, and demonstrate how knowledge of coupled actions can help palpation of scapular rotator muscles.
14. Explain, give an example of, and demonstrate how to use reciprocal inhibition to palpate a target muscle.
15. Explain the importance of using appropriate pressure, and give examples of when using light pressure is preferable and when using deep pressure is preferable.
16. Discuss the importance of slow palpation and the client's breathing pattern when palpating deeper muscles.
17. Explain and give an example of using one muscle as a landmark to locate and palpate another muscle.
18. Discuss why it is important to relax and passively slacken a target muscle when palpating its bony attachments.
19. Explain why it can be helpful for therapists to close their eyes when palpating.

Continued

2

20. Explain why it can be helpful for the therapist to construct a mental image of the client's anatomy under the skin.
21. Describe an approach that can be tried to lessen the sensitivity of a client who is ticklish.

22. Explain the importance of having short and smooth fingernails.
23. Discuss the relationship between using the optimal client position for target muscle palpation and treating the client.

Key Terms

ADD resistance
alternately contract and relax
appropriate pressure
art of muscle palpation
baby steps
coupled actions

isolated contraction
look before you touch
optimal palpation position
palpation hand
reciprocal inhibition
science of muscle palpation

stabilization hand
strumming perpendicularly
target muscle
target structure
visual observation

Introduction

As described in Chapter 1, palpation of the client's body involves the location and assessment of a structure termed the target structure. The first step of palpation is to accurately locate the target structure. Once located, the second step is to assess its health. When the target structure is a bone or bony landmark, the process of palpation is relatively easy because the skeleton is a hard tissue that is surrounded by soft tissues. Therefore bones and bony landmarks stand out. However, when the target structure is a muscle, palpation can be more difficult because a muscle is a soft tissue that is usually surrounded by other soft tissues; this makes the discernment of one muscle from all the adjacent muscles and other soft tissues more challenging.

Given that massage therapists and many other bodyworkers work primarily on the muscles, accurate palpation of the musculature is of the utmost importance; this is especially true when working clinically. The emphasis of this chapter is to learn how to carry out the first step of muscle palpation; that is, to learn how to locate a target muscle. When we speak of palpating a muscle, as a rule we are referring to the location of the muscle. Toward this end, 20 guidelines are offered in this chapter that will help increase palpatory literacy of the musculature of the body. This chapter should be read in its entirety before attempting the palpations of the skeletal muscles covered in Chapters 10 to 20.

 Refer to the DVD 1 for a demonstration of how to palpate.

The Science of Muscle Palpation

Guideline #1: Know the Attachments of the Target Muscle

When a target muscle is superficial, it is usually not difficult to palpate. If we know where it is located, we can simply place our hands there and feel for it. Unless there is a great deal of subcutaneous fat in that region of the body, apart from the client's skin, we will be directly on the muscle. Therefore the first step of muscle palpation is to know the attachments of the target muscle. For example, if we know that the deltoid is attached to the lateral clavicle, acromion

Figure 2-1 The deltoid is a superficial muscle and can be palpated by simply placing our palpating hand on the muscle between its attachments. Therefore knowing the attachments of the target muscle is the first necessary step when looking to palpate it.

process, spine of the scapula, and deltoid tuberosity of the humerus, then we need simply place our palpating hand there to feel it (Figure 2-1).

Guideline #2: Know the Actions of the Target Muscle

Often, even if a target muscle is superficial, it can be difficult to discern the borders of the muscle. If the target muscle is deep to another muscle, it can be that much harder to palpate and discern from superficial and other nearby muscles. To better discern the target muscle from all adjacent musculature and other soft tissues, it is helpful to ask the client to contract the target muscle by doing one or more of its actions. If the target muscle contracts, it will become palpably harder. As-

YOU ARE HERE

the action chosen is shared with an adjacent muscle, then it will also contract, making it very difficult to discern the target muscle from the adjacent muscle.

For this reason, knowing which joint action to ask the client to perform is where the therapist needs to be creative and think critically. This is where the art of muscle palpation begins. It requires knowledge of not only of the actions of the target muscle, but also the actions of all adjacent muscles. With this knowledge, the client can be asked to perform the best joint action for the palpation of the target muscle.

BOX 2-1

The goal when engaging the target muscle to contract is to have an isolated contraction of the target muscle. This means that the target muscle must be the only muscle that contracts, and every other muscle must remain relaxed. Although this is the ideal, it is not always possible to achieve.

BOX 2-2

There are times when the client is not able to perform only the action that is asked for by the therapist; this is especially true with motions of the toes, because we do not usually develop the coordination necessary to isolate certain toe actions. For example, if the target muscle is the extensor digitorum longus (EDL) and the client is asked to engage this muscle by extending toes two through five at the metatarsophalangeal and interphalangeal joints, the client may be unable to extend these toes without also extending the big toe (toe one) at the same time. This poses a problem because extending the big toe will also engage the extensor hallucis longus (EHL) muscle. When this happens, it is tempting to isolate extension of toes two through five by holding down the big toe of the client so that it does not move into extension. However, the goal of engaging the target muscle is for it to be the only muscle that contracts. If the big toe is held down in this scenario, even though the big toe is not moving, the EHL muscle is still contracting; it is simply contracting isometrically instead of concentrically. This will still cause the EHL to contract and harden, making it harder to palpate and discern the EDL. For this reason, any time that a client contracts a muscle that he or she is not supposed to, preventing the body part from moving does not help the palpation. It is the *contraction* of any muscle other than the target muscle that is undesirable, not the movement of a client's body part.

Figure 2-2 The precise location of the deltoid is more easily palpated if the deltoid is contracted. In this figure, the client is asked to abduct the arm at the shoulder against the force of gravity. When a muscle contracts, it becomes palpably harder and is easier to distinguish from the adjacent soft tissues. Therefore knowing the actions of the target muscle is the second necessary step when looking to palpate a muscle.

suming that all the adjacent muscles stay relaxed and therefore palpably soft, the difference in tissue texture between the hard target muscle and the soft adjacent muscles will be clear. This will allow an accurate determination of the location of the target muscle. Therefore the second step of muscle palpation is to know the actions of the target muscle (Figure 2-2).

Guidelines one and two of muscle palpation involve knowing the "science" of the target muscle; in other words, knowing the attachments and actions of the muscle that were learned when the muscles of the body were first learned. Armed with this knowledge, the majority of muscle palpations can be reasoned out instead of memorized. Using the attachments and actions to palpate a target muscle can be thought of as the science of muscle palpation.

Beginning the Art of Muscle Palpation

Guideline #3: Choose the Best Action of the Target Muscle to Make It Contract

Applying knowledge of the attachments and actions of a target muscle to palpate it is a solid foundation for palpatory literacy. However, effective palpation requires not only that the target muscle contracts, but that an isolated contraction of the target muscle occurs. This means that the target muscle needs to be the only muscle that contracts, and all muscles near the target muscle must remain relaxed. Unfortunately, because adjacent muscles often share the same joint action with the target muscle, it is usually not enough to simply place our hands on the location of the target muscle and then choose any one of the target muscle's actions to contract it. If

For example, if the flexor carpi radialis of the wrist flexor group is the target muscle, then asking the client to flex the hand at the wrist joint will engage not only the flexor carpi radialis, but also the other two wrist flexor group muscles, the palmaris longus and flexor carpi ulnaris. In this case, to palpate and discern the flexor carpi radialis from the adjacent palmaris longus and flexor carpi ulnaris, the client should be asked to do radial deviation of the hand at the wrist joint instead of flexion of the hand at the wrist joint. This will isolate the contraction to the flexor carpi radialis. It becomes palpa-

Figure 2-3 The flexor carpi radialis (FCR) muscle is being palpated. To make the FCR easier to palpate, the client is asked to do one of its actions. If the client is asked to flex the hand at the wrist joint as shown in **A**, the FCR will contract, but so will the adjacent palmaris longus (PL) muscle, making it difficult to discern the FCR from the PL. However, if the client is asked to radially deviate the hand at the wrist joint as shown in **B**, the contraction is isolated to the FCR while the adjacent PL remains relaxed. This makes it easier to palpate and discern the FCR.

bly harder than the relaxed and palpably softer palmaris longus and flexor carpi ulnaris muscles, which facilitates palpating and locating the flexor carpi radialis (Figure 2-3).

Perfecting the Art of Muscle Palpation

Knowing the attachments and actions of the target muscle are the first two steps of learning the science of muscle palpation. Determining which joint action to ask the client to perform is the beginning of learning the art of muscle palpation. However, perfecting the art of muscle palpation involves the knowledge and application of many more guidelines. These additional guidelines are presented in the following pages. After discussing each of the guidelines, a summary list of all 20 muscle palpation guidelines is given. It is difficult if not impossible to memorize a list this long; rather these guidelines need to be learned by using them as the palpations of the skeletal muscles of the body are covered in Chapters 10 to 20 of Part III of this book. With practice, these guidelines will become familiar and comfortable to you and will enhance the art and science of your muscle palpation technique.

Guideline #4: Add Resistance to the Contraction of the Target Muscle

When a client is asked to do one of the joint actions of the target muscle to make it contract, harden, and stand out, there are times when this contraction is not forceful enough to make it easily palpable. This is especially true if the joint action does not require a large body part to be moved and/or if the body part that is moved is not moved against gravity. When the client's contraction of the target muscle is not forceful enough, it might be necessary for the therapist to add resistance, so that the target muscle contracts harder and stands out more. A good example is when the target muscle is the pronator teres and the client is asked to pronate the forearm at the radioulnar joints. Because the forearm is not a very large body part and pronation does not occur against gravity, the pronator teres muscle will contract, but most likely not forcefully enough to make it stand out and be easily palpable. In this case, the therapist can add resistance to the client's contraction by resisting the forearm during pronation. This will require a more forceful contraction of the pronator teres, making it easier to palpate and discern from the adjacent musculature (Figure 2-4).

> **BOX 2-3**
>
> When palpating, the hand of the therapist that is doing the palpation is called the palpation hand. The other hand, in this case offering resistance, is called the stabilization hand.

Resisting a client's target muscle contraction is not a battle between the therapist and client to see who is stronger. The role of the therapist is simply to oppose the force of the client's muscle contraction, not overpower the client. The degree that the client is asked to contract the target muscle can vary. Ideally, it should be the lightest amount necessary to bring out the target muscle's contraction so that it is palpable. However, there are times when a forceful contraction might be needed to achieve this. A good guideline is to begin with a gentle resistance as you try to palpate the target muscle. If it not successful, then gradually increase the force of the resistance as necessary.

> **BOX 2-4**
>
> When you ask the client to contract the target muscle or to contract it against your resistance during palpation, remember to give the client a rest every few seconds or so. Holding a sustained isometric contraction can become uncomfortable and painful. It is more comfortable for the client and actually better for our palpation procedure if the client is asked to alternately contract and relax the target muscle instead of holding a sustained isometric contraction (see Guideline #9 for more on alternately contracting and relaxing the target muscle).

Whenever resistance is added to the contraction of the target muscle by the client, it is extremely important that the therapist does not cross any additional joints with the placement of the stabilization hand. The goal of having a client contract the target muscle during palpation is to limit contrac-

Figure 2-4 To create a more forceful contraction of the pronator teres muscle, the therapist can hold on to the client's distal forearm and resist forearm pronation at the radioulnar joints. Adding resistance increases the contraction force of the client's target muscle. The muscle "pops out" and is easier to palpate. Note that the stabilization hand resisting the client's forearm pronation is placed on the distal forearm and does not cross the wrist joint to hold the client's hand. Otherwise additional muscles are likely to contract, and the target muscle contraction will not be isolated.

tion to the target muscle. This way, it will be the only muscle that is palpably hard and can be discerned from the adjacent relaxed and palpably soft muscles. However, if the therapist's stabilization hand does cross other joints, it is likely that muscles crossing these joints will also contract. This will defeat the purpose of having an isolated contraction of the target muscle.

For example, in the case of the pronator teres palpation, when resistance to forearm pronation is added, it is important that the therapist's stabilization hand does not cross the wrist joint and hold the client's hand. If the stabilization hand holds the client's hand, then other muscles that cross the client's wrist joint, such as the muscles of the wrist flexor group that move the hand at the wrist joint, or flexor muscles of the fingers, will likely also contract, making it difficult to discern the pronator teres from these adjacent muscles. Therefore the resistance hand should be placed on the client's forearm (see Figure 2-4). Ideally, placing the resistance hand on the distal end of the forearm affords the best leverage force so that the therapist does not have to work as hard.

Generally, if the therapist is resisting an action of the arm at the shoulder joint, the therapist's stabilization hand should be placed just proximal to the elbow joint and not cross the elbow joint to grasp the client's forearm. If the therapist is resisting an action of the forearm at the elbow joint, the therapist's stabilization hand should be placed on the distal forearm and not cross the wrist joint to grasp the client's hand. If the therapist is resisting an action of the hand at the wrist joint, the therapist's stabilization hand should be placed on the palm of the hand and not cross the metacarpophalangeal joints to grasp the client's fingers. The same reasoning can be applied to the lower extremity and the axial body.

Guideline #5: Look Before You Palpate

Even though palpation is done via touching, **visual observation** can be a valuable tool for locating a target muscle. This is especially true for muscles that are superficial and whose contours show through the skin. Very often, a target muscle visu-

ally screams, "Here I am!" yet the therapist doesn't see it because the palpating hand is in the way. This may be true when the target muscle is relaxed, but is even more likely to be true when the target muscle is contracted (especially if it contracts harder from increased resistance), because when it contracts and hardens, it often pops out visually. For this reason, whenever attempting to palpate a target muscle, look first; then place your palpating hand over the muscle to feel for it.

For example, when palpating the palmaris longus and flexor carpi radialis muscles of the wrist flexor group, before placing your palpating hand on the client's anterior forearm, first look for the distal tendons of these two muscles at the anterior distal forearm near the wrist joint. They may be fully visible, aiding you in finding and palpating them (Figure 2-5, A). If they are not visible, ask the client to flex the hand at the wrist joint and add resistance if you would like. Now look again before placing your palpating hand on the client. When contracted, it is even more likely that these distal tendons will tense and visually pop out, helping you to locate and palpate them (Figure 2-5, B). There are many muscles whose visual information can help with their palpation. For this reason, it is a good rule to always look before you touch.

BOX 2-5

It should be noted that the palmaris longus muscle is often missing, either unilaterally or bilaterally, in many individuals.

Guideline #6: First Find the Target Muscle in the Easiest Place Possible

Once a target muscle has been found, it is much easier to continue to palpate along its course than it is to locate it in the first place. For this reason, a good palpation guideline is to always feel for the target muscle wherever it is easiest to first

A   B

Figure 2-5 It is important to visually look for the presence of the target muscle before placing your palpating hand over the target muscle and blocking possibly useful visual information. **A** shows that the distal tendon of the flexor carpi radialis (FCR) muscle might be visible even when it is relaxed. **B** shows that when contracted (in this case against resistance), its distal tendon tenses and becomes even more visually apparent. Note: the palmaris longus (PL) and flexor carpi ulnaris (FCU) tendons are also visible.

find. Once located, then you can continue to palpate it toward one or both of its attachments. For example, using the flexor carpi radialis as an example, if the distal tendon is visually apparent (see Figure 2-5), then begin your palpation there. Once it is clearly felt, then continue to palpate toward its proximal attachment on the medial epicondyle of the humerus.

Guideline #7: Strum Perpendicularly Across the Target Muscle

When first locating a target muscle or when following a target muscle that has already been found, it is best to strum perpendicularly across its belly or tendon. Strumming perpendicularly across a muscle belly or its tendon is like strumming or twanging a guitar string; you begin on one side of the belly or tendon, then you rise up onto its prominence, and then fall off the other side of it. This change in contour is much more palpably noticeable than if your palpating fingers simply glide longitudinally along the muscle (which offers little change in contour and thus does not help to define the location of the target muscle).

It is important to note when strumming perpendicularly across a muscle's belly or tendon that the movement of your palpating fingers is not a short vibration motion; rather it must be large enough to begin off one side of the target muscle, rise onto it, go all the way across it, and end off the other side of it. This means that the length of excursion of your strumming

Figure 2-6 The pronator teres is being palpated by strumming perpendicularly across its belly. It is important that the excursion of the strumming motion is large enough to begin off the muscle on one side and end off the muscle on its other side. (Muscolino JE: *Kinesiology: the skeletal system and muscle function*, enhanced edition, St Louis, 2007, Mosby.)

motion must be fairly long. Figure 2-6 illustrates the belly of the pronator teres being strummed perpendicularly.

Guideline #8: Use Baby Steps to Follow the Target Muscle

Once a target muscle has been found in the easiest place possible by strumming perpendicular to it, it should then be followed all the way to its attachments. This should be done in baby steps. Using baby steps to follow a muscle means that each successive "feel" of the muscle should be immediately after the previous feel so that no geography of the muscle's contour is skipped. If you feel the target muscle in one spot, then you should not skip a couple of inches down the muscle to feel it again. The farther down you skip, the more likely it is that you will no longer be on the muscle and will lose the course of its palpation. Figure 2-7 illustrates the idea that once a target muscle has been located, baby steps should be used to follow it toward its attachments.

Guideline #9: Alternately Contract and Relax the Target Muscle

It has already been stated that it can be uncomfortable for the client to hold a sustained isometric contraction of the target muscle while it is being palpated; therefore it is better for the client to alternately contract and relax it. In addition, having the client alternately contract and relax the target muscle while the therapist follows its course with baby steps aids in successful palpation. At each baby step of the palpation process, if the target muscle alternately contracts and then relaxes, the therapist can feel its change in texture from being soft when it is relaxed, to being hard when it is contracted, to being soft when it is relaxed again. This assures the therapist that he or she is still on the target muscle. If the therapist does accidentally veer off the target muscle onto other tissue, it will be evident because the tissue texture change from soft to hard

to soft (as the target muscle contracts and then relaxes) will not be felt.

When the therapist does veer off course, the palpating fingers should be placed back at the last spot where the target muscle was felt clearly and then make the next baby step in a slightly different direction to relocate the course of the target muscle as the client is asked once again to alternately contract and then relax the target muscle.

Guideline #10: When Appropriate, Use Coupled Actions

There are certain instances in which knowledge of coupled actions can help isolate contraction of a target muscle so that its palpation is facilitated. Most of these instances involve rotation of the scapula at the scapulocostal joint, because scapular rotation cannot occur on its own; rather the scapula can only rotate when the arm is moved at the shoulder (glenohumeral) joint. For example, if the target muscle to be palpated is the pectoralis minor, even though it has a number of actions that could be used to make it contract, most of these actions would also cause the pectoralis major to contract, which would block palpation of the pectoralis minor. The only effective action that would isolate contraction of the pectoralis minor in the anterior chest is downward rotation of the scapula. However, this rotation will occur only in conjunction with extension and/or adduction of the arm at the shoulder joint. Therefore, to create downward rotation of the scapula to engage the pectoralis minor, ask the client to extend and adduct the arm at the shoulder joint. This can be accomplished by having the client first rest the hand in the small of the back; then, to engage the pectoralis minor, have the client move the arm further into extension by moving the hand posteriorly away from the small of the back. This will immediately engage the pectoralis minor, allowing it to be easily palpated through the pectoralis major (Figure 2-8). This same procedure can be used to palpate the rhomboid muscles through the middle trapezius (see Figures 10-15 and 10-16).

Figure 2-7 The pronator teres muscle is palpated in "baby steps" toward its distal attachment. Palpating in baby steps means that the muscle is palpated with successive feels, each one immediately after the previous one. This helps ensure that the therapist will successfully follow the course of the target muscle.

YOU ARE HERE

2

Figure 2-8 When the client moves the hand posteriorly away from the small of the back, extension of the arm occurs. This requires the coupled action of downward rotation of the scapula at the scapulocostal joint, which engages the pectoralis minor muscle so that it can be easily palpated through the pectoralis major muscle. Knowledge of the coupled actions of the arm and scapula can be very helpful when palpating muscles of scapular rotation, such as the pectoralis minor.

BOX 2-7

Knowledge of coupled actions can also be used with reciprocal inhibition to palpate a target muscle. For example, when palpating the levator scapulae, the client's arm is extended and adducted at the shoulder joint by placing the hand in the small of the back. This requires the coupled action of downward rotation of the scapula at the scapulocostal joint, which then reciprocally inhibits and relaxes the upper trapezius (because it is an upward rotator of the scapula). With the upper trapezius relaxed, palpation of the levator scapulae through it can now be done. For a fuller explanation of this, see the discussion on reciprocal inhibition, Guideline #11.

Guideline #11: When Appropriate, Use Reciprocal Inhibition

Reciprocal inhibition is a neurologic reflex that causes inhibition of a muscle whenever an antagonist muscle is actively contracted. This neurologic reflex can be used to great advantage when palpating certain target muscles. For example, if our target muscle is the brachialis and we want to make it contract so that it hardens and is easier to feel, we have no choice but to ask the client to flex the elbow joint, because that is the only action of the brachialis. The problem with this is that if the client flexes the forearm at the elbow joint to contract the brachialis, the biceps brachii will also contract. This makes it difficult to palpate the brachialis because the biceps brachii overlies the brachialis in the anterior arm. Given that it is always the goal of a muscle palpation to have an isolated contraction of the target muscle (in this case, we want only the brachialis to contract), the biceps brachii needs to remain relaxed. Even though the only action of the brachialis (elbow joint flexion) is an action of the biceps brachii, it is possible to achieve this if we use the principle of reciprocal inhibition (Figure 2-9). To do this, we ask the client to flex the forearm at the elbow joint while the forearm is in a position of full pronation. Because the biceps brachii is also a supinator of the forearm, having the forearm pronated will reciprocally inhibit it from contracting, so it will remain relaxed as the brachialis contracts to flex the forearm at the elbow joint. Thus we have achieved the goal of having an isolated contraction of our target muscle, the brachialis.

Figure 2-9 The principle of reciprocal inhibition is used to inhibit and relax the biceps brachii muscle as the brachialis muscle contracts to flex the forearm at the elbow joint. The biceps brachii, which is also a supinator of the forearm, is reciprocally inhibited because the forearm is pronated (as it is flexed). It is important that flexion of the forearm at the elbow joint is not performed forcefully or the reciprocal inhibition of the biceps brachii might be overridden and permit the unwanted contraction. (Muscolino JE: *Kinesiology: the skeletal system and muscle function*, enhanced edition, St Louis, 2007, Mosby.)

Another example of using the principle of reciprocal inhibition to isolate the contraction of a target muscle is palpating the scapular attachment of the levator scapulae. If we ask the client to elevate the scapula to contract and palpably harden the levator scapulae, the problem is that the upper trapezius will also contract and harden, making it impossible to feel the levator scapulae at its scapular attachment deep to the upper trapezius. To stop the upper trapezius from contracting, ask the client to place the hand in the small of the back. This position of humeral extension and adduction requires downward rotation of the scapula at the scapulocostal joint. Because the upper trapezius is an upward rotator of the scapula, it will be reciprocally inhibited and stay relaxed. This allows for an isolated contraction of and a successful palpation of the levator scapulae when the client is asked to elevate the scapula (Figure 2-10).

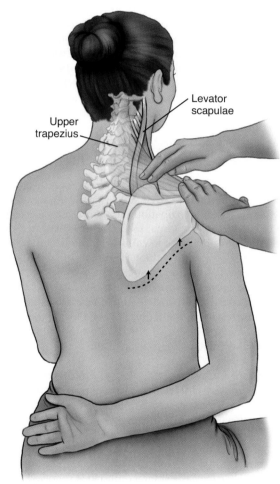

Figure 2-10 The principle of reciprocal inhibition is used to inhibit and relax the upper trapezius so that the scapular attachment of the levator scapulae can be more easily palpated as it contracts to elevate the scapula at the scapulocostal joint. The upper trapezius, which is also an upward rotator of the scapula, is reciprocally inhibited because the scapula is downwardly rotated (as it is elevated) because of the position of the hand in the small of the back. It is important that elevation of the scapula at the scapulocostal joint is not performed forcefully or the reciprocal inhibition of the upper trapezius might be overridden, resulting in a contraction of the upper trapezius.

BOX 2-8

The downward rotation of the scapula at the scapulocostal joint when palpating the levator scapulae not only aids palpation of the levator scapulae by reciprocally inhibiting the upper trapezius, but also increases the contraction strength of the levator scapulae, because downward rotation of the scapula is another one of its actions.

There is one important caution when using the principle of reciprocal inhibition for a muscle palpation. When the client is asked to contract and engage the target muscle, the force of its contraction must be small. If the contraction is forceful, the client's brain will override the reciprocal inhibition reflex in an attempt to recruit as many muscles as possible for the joint action. This will result in a contraction of the muscle that was supposed to be reciprocally inhibited and relaxed. Once this other muscle contracts, it will likely block successful palpation of the target muscle. For example, when palpating for the brachialis, if flexion of the forearm at the elbow joint is performed forcefully, the biceps brachii will be recruited, making palpation of the brachialis difficult or impossible. Another example is palpating for the levator scapulae: if elevation of the scapula at the scapulocostal joint is performed forcefully, the upper trapezius will be recruited, making palpation of the levator scapulae at its scapular attachment difficult or impossible.

Guideline #12: Use Appropriate Pressure
The concept of using appropriate pressure has already been discussed in Chapter 1; however, the use of appropriate pressure is so critical to muscle palpation that the key points are repeated here (for a more complete discussion of palpation pressure, please see Chapter 1, page 3). It is important to not be too heavy handed; sensitivity can be lost with excessive pressure. On the other hand, it is important to not be too light with your pressure either; some muscles are quite deep and require moderate to strong pressure to feel. Generally, when most new students have a difficult time palpating a target muscle, it is because their pressure is too light. Appropriate pressure means applying the optimal palpation pressure for each target muscle palpation.

BOX 2-9

There are occasional times when a deep muscle palpation is facilitated by extremely light pressure. If a muscle is so deep that its borders cannot be felt, then its location must be determined by feeling for the vibrations of its contraction through the tissues. This can only be felt with a very light touch. One example of this approach is palpation of the extensor hallucis longus muscle in the leg deep to the tibialis anterior and extensor digitorum longus muscles.

Guideline #13: For Deep Palpations, Sink Slowly into the Tissue and Have the Client Breathe

All deep muscle palpations should be done slowly. Although deep pressure can be uncomfortable for many clients, it is often accomplished quite easily if we work with the client as we palpate. This can be accomplished by sinking slowly into the client's tissues and having the client breathe with the palpation process in a slow and rhythmic manner. An excellent example of this is palpating the psoas major in the abdominopelvic cavity. The psoas major must be palpated from the anterior perspective. This requires firm pressure to reach through the abdominal viscera, because the psoas major lies against the spinal column and forms part of the posterior abdominal wall. For the client to remain comfortable, the therapist needs to sink into the client's tissues very slowly as the client breathes slowly and evenly. To begin the palpation, ask the client to take in a moderate to deep breath; then as the client slowly exhales, slowly sink in toward the psoas major. It is not necessary to reach the psoas major at the end of the client's first exhalation. Instead, ease off slightly with your pressure and ask the client to take in another moderate-sized breath; then continue to slowly sink in deeper as the client slowly exhales again. This process may need to be repeated a third time to reach the psoas major; a deep muscle can usually be accessed in this manner with two or three breaths by the client. What is most important to remember is that firm deep pressure must be applied slowly.

BOX 2-10

When having a client breathe with your palpation as you sink slowly and deeply in the client's tissues to access a deep muscle, it is important that the client's breath is not quick and shallow. However, the breaths do not need to be very deep either; a very deep breath may push your palpating hands out, especially if you are palpating in the abdominal region. More important than the depth of the breath is its pace. The client's breathing should be slow, rhythmic, and relaxed. This type of breathing on the part of the client is facilitated if you breathe in a similar manner.

Guideline #14: Use Muscles as Landmarks

Once the bones and bony landmarks of the skeleton have been learned, it is common to use a bony landmark to help locate and palpate a target muscle. However, once the palpation of one muscle has been learned, it can also be a useful landmark for locating another adjacent muscle. For example, if palpation of the sternocleidomastoid (SCM) has been learned, then it is a simple matter to palpate the scalene muscles (see page 190). All that is required is to locate the lateral border of the clavicular head of the SCM and then drop off it immediately laterally and you will be on the scalene group. This is a much easier way to locate the scalenes than to first try to palpate the anterior tubercles of the transverse processes of the cervical vertebrae. Similarly, the SCM can also be used to locate and palpate the longus colli muscle (see page 194). First locate the medial border of the sternal head of the SCM and then drop off it just medially and sink in toward the spinal column. There are countless other examples wherein the knowledge of one muscle's location can help the therapist locate another muscle that might otherwise be more difficult to find.

Guideline #15: Relax and Passively Slacken the Target Muscle When Palpating Its Bony Attachment

It is always desirable to palpate as much of a target muscle as possible; preferably it should be palpated all the way from one bony attachment to its other bony attachment. However, there are times when it is difficult to follow a target muscle all the way to its bony attachment. This is especially true if the client is contracting the target muscle, because this tenses and hardens its tendon, making it difficult to discern from its bony attachment. Ironically, even though contracting the target muscle helps us discern its belly from adjacent soft tissue because the muscle belly becomes hard, contracting the target muscle tenses and hardens the tendon of the muscle too; and that makes it harder to discern the hard tendon from the adjacent hard bony tissue of its attachment. In other words, contracting a target muscle helps to discern it from adjacent soft tissue, but makes it more difficult to discern from adjacent hard tissue, such as its bony attachments. Therefore one guideline that can help the therapist follow a target muscle all the way to its bony attachment is to have the client relax the target muscle and have it passively slackened as the therapist reaches its bony attachment. Examples that use this guideline are palpating the proximal attachment of the rectus femoris muscle on the anterior inferior iliac spine (AIIS) of the pelvis (see Figure 18-30), and palpating the distal attachment of the subscapularis muscle on the lesser tubercle of the humerus (see Figure 10-60).

Guideline #16: Close Your Eyes When You Palpate

Although it is important to visually inspect the palpation region when beginning palpation of the target muscle (see Guideline #5), once the visual inspection is done, it is often not necessary for a therapist to continue looking at the client's body as the palpation procedure continues. In fact, it can be greatly beneficial if the therapist closes his or her eyes when palpating. By closing the eyes, the therapist can block out extraneous sensory stimuli that might otherwise distract from what is being felt in the palpation fingers. Closing the eyes allows the therapist to focus all attention on the palpating fingers, thereby increasing their sensory acuity.

Guideline #17: Construct a Mental Picture of the Client's Anatomy Under the Skin as You Palpate

As the therapist's eyes are closed during palpation, it can be further beneficial to picture the target muscle and other adjacent anatomic structures under the client's skin. Creating this mental picture of the client's anatomy under the skin can facilitate correct initial location of the target muscle and facilitate use of baby steps as the target muscle is followed toward its attachments.

Guideline #18: If a Client Is Ticklish, Have the Client Place a Hand Over Your Palpating Hand

Unfortunately, when clients are ticklish, it often makes it difficult if not impossible to palpate them because touching causes them to pull away. This is especially true if we touch the client lightly. Therefore it is usually best to palpate ticklish clients with firm pressure. However, some clients are extremely ticklish whether we touch them lightly or firmly. This can interfere with palpation assessment and also with treatment. One thing that can be done to help lessen the sensitivity of a ticklish client is to ask the client to place one of his or her hands over the therapist's palpating hand. Ticklishness is a perceived invasion of one's space by another individual; this is why a person cannot tickle himself or herself. Therefore if the client's hand is placed over our palpating hand, the client will subconsciously have a sense that he or she is in control of this space and will tend to be less ticklish. Using this guideline does not work with everyone in every circumstance, but is often successful and worth trying.

Guideline #19: Keep Fingernails Short and Smooth
For some muscle palpations, the therapist's fingernails need to be very short (Figure 2-11, A). This is especially true when it comes to deeper palpations; for example, when palpating the subscapularis muscle (see page 165), quadratus lumborum muscle (see page 365), or the vertebral attachments of the scalene muscles (see page 190). Unfortunately, it seems that everyone has a different sense of what *short* means when it comes to the length of fingernails. As a result, some therapists allow their nails to be too long. Consequently they are unable to comfortably palpate some muscles and either

A

B

Figure 2-11 Fingernails need to be very short for muscle palpations, especially of deep muscles. **A** shows the proper length for fingernails when palpating and working deeply. An easy way to check that fingernail length is short enough for deeper palpations is seen in **B**. See if you can catch the fingernails of your palpating hand (when the pads are oriented away from you) with a fingernail of your other hand. If you can, that fingernail may be too long.

cause pain and leave fingernail marks on the client or, just as bad, avoid adequately palpating or working musculature of the client that is in need of treatment because they are afraid of hurting the client with their nails. The exact fingernail length that is necessary will vary from one palpation to another. A good way to check for appropriate fingernail length is to place the pads of your palpating hand fingers away from you and try to catch the fingernails of your palpating hand with a fingernail of your other hand (Figure 2-11, B). If you can, then the fingernails are likely too long. If you cannot, then the length of your fingernails are short enough for deep palpations.

It is just as important that fingernails are smooth (i.e., their edges are not sharp). When filing fingernails, it is important to finish with a fingernail file that buffs and smoothes the edges of the nails. Short nails that are sharp can be just as uncomfortable or painful to the client as long fingernails.

Guideline #20: Use the Optimal Palpation Position
The optimal palpation position is simply the client position that is most effective for the palpation of a particular target muscle. It is important to realize that the optimal position in which to palpate a certain target muscle might not be the position that a client is usually in when that muscle is being treated. Clients are usually treated in the prone or supine position. However, some muscles are optimally palpated with the client side lying, standing, or seated. For example, the pectoralis minor is most often treated with the client supine. However, the optimal client position in which to palpate the pectoralis minor is probably seated. This is because the seated position better allows the client to first place the hand in the small of the back and then move the hand posteriorly away from the small of the back (creating downward rotation of the scapula to engage the pectoralis minor) (see Figure 10-80). For this reason, even though it is usually preferred to not have the client change positions in the middle of a treatment session, if accurate palpation is critical to the assessment and treatment of the client, it might be necessary to do so. To avoid this interruption to the flow of a treatment session, the therapist may choose to do all palpation assessments at the beginning of the session before commencing with treatment.

BOX 2-11

Often the client can be placed in more than one position to palpate a particular target muscle. Although one position might generally be considered optimal for palpation of that target muscle, some therapists may prefer an alternative position. Even if one client position and palpation procedure is the favorite approach, an alternative position and procedure might work better for certain clients. For this reason, it is always desirable to be creative and flexible when approaching muscle palpation. The more palpation positions and methods you are comfortable with, the more likely it is that you will be successful when working with your clients. For each muscle palpation given in Part III of this book, alternative client positions are given whenever applicable. Alternative palpation methods are also often presented.

YOU ARE HERE

2

Summary List of Muscle Palpation Guidelines

Each of the following muscle palpation guidelines has already been discussed in this chapter. All 20 are summarized in list form here.

1. Know the attachments of the target muscle to know where to place your hands.
2. Know the actions of the target muscle. The client will most likely be asked to perform one of them to contract the target muscle so that it can be discerned from the adjacent musculature (make sure that the client is not asked to hold the contraction too long or the target muscle may fatigue and the client may become uncomfortable).
3. Think critically to choose exactly which joint action of the target muscle will best isolate its contraction.
4. If necessary, add resistance to the client's contraction of the target muscle (when resistance is added, do not cross any joints that do not need to be crossed; in other words, be sure to resist only the action of the target muscle that is desired).
5. Look before placing your palpating hand on the client (this is especially important with superficial muscles).
6. First find and palpate the target muscle in the easiest place possible.
7. Strum perpendicularly across the belly or tendon of the target muscle.
8. Once located, follow the course of the target muscle in small successive baby steps.
9. At each baby step of palpation, have the client alternately contract and relax the target muscle and feel for this tissue texture change as the muscle goes from relaxed and soft, to contracted and hard, to relaxed and soft again.
10. Use knowledge of coupled actions to palpate target muscles that are scapular rotators.

11. Use reciprocal inhibition whenever needed to aid palpation of the target muscle (when reciprocal inhibition is used, do not have the client contract the target muscle too forcefully, or the muscle that is being reciprocally inhibited may be recruited anyway).
12. Use appropriate pressure. Appropriate pressure is neither too heavy nor too light.
13. When using deep palpation pressure, sink slowly into the client's tissues as the client breathes slowly and evenly.
14. Once the palpation of one muscle is known, it can be used as a landmark to locate other muscles.
15. Relax and passively slacken the target muscle when palpating it at its bony attachment.
16. Close your eyes when you palpate to focus your attention on your palpating fingers.
17. Construct a mental picture of the client's anatomy under the skin as you palpate.
18. If the client is ticklish, use firm pressure and have the client place a hand over your palpating hand.
19. Fingernails need to be very short and smooth.
20. Place the client in a position that is optimal for the muscle palpation.

Conclusion

Although the science of muscle palpation begins with a solid knowledge of the attachments and actions of the target muscle, turning palpation into an art requires much more. The art of muscle palpation involves weaving the knowledge of the attachments and actions of the target muscle and all adjacent musculature, as well as the many guidelines listed in this chapter, into a cohesive approach that allows the target muscle to be discerned from adjacent tissues. Overall, what are necessary are sensitive hands, critical thinking, and a willingness to be creative.

Chapter 3

Draping and Basic Massage Strokes

Sandy Fritz, Susan Salvo, and Joseph E. Muscolino

Overview

This chapter covers two topics: draping and massage strokes. The first half of the chapter begins by discussing principles of draping. A compendium of draping techniques is then given that describes and illustrates how to drape each of the major body parts. The second half of the chapter discusses massage strokes. The fundamental characteristics of touch that underlie all massage strokes are discussed first. The major massage strokes are then defined and described with illustrations.

Chapter Outline

Draping, 20
Draping Methods, 20
Compendium of Draping Techniques, 20

Massage Strokes, 23
Characteristics of Touch, 23
Compendium of Massage Strokes, 24

Chapter Objectives

After completing this chapter, the student should be able to perform the following:

1. Define the key terms of this chapter.
2. Explain the purposes and principles of draping.
3. Describe the two major draping methods.
4. Describe how to drape each major body part.
5. List and describe the seven characteristics of touch.
6. List and describe the six major types of massage strokes.

Key Terms

compression
contoured draping
depth of pressure
direction
drag
draping
duration

effleurage
flat draping
frequency
friction
gliding
kneading
oscillation

percussion
petrissage
rhythm
speed
tapotement
vibration

19

Draping

Introduction to Draping

Draping is essentially covering the body with cloth, and it allows the client to be undressed while receiving massage. Draping serves two major purposes: (1) to maintain the client's privacy and sense of security, and (2) to provide warmth. The most frequently used draping materials are sheets and towels.

Principles of Draping

Many different draping methods exist; however, the following principles consistently apply:

o All reusable draping material must be freshly laundered for each client. Disposable linens must be fresh for each client and then disposed of properly.

o Only the area being massaged is undraped. In most circumstances, after moving the draping material to expose the area to be massaged, the draping material stays where it is placed.

o Always use a bottom drape (usually a sheet) under the client.

o Draping may be secured by tucking it underneath the client's body.

o If placing the drape in position feels invasive to the client, especially if tucking the drape under or around a body part, have the client assist in placement of the drape to preserve the client's modesty.

o Draping methods should keep the client covered in all positions, including the seated position.

o The genital area is never undraped.

o The breast area of women is not undraped during routine wellness massage. Specific breast massage under the supervision of a licensed physician may require special draping procedures.

Draping Methods

The two basic types of draping are flat draping and contoured draping.

Flat Draping Methods

With flat draping, a top drape, usually a sheet, is placed over the client. The top drape, and sometimes the bottom drape, is moved in various ways to cover and uncover the area to be massaged.

Contoured Draping

Contoured draping can be done with two towels or with a sheet and a towel (a pillow case may substitute for a towel). These drapes are wrapped and shaped around the client. This type of draping is very effective for securely covering and shielding the genital region and buttocks. For women, a separate chest drape (usually a towel or pillowcase) can be used to drape the breast area when accessing the abdomen.

Alternative to Draping

As an alternative to draping, the client can wear a swimsuit or shorts and a loose shirt. A bottom drape (sheet) is placed over the table or mat. A top drape is available if the client becomes chilled during massage.

Compendium of Draping Techniques

Table 3-1 demonstrates a compendium of draping techniques. A description and illustration of how to drape each major body part are given.

TABLE 3-1

Draping Techniques

Position	Description	
Prone back	The client is in the prone position and the top sheet is folded over to expose the back (Figure 3-1).	

Figure 3-1

TABLE 3-1

Draping Techniques—cont'd

Position	Description
Prone buttock and lower extremity	The buttock and lower extremity in the prone position are undraped by folding the top sheet up and around to the inside of the lower extremity and secured under the lower extremity to be massaged. The flat sheet on the bottom can be folded up for additional coverage to maintain warmth (Figure 3-2). **Figure 3-2**
Prone upper extremity	The top flat sheet is folded back on a diagonal to access the upper extremity in the prone position (Figure 3-3). **Figure 3-3**
Supine lower extremity	In the supine position the lower extremity is undraped by folding the top sheet up and over and then wrapping it around the inside of the lower extremity (Figure 3-4, A). **Figure 3-4, A** A variation to secure the groin area is to contour the top sheet through the thighs and up and under the buttocks (Figure 3-4, B). **Figure 3-4, B**

Continued

TABLE 3-1

Draping Techniques—cont'd

Position	Description
Supine upper extremity	The upper extremity in the supine position is exposed by lifting it up and out from under the top sheet and then placing on top of the sheet (Figure 3-5).

Figure 3-5

Supine abdomen	The abdominal area is exposed on the female client who is in the supine position. The therapist uses a towel or pillowcase (king size may be preferable) folded horizontally as a bikini top. The top drape over the lower body in this image stops at the anterior superior iliac spines (Figure 3-6).

Figure 3-6

Supine neck and shoulder	The top sheet is folded down just below the clavicles to expose the inferior attachments of the sternocleidomastoid muscles and to keep the female breasts draped. Note: In this image, the therapist is taking advantage of this draping technique to address trigger points in these muscles while supporting the base of the skull with the opposite hand (Figure 3-7).

Figure 3-7

Side lying back	To expose the back of a side lying female client, the therapist uses contoured draping. To keep the sheet in place and cover the female breasts, the therapist incorporates a towel folded horizontally to anchor the top edge of the sheet. A cushion or rolled-up towel is placed under the head to maintain the spine in neutral alignment. The client may also be given a pillow to place in front of the trunk and "hug." This provides further security and privacy (Figure 3-8).

Figure 3-8

Side lying upper extremity	To access the upper extremity of a side lying female client, pull the upper extremity from under the sheet, then arrange the sheet to cover the breasts. The exposed upper extremity can be placed on a draped cushion for client comfort. Note that the neck is placed on a cushion to maintain the spine in a neutral alignment (Figure 3-9).

Figure 3-9

YOU ARE HERE

3

TABLE 3-1

Draping Techniques—cont'd

Position	Description
Side lying lower extremity (that is away from the table)	To access the lower extremity that is away from the table of a side lying client, undrape the area, gather the fabric, and then tuck the sheet around the upper part of the thigh. Be sure the knee joint is flexed approximately 90 degrees. The undraped lower extremity can be placed on a draped cushion for client comfort (Figure 3-10).

Figure 3-10

Position	Description
Side lying lower extremity (that is closer to the table)	To access the lower extremity that is next to the table of a side lying client, undrape the area, gather the fabric, and then tuck the sheet around the upper part of the thigh. The knee joint is slightly flexed. A rolled-up towel can be placed under the ankle for client comfort. Note that the other lower extremity remains draped and supported by a draped cushion (Figure 3-11).

Figure 3-11

Massage Strokes

Introduction to Massage Strokes

Massage application involves touching the body to manipulate soft tissues, influence body fluid movement, and stimulate neuroendocrine responses. During a massage session, many different strokes are often employed. However, more fundamental than the strokes themselves are the characteristics of the touch of the strokes. Following the classification of massage by pioneer Gertrude Beard, as well as current trends in therapeutic massage, the touch of a massage stroke can be characterized by the following seven characteristics: depth of pressure, drag, direction, speed, rhythm, frequency, and duration. Each of these seven characteristics is described. Following their description, a compendium of the major treatment strokes employed in massage therapy is presented with a brief description and illustration of each stroke.

Characteristics of Touch

Depth of Pressure

Depth of pressure, or the compressive force of massage, can be light, moderate, or deep.

Most areas of the body consist of four major tissue layers. These layers are the skin, superficial fascia, layers of musculature, and various fascial sheaths. Soft tissue dysfunction can develop in any or all of these layers. When dysfunction is present more superficially, the depth of pressure necessary is usually light. When dysfunction is present in deeper layers, deeper pressure is usually necessary. Pressure should be delivered through each successive layer, reaching deeper layers without damage and discomfort to superficial tissues. The deeper the pressure, the broader the base of contact required on the body's surface. To treat any soft tissue dysfunction, such as a trigger point or spasm, the therapist applies the proper level of pressure to reach the location of the dysfunction. It should be noted that pressure, by virtue of compressing tissues, also alters the circulation of fluids within the body.

Drag

Drag describes the amount of pull (stretch) on the tissue. Drag is a component of connective tissue massage wherein one layer of tissue is dragged/pulled along an adjacent layer, helping to break up patterns of adhesions. Drag is also used during palpation assessment of various soft tissue dysfunctions to identify areas of ease and bind within the tissues. *Ease* occurs when tissue moves freely and easily; *bind* occurs when tissue feel stuck, leathery, or thick.

Direction

Direction can move out from the center of the body (centrifugal) or in from the extremities toward the center of the body (centripetal). Furthermore, direction can proceed longitudinally, along a muscle following the direction of its fibers; transversely, across the direction of the fibers; or circularly. Direction is a factor in broadening and lengthening tissues containing soft tissue dysfunctions or in the methods that influence blood and lymphatic fluid movement.

Speed

Speed is the rate that massage methods are applied. The speed of a stroke can be fast, slow, or variable, depending upon the demands of the tissues being addressed and the state of the client (faster and more energizing in situations where stimulation is called for, slower and more rhythmic where calming influences are needed).

Rhythm

Rhythm refers to the regularity of technique application. If the method is applied at regular intervals, it is considered even, or rhythmic. If the method is disjointed or irregular, it is considered uneven, or arrhythmic. Rhythmic stroking tends to be more calming, especially if applied slowly and with mild to moderate pressure. Arrhythmic strokes, especially arrhythmic jostling and shaking, tend to be more stimulating.

Frequency

Frequency is the number of times that a treatment method is repeated in a given time frame. This aspect relates to how many repetitions of a stroke, such as a compression or gliding stroke, are performed. In general, the massage practitioner repeats each stroke three to five times before moving or switching to a different one. Although every application of a stroke is therapeutic, the therapist should also be assessing the health of the client's tissues as they are treated with the strokes. If the final stroke indicates remaining dysfunction, then the frequency can be increased and more strokes performed on that tissue.

Duration

Duration has two aspects. It can mean the length of time the session lasts or the length of time that a particular stroke or other treatment application, such as a stretch, is used in the same location. Typically, duration of a specific stroke application is approximately 30 to 60 seconds. Certain treatment protocols may call for less or more time.

Compendium of Massage Strokes

Following is a description of the six major types of massage therapy strokes: gliding, kneading, friction, compression, percussion, and vibration.

Gliding

A gliding stroke (historically known as effleurage) is a long, broad stroke that is usually applied along the direction of the muscle fibers. It can also be applied across the muscle fibers; when this is done, it is often called *stroking*.

In this example of gliding (Figure 3-12), the therapist starts at the top of the client's back and applies pressure using the palms of her hands on both sides of the spinous processes until she arrives at the sacrum. The hands then separate and slide back toward the top of the back using just the weight of the hands. Contact with the client's skin is maintained when moving from pushing to pulling and between repetitions.

Figure 3-12 Gliding example #1: Long stroke gliding along the back.

In Figure 3-13, the client is supine with her head and neck rotated to one side. Pressure is applied with the fist from the occiput to the acromion process and then back to the occiput. While on the cervical vertebrae, the pressure is focused over the laminar groove. While on the top of the shoulder, the pressure is focused on the thickest portion of the upper trapezius.

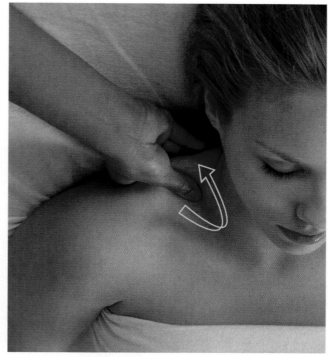

Figure 3-14 Kneading stroke example #1: One-handed kneading of the upper trapezius.

In Figure 3-15, the client is lying supine while the therapist kneads the client's left thigh. The hands move in opposite directions; one hand applying a force forward while the other is pulling back. The tissue under the therapist's hands is compressed, twisted, and squeezed. The hands cross each other midstroke.

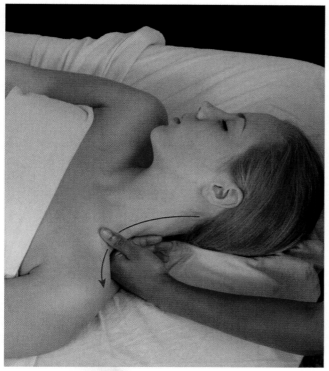

Figure 3-13 Gliding example #2: Gliding along the neck and shoulder.

Kneading

A **kneading** stroke (historically known as **petrissage**) lifts the tissue, and then the full hand is used to squeeze the tissue as it rolls out of the hand, while the other hand prepares to lift additional tissue and repeat the process. Skin rolling is a variation of a kneading stroke.

The therapist positions herself between the client's head and shoulder; this helps keep her wrist joint as straight as possible. The upper trapezius is compressed, lifted, and then released (Figure 3-14).

Figure 3-15 Kneading stroke example #2: Two-handed kneading of the anterior thigh.

Compression

A **compression** stroke directs pressure downward into the tissues at a 90-degree angle to the contour of the surface of the body part being worked (Figure 3-16). A compression stroke spreads or displaces surface layers of tissues. It is often applied with a "pumping" action in which the pressure is gradually increased as the compression is applied.

Compression can be applied with two hands moving simultaneously. In this example, the clothed client lies prone on a draped floor mat; her right hip joint is laterally rotated to shorten the targeted muscles. The therapist positions herself above the client so that she can use her body weight. She places her hands onto the gluteal musculature and leans in, applying rhythmic compression strokes to broaden the muscles.

Figure 3-16 Compression stroke example #1: Two-handed compression of the gluteal region.

In Figure 3-17, compression is applied down into the musculature of the medial thigh at a 90-degree angle. The therapist leans forward and uses forearm compression into the musculature.

Figure 3-17 Compression stroke example #2: Forearm compression to the medial thigh.

Friction

A **friction** stroke moves tissue under the skin. The movement is produced by beginning with a specific and moderate-to-deep compression. The surface tissues are moved back and forth across the fibers of deeper tissues for transverse or cross-fiber friction; or the tissues are moved in a circle to produce circular friction.

In Figure 3-18, the therapist braces (double supports) her finger pads and applies friction to the tissues near the medial border of the scapula.

Figure 3-18 Friction example #1: Double-supported hand contact, friction to the back.

In Figure 3-19, friction is being applied with a broader but still focused contact; the therapist is using the ulnar side of her forearm. The client is in a side lying position and friction is being applied to the latissimus dorsi muscle.

Figure 3-19 Friction example #2: Forearm contact, friction to the back.

Percussion

A percussion stroke (historically called tapotement) is a controlled flailing of the arms or forearms as the wrists snap back and forth and the hands strike the client's tissues. Various methods include slapping, tapping, hacking, pounding, and beating. Percussion can also be classified as oscillation movements.

In Figure 3-20, the ulnar surface of one hand is seen striking the client's upper back. The fingers are slightly spread while lifted. On contact, the momentum of the stroke causes each finger to contact the one above it, creating a slight vibratory effect. Two hands can be used instead of one.

In Figure 3-21, the therapist is standing to the side of a prone client and using the ulnar sides of both loosely closed fists to pound the client's upper back. The knuckles of a loosely closed fist can also be used to percuss the back.

Figure 3-20 Percussion stroke example #1: Hacking the upper back.

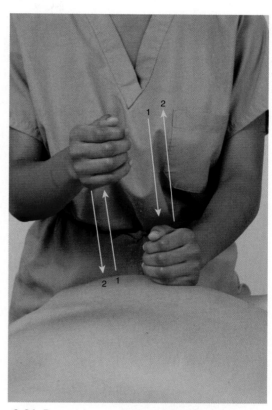

Figure 3-21 Percussion stroke example #2: Loose-fist percussion of the upper back.

3

Vibration

A **vibration** stroke begins with compression. After the depth of pressure has been achieved, the hand trembles/vibrates and transmits the action to the surrounding tissues. Shaking is a larger, more abrupt movement and is usually applied to the limbs of the client. Vibration can also be classified as oscillation movements.

In Figure 3-22, the client is lying supine and a draped bolster is placed under the knee joint. Repetitive vibratory shaking movements are used to relax the thigh muscles. The therapist uses the entire palmar surface of her hand to slightly compress and lift the client's tissue before beginning the vibratory shaking motions.

In Figure 3-23, the client is lying supine and the therapist is standing to her side. To access the abdomen, a sheet drapes her lower body and a pillowcase folded horizontally drapes the breast region. Vibratory movements are begun in the therapist's arms and are transmitted to the client's tissues via the tips of the last three fingers. Vibration to the abdomen may help stimulate intestinal peristalsis.

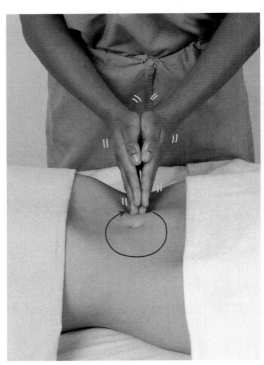

Figure 3-23 Vibration stroke example #2: Abdominal vibration.

Figure 3-22 Vibration stroke example #1: Vibrating the thigh.

Photos in this chapter are from Salvo S: *Massage therapy: principles and practice,* ed 3, St Louis, 2008, Saunders, and Fritz S: *Mosby fundamentals of therapeutic massage,* ed 4, St Louis, 2009, Mosby.

Chapter 4

Body Mechanics for the Manual Therapist*

Overview

This chapter offers a set of 10 guidelines designed to create healthy body mechanics when delivering massage or other forms of bodywork. These guidelines help us to maximize our efficiency while working by showing and explaining how to use the laws of physics to work for us instead of having them work against us. These 10 guidelines are divided into 3 major categories: (1) equipment, (2) positioning the body, and (3) performing the massage stroke.

The section on equipment discusses the importance of the height and width of the table, as well as the quality and quantity of the lubricant used. Our discussion on positioning the body addresses how to properly bend the body, align the feet, align the head, and stack the joints of the upper extremity. And the section on performing the massage stroke explains the importance of generating force from the larger proximal muscles of the body instead of the smaller distal ones, how to determine the optimal direction for the line of force, and the advantages of using a larger contact whenever possible as well as double-supporting the contact. The purpose of these guidelines is to help the manual therapist to work smarter instead of work harder.

Chapter Outline

Chapter Objectives

After completing this chapter, the student should be able to perform the following:

1. Define the key terms of this chapter.
2. Explain the importance of table height and table width to the efficient delivery of force.
3. Discuss using internal versus external forces when generating pressure.
4. Explain the importance of the lubricant to the delivery of force.
5. Compare and contrast the relative merits of the stoop and squat bends.
6. Discuss the concept of core alignment to the delivery of force.
7. Discuss the relationship between foot position and delivery of force.
8. List and discuss the three positions of the feet.
9. Discuss the importance of the posture of the neck and head.
10. Explain the importance of stacking the joints when performing massage.
11. Discuss the importance of proximal versus distal generation of force.
12. Discuss the importance of the direction of force of a massage stroke.
13. Discuss the importance of using larger versus smaller contacts on the client.
14. Explain why double-supporting the contact is helpful.

---

*This chapter is modified from Muscolino JE: Work smarter, not harder: body mechanics for massage therapists, *Massage Ther J* Winter:2-16, 2006. Photos by Yanik Chauvin.

4

Key Terms

body mechanics	feet staggered position	proximal generation of force
bracing the contact	head position	self-support
closed-packed position	internal force	squat bend
contact	joint compression forces	squat bend with the trunk inclined forward
core alignment	line of force	squat bend with the trunk vertically positioned
direction of force	longitudinal stance	stacked joints
distal generation of force	lubricant	stoop bend
double-support the contact	open-packed position	transverse stance
external force	pressure	weight
feet aligned position		

Introduction

Regardless of the technique employed, the essence of all forms of physical bodywork is the delivery of pressure—in other words, force—into the tissues of our clients. The efficiency with which we achieve this is crucial, not only to the quality of therapeutic care that we give our clients, but also to our own health and longevity in the field. To examine the efficiency with which our body works, we must study the mechanics of our body; therefore this field is called body mechanics.

Understanding and applying the fundamentals of good body mechanics is simple. We need to apply the laws of physics to our body. The same laws of physics that rule all physical matter including the moon and stars governs the forces that our body generates and to which our body is subjected. If we work with these laws of physics, we can generate greater forces with less fatigue, effortlessly working on our clients, and subject our body to less force. But if we work against the laws of physics, it will be more fatiguing to generate the power necessary to do our work, and our body will be subjected to greater forces that may injure us.

Unfortunately, the study of body mechanics is often given insufficient attention in the world of manual therapy. As a result, many new graduates and established therapists alike are often ill-equipped to do deep tissue work without *muscling* the massage via excessive effort. Instead of working smarter, they work harder, resulting in a high number of injuries. Many of these injuries force otherwise able and successful therapists to prematurely leave the field. Furthermore, many therapists leave the field not because of overt injuries, but because of the physical burnout that occurs from the physicality of doing massage on a regular basis. Giving massage and engaging tissue can be hard work, especially when done with poor technique!

The goal of this chapter is to offer a set of 10 guidelines designed to create healthy body mechanics. Using good body mechanics is important all the time; however, it is crucial when performing deep tissue work, which requires a greater production and delivery of pressure. For this reason, these guidelines are especially recommended to bodyworkers who do deep tissue work on a regular basis. Although this chapter does not address all aspects and facets of body mechanics for bodyworkers, it does provide a number of essential basics. As much as following rules and guidelines is important, keep in mind that bodywork is not only a science, it is also an art. Therefore the following guidelines need to be incorporated into the particular style of the therapist.

Category 1: Equipment

Guideline #1: Lower Table Height

Table height is probably the number one factor determining the efficiency of the therapist's force delivery. The proper height of the table is determined by a combination of factors, including the following:

o Height of the therapist
o Size of the client
o Positioning of the client on the table (supine, prone, or side lying)
o Technique being employed

When it comes to the production and delivery of force with less effort, the table must be low. Setting the table low allows the therapist to use his/her body weight to create force. Weight is merely a measure of the force that gravity exerts upon mass; given that gravity is an external force that never tires, why not take advantage of it?

When a therapist generates force to work on a client, that force can be created in two ways, internally within the body by muscles, or externally from gravity. Creation of internal force by musculature requires effort on our part, and can be fatiguing. However, the creation of force by gravity requires no effort. If the goal is to create force with the minimum effort possible, it is desirable to use gravity as much as possible. However, gravity does not work horizontally or diagonally; it only works vertically, or downward. Therefore it only works if the therapist's body weight is literally above the client. This requires the client to be placed below the therapist; hence the necessity of low table height.

BOX 4-1

Although there is not one exact proper height of a table, as a rule for deep work, the top of the table should be no higher than the top of the therapist's patella (knee joint).

With the client located below the therapist, the therapist does not need to expend much effort; rather it is only necessary to *lean into* the client, letting the therapist's body weight generate forceful deep pressure (Figure 4-1). Given that the greatest weight of the body is located in the core (i.e., the trunk and pelvis) of the body, it is the trunk and pelvis that must be positioned above the client when the therapist leans in.

Figure 4-1 Illustration of a therapist working on a client with the table set at three different heights. In each photo, the blue arrow represents the force through the therapist's upper extremity into the client, and the green vertical arrow represents the component of that force that is due to gravity (the green horizontal arrow represents the force of body weight of the therapist that is lost because it is not purely vertical). Note that the vertical component vector is least when the table is set high (**A**), and is greatest when the table is set low (**C**). Ideally, if the line of force of the therapist is almost purely vertical as in **C**, nearly all the force can be delivered via gravity, and little effort needs to be expended by the therapist's musculature. A good guideline to determine proper table height for deep tissue work is to have the top of your table be no higher than the top of the patella (the knee joint).

When generating deep pressure by leaning into the client, it is important for the therapist to maintain a position of self-support. This means that even though the therapist is leaning into the client, if the client moved or the therapist needed to remove the pressure from the client, the therapist could quickly stop leaning on the client and regain balance and be

BOX 4-2

To test at home the principle of table height, place a bathroom scale on a chair or massage table at various heights. At each height, simply lean into the scale and read the force that you are generating on the scale (Figure 4-2). If the scale is low enough that you are directly above it, note how much pressure you can effortlessly generate by passively leaning into the scale. Try to create the same reading on the scale through muscular effort when the scale is located on a higher surface. The difference in effort required is the difference in work that the therapist must do. Multiply this by how many minutes or hours the therapist works per week/month/year, and the cumulative effect of a table set too high can be appreciated.

Figure 4-2 Demonstration of an easy method using an ordinary bathroom scale to determine how much effort is necessary at different heights to generate force in a client's body. By placing the scale lower and simply leaning into it, the greatest pressure with least effort is obtained.

able to support his or her body again. Working from a position of self-support maintains the therapist's control and balance, increasing the effectiveness of the session as well as the client's comfort. This self-support can be maintained via a strong and stable stance of the lower extremities (this will be discussed more fully in Guideline #5).

In addition to the height of the table, the table width must also be considered. The wider the table, the more difficult it is for the therapist to position body weight over the client; if the client is located at the center of the table, the client is farther away from the therapist. For this reason, a narrow table is more desirable when it comes to using body weight.

Electric Lift Table

When working with a table set lower, there is another factor to consider. A low table height is ideal when deep pressure is desired; however, it is actually easier to work with a higher table height when light pressure is being applied. It requires less effort for lighter pressure if you stand straighter and apply pressure into the client with strokes that are more horizontally oriented. If the table is set low in this scenario, you either must bend to reach lower or must widen the stance of the lower extremities to bring the upper body down to the height of the client. Between these two choices, widening the stance is preferable; however, it requires greater effort than simply standing upright. For this reason, ideal table height will vary during a treatment session based upon the work that is being done. The solution to this dilemma for anyone who combines deep tissue work and lighter work on a regular basis is to use an electric lift table. Although electric lift tables are viewed as extravagant by many in the bodywork profession, in my opinion, they are a necessity. Being able to change the height of the table during a session by merely pressing on a foot pedal enables deeper pressure to be delivered with less effort on a low table, and allows you to stand straighter when doing lighter work with the table set higher. This allows for better sessions therapeutically for the client and healthier and less fatiguing sessions for the therapist. In the long run, the benefits of an electric lift table far outweigh the increased cost of the initial purchase.

Guideline #2: Use Less Lubricant

For beginning bodyworkers, the amount of lubricant used is often part of the problem. The point of using a lubricant is to allow the therapist's hands to glide along the client's skin without excessive friction. However, the more lubricant that is used, the more the therapist's pressure translates into slipping and sliding *along* the client's skin instead of delivering pressure *into* the client's tissues. The general guideline for lubricant is to use the least amount necessary for the client's comfort. Any amount greater than this decreases the efficiency of pressure delivery into the client. Besides the amount of lubricant, the type of lubricant can also make a difference. Generally, oil-based lubricants tend to create more slide and are not as efficient as water-based lubricants for deep tissue work.

Category 2: Positioning the Body

Guideline #3: Bend Properly

Although the ideal body posture for delivering deep pressure with maximal efficiency is for you to be positioned directly above the client and delivering the force directly downward, this body posture is not usually possible to attain without

BOX 4-3

To Shrug or Not to Shrug?

It seems universally accepted that when doing massage therapy, it is bad body mechanics to work with our shoulders up at our ears—in other words, the scapulae elevated at the scapulocostal joints—giving what could be called "shrugged shoulders." I must admit that I accepted this sacred cow of body mechanics for many years. After all, we always tell our clients that they should relax and let their shoulders drop. And who doesn't have tight muscles of scapular elevation (upper trapezius, levator scapulae, and rhomboids), most likely due to our stress patterns of holding our shoulders up in an uptight posture? Therefore it seems perfectly reasonable that when we see massage therapy students or practicing therapists with their shoulders up at their ears while working on their clients, we instinctively tell them to relax and let their shoulders down.

But recently, I started noticing that my shoulders were often up high when working on clients. This puzzled me because I felt relaxed while doing these massages. Yet, I told myself that shrugged shoulders could not be right, so I brought them down and continued with the massage. However, I soon found myself with my shoulders elevated again. So, a doubt began to enter my mind, but remained in the shadows. Once in a while I would think about it for a minute or two, but I never actually came out and said to anyone that shrugged shoulders could be okay. It was when I was demonstrating proper body posture/mechanics while teaching a deep tissue workshop in Tucson, Arizona, that a particularly astute participant pinned me down with the question, "Is working with elevated shoulders always bad?" I was a bit shocked to hear myself answer, "No." It was the first time I ever said that out loud. It seemed heretical and I am sure that a number of readers right now are shaking their heads and wondering how I could be saying this.

What I realized at that moment is that working with shrugged shoulders is not necessarily right or wrong. It depends on why our shoulders are up there. Most of the time, it is likely that our shoulders are shrugged because our table is set too high (see Guideline #1), and we are trying in vain to get over our client. In this scenario, we actively contract our scapular elevators to raise our shoulders. Staying like this for more than a moment or two will certainly lead to tight and painful muscles of scapular elevation. In this circumstance, working with shrugged shoulders is definitely bad. However, when the table is set low and we are directly over the client, if we simply lean into the client and relax our scapular muscles, then our shoulders will naturally be pushed up toward our ears.

As a law of physics states, "For every action, there is an equal and opposite reaction." If we are pressing down on our client, our client is pressing back up on us, pushing our shoulders up. In this scenario, if we do not want our shoulders to rise in the air, then we would have to exert muscular effort to hold them down, whereas letting them elevate would be the more relaxed and effortless posture to assume, and (dare I say it…?) good body mechanics!

The one potential drawback to allowing the shoulders to passively rise is that the shoulder girdle will be slightly less rigid, and as such, a small amount of pressure and control might be lost when transmitting force from the core through the shoulder girdle to the client. However, I believe this loss is negligible and, depending upon the circumstance, would likely be outweighed by the benefit of having relaxed musculature. Furthermore, having a relaxed shoulder girdle creates a more fluid base from which to work, decreasing the possibility that the client may sense rigidity in our technique.

When working on your clients, examine your own shoulder posture (having a mirror in the massage room is an excellent way to monitor your posture). If your shoulders are up high, feel whether you are actively working to keep them up there or whether you are relaxed. If you are working hard to hold them up there, then I recommend that you lower your table and relax your shoulders. However, if they are comfortably relaxed up there, then maybe there is nothing wrong with letting them be there!

some bending. The manner in which the therapist bends is extremely important, because bending tends to create postural imbalances that require effort to maintain and places stress upon the therapist's body. Bending postures can be divided into two general categories: the stoop bend and the squat bend.

Stoop Bend

The stoop bend, which involves flexing the trunk at the spinal joints to bring the body over the client, is less healthy for the therapist. This is because it unbalances the therapist's body by moving the center of weight of the trunk from being balanced directly over the pelvis to being unsupported (Figure 4-3, A). In this position, the only reason that the therapist's trunk does not fall into full flexion is that the spinal extensor musculature must contract isometrically to maintain the partially flexed and imbalanced trunk posture. Furthermore, a stooped posture of spinal flexion places the spinal joints in their open-packed position. The open-packed position of a joint is its least stable position; therefore greater muscular contraction is necessary to stabilize the joints. The result is greater effort on the part of the spinal extensor musculature to maintain the stooped posture.

Squat Bend

A better alternative is the squat bend, which is achieved by flexing the hip and knee joints instead of the spinal joints. In a squat bend, the spine stays erect in its closed-packed position, which is its most stable position. This requires less stabilization contraction effort by the spinal extensor musculature and is healthier for the spine.

BOX 4-4

In addition to flexion of the hip joints and knee joints, the squat bend also requires the ankle joints to dorsiflex (the dorsum of the legs move toward the dorsum of the feet).

YOU ARE HERE

4

Figure 4-3 A shows the stoop bend, in which the therapist bends by flexing the spinal joints of the trunk. Of the three methods of bending, the stoop bend is least healthy for the therapist. **B** shows the squat bend with the trunk inclined forward, and **C** shows the squat bend with the trunk vertical. The squat bend with the trunk vertical is biomechanically the least stressful on the therapist's body and should generally be used whenever bending over a client.

BOX 4-5

The closed-packed position of a joint is the position in which it is most stable. This is usually a combination of the joint surfaces having maximal contact and the ligaments and joint capsules being most taut.

There are two squat bend methods:
1. Squat bend with the trunk inclined forward
2. Squat bend with the trunk maintaining its vertical posture

Between these two, maintaining a vertically positioned trunk is preferable, because a squat bend with the trunk inclined forward still places the trunk in an imbalanced posture in which its center of weight is unsupported (Figure 4-3, B). This requires spinal extensor musculature contraction to prevent the trunk from falling into flexion, as well as hip joint extensor musculature contraction to maintain the flexed anterior tilt posture of the pelvis at the hip joints.

The squat bend with the trunk vertically positioned maintains the trunk in a balanced posture, such that its center of weight is aligned and supported over the pelvis (Figure 4-3, C). This eliminates the need for spinal extensor musculature contraction to keep the trunk from falling into flexion and hip joint extensor musculature to maintain pelvic posture.

The key to creating a vertical squat bend instead of an inclined squat bend is the degree of knee joint flexion. As the hip joints are flexed to achieve the squat bend position, the pelvis anteriorly tilts, inclining the trunk forward. However, the more the knee joints are flexed as the hip joints are flexed, the easier it is to keep the trunk vertical. This is "bending with the knees" as we often hear. Hence, a squat bend with the trunk vertically aligned maintains the spine in its most stable closed-packed posture, and maintains the trunk in a balanced and supported posture over the lower body. This allows the therapist to work and deliver pressure efficiently while maintaining a healthy spine.

BOX 4-6

It is interesting that even though most everyone knows that it is healthier for our back if we bend with our knees, so many people do not follow this advice and instead fall into a stoop bend. There must be a reason for this. As it turns out, although the squat bend is healthier for the back, it requires more energy expenditure than the stoop bend. Furthermore, even though the squat bend is healthier for the back, it does place a greater stress on the knee joints. All things being equal, it is usually more important to protect the spinal joints. However, when applying these bending guidelines to each therapist's needs, the stress upon the knee joints must be factored in. If a therapist has unhealthy knee joints, a stoop bend may be the lesser of two evils.

Guideline #4: Align the Core
It has been stated that the key to delivering a strong force is for the therapist to use the weight of the core as much as possible. The importance of core (i.e., trunk and pelvis) positioning was discussed in Guideline #1. However, the orientation and alignment of the core, not just the position, are also critically

important to efficiently delivering pressure. As a rule, for body weight to be behind the pressure that is being delivered to the client, your trunk and pelvis must face the same direction as that of the pressure being applied. An easy way to determine your core alignment is to look at your navel. Whatever direction your navel is facing, your core is facing.

BOX 4-7

Some therapists prefer to look at where their sternum or anterior superior iliac spines (ASISs) are facing instead of where their navel is facing to determine the alignment of their core.

For example, if the force of a soft tissue stroke is being applied across the client's body, then your navel should be facing across the client's body in the identical direction. If, on the other hand, the force of the soft tissue stroke is being applied longitudinally along the length of the client's body, then your navel should be similarly oriented. Figure 4-4 demonstrates a few examples of proper orientation and alignment of the core. In these examples, note the change in orientation and alignment of the therapist's core to match the direction of force delivery. Furthermore, note that when working from a seated position, the therapist's elbow is tucked in front of the core of his body. This is best accomplished by laterally rotating the arm at the shoulder joint. This naturally brings the elbow in front of the core of the pelvis, where it can be tucked inside the anterior superior iliac spine (ASIS). When the therapist now leans in with his core, his body weight is transmitted right through his forearm and hand into the client.

BOX 4-8

Aligning the core along the direction of force is largely a matter of proper positioning of the feet. This is discussed in more detail in Guideline #5.

Guideline #5: Position the Feet
Thus far, much has been said about the importance of the positioning, orientation, and alignment of your core. However, there is an old adage in tennis that says, "It's all in the footwork." This is no less true when doing bodywork. Your footwork is crucially important, for both aligning and positioning the core, and also for pushing off to generate pressure. To achieve all these things, let's look at the placement of the feet. Generally, the direction that the feet are facing is the direction that the core is facing. Therefore, if it is desired to change the orientation of the core, the easiest way to accomplish this is to change the orientation of the feet. Furthermore, if the feet are not positioned correctly, it is not possible to generate force from a lower extremity by plantarflexing a foot against the ground to push the body weight into the client.

Positioning of the feet can be divided into two general categories—transverse stance and longitudinal stance. Squaring off the feet perpendicular to the length of the table is called the transverse stance, and orienting the feet parallel to the length of the table is called the longitudinal stance. The transverse stance is effective for delivering pressure transversely across the client's body because it orients your core in that direction (Figure 4-5, A); however, it is ineffective when working longitudinally up the client's body because the core is not facing that direction. On the other hand, the longitudinal stance is effec-

4

Figure 4-4 Demonstration of the importance of the orientation and alignment of the therapist's core (trunk and pelvis). **A** illustrates a long massage stroke along the spine on the paraspinal musculature. For the body weight of the core to be behind the stroke, the alignment of the core must be identical to the line of force of the stroke. **B** and **C** illustrate core alignment during the application of force to a client's neck, with the therapist working from a seated position. In **B**, the therapist is working the client's lower neck. In **C**, the therapist is working the client's upper neck. In these examples, note the change in orientation and alignment of the therapist's core to match the direction of force delivery.

Figure 4-5 The two positions of the therapist's feet relative to the table, and therefore the client's body, when doing bodywork. **A** is the transverse stance and is optimal when delivering force transversely across the client's body. **B** is the longitudinal stance and is optimal when delivering pressure longitudinally up or down the client's body. The importance of the orientation of the feet is that the trunk and pelvis, and therefore core body weight, are usually oriented in the direction that the feet are pointed.

tive for delivering pressure longitudinally along the client's body because it orients your core to face that way (Figure 4-5, B); however, it is ineffective when working transversely across the client's body because the core is not facing that direction.

Further discussion is warranted regarding the precise orientation of your feet relative to each other. There is a great deal of argument over optimal positioning of the feet. In the feet aligned position, they are located next to each other; in the feet staggered position, one foot is farther anterior than the other. When the feet are staggered, there are then two choices for the orientation of the rear foot. Overall, there are three possible positions of the feet relative to each other:
1. Feet aligned position (next to each other and parallel)
2. Feet staggered position, with both feet facing approximately the same direction (i.e., approximately parallel)
3. Feet staggered position, with the rear foot oriented approximately perpendicular to the front foot

An inherent weakness with the aligned position of the feet (Figure 4-6, A) is that the base of support created by the feet is not very long in the sagittal plane from anterior to posterior. This makes it difficult to maintain balance of the upper body over the feet with movements of the pelvis and trunk in the sagittal plane as you lean forward into the client. For example, if you try to lean into the client by bringing the pelvis and

trunk forward (bending at the hip joints), your body weight will be projected anterior to the base of the feet and will not be supported and balanced. If you compensate for the anterior weight shift of the trunk by shifting the weight of the pelvis posteriorly in an effort to counterbalance the body, then your overall body weight shifts posteriorly and is no longer sufficiently anterior to be over the client's body. In this position, body weight cannot be used effectively to generate force.

Similarly, the therapist is unbalanced and unsupported in this position if the core of the body is propelled forward by pushing off from the feet. Either staggered position of the feet is superior in this regard, because the rear foot can be used to push off the ground and project the therapist's body weight forward, while the therapist's body weight will still be balanced and supported over the front foot. Hence, a staggered position of the feet provides a wide sagittally oriented stance allowing for balance of the body between the rear foot and front foot. This is especially valuable when performing strokes of any length.

Between the two choices of staggered positioning of the feet, having the rear foot facing approximately the same direction as the front foot (Figure 4-6, B) is the superior position because it places the powerful sagittally oriented ankle joint plantarflexor musculature (soleus, gastrocnemius, tibialis posterior, flexors digitorum and hallucis longus, and fibularis

4

Figure 4-6 Illustration of three positions of the therapist's feet. In **A**, both feet are aligned and parallel to each other. This position is least efficient at generating a forward force into the client. In **B** and **C**, the feet are staggered, with one foot in front and one in back. In **B**, they are both facing approximately forward. In **C**, the rear foot is pointed nearly perpendicular to the front foot. The staggered position of **B** with both feet facing forward is the most efficient at generating a forward force into the client.

BOX 4-9

An advantage to having the two feet oriented in opposite directions, such as in Figure 4-6, C, is that it allows the therapist to easily change the direction that the body is facing. Being able to change the direction of the body is extremely important in martial arts; this is why this position is so often employed there. However, for delivering pressure during bodywork, this advantage does not outweigh the disadvantage of losing the strength possible when the feet are oriented in the same direction.

---

longus and brevis), knee joint extensor musculature (quadriceps femoris), and hip joint extensor muculature (hamstrings, adductor magnus, and posterior gluteals) in line with the direction of the stroke.

The position in Figure 4-6, C, wherein the rear foot is oriented markedly differently than the front foot (and indeed the entire body), loses the orientation of the powerful sagittally oriented musculature just mentioned and also places the two lower extremities at odds with each other during force generation because they face in different directions.

There is one final aspect of feet placement that should be addressed. There is no rule that states the feet must be planted at the beginning of a stroke and stay in that planted position for the entire stroke; the feet can be moved. With a short stroke or compression applied to one location, there is little or no need to move the feet. However, with a longer stroke, if the feet are not moved, you will have to reach out horizontally farther away from the initial base of support of the feet. Support and balance will be lost, the trunk cannot be maintained vertically, and therefore body weight can no longer be used as effectively to generate force downward with gravity. To prevent this, especially during longer strokes, it is important to move the feet.

Guideline #6: Position the Head
An often overlooked aspect of body mechanics is the head position of the therapist, or more specifically, the position of the therapist's neck and head. The position of the neck and head has little to do with the direct generation and delivery of force while performing a massage. Therefore it makes sense that the therapist should posturally hold the neck and head in whatever position is least stressful. The healthiest posture is to hold

4

Figure 4-7 Two postures of the therapist's head during bodywork. In **A**, the therapist is flexing the neck and head to look at the client as the stroke is being performed. In **B**, the therapist is holding the head in a more balanced posture over the trunk. This posture is least stressful to the body.

the head over the trunk so that the center of weight of the head is balanced over the trunk. This position requires little or no muscular effort by neck muscles to support it. Unfortunately, many therapists have a habit of flexing the neck and head at the spinal joints to look down at their client while they work. This unbalances the posture of the head and requires isometric contraction of the extensor musculature of the neck to keep the head from falling anteriorly into flexion. Over time, this leads to pain and spasm in the posterior neck musculature. If it is necessary for you to look at the client during a stroke, then this posture is necessary and correct to assume. However, most of the time there is little or no need for it; you even can close your eyes and visualize the structure of the client under your hands. So it is a good reminder for you to occasionally focus on the posture of your neck and head to be sure they are in a posture that is as easy and relaxed as possible (Figure 4-7).

Guideline #7: Stack the Joints
Whether the force behind the stroke is created by muscular effort on your part or is due to using body weight, this force must be transmitted through your upper extremity joints (elbow, wrist, fingers, thumb). For this force to travel through the upper extremity joints without loss of strength, it is important that the joints are stacked. Stacked joints are extended and placed in a straight line as seen in Figure 4-8, A. This is usually best accomplished by laterally rotating the arms at the shoulder joints, bringing the elbows in front of the core of the body. In this manner, you can deliver pressure for the stroke in a

straight line from the core of the body through the stacked joints of the upper extremity to the contact with the client.

If you do this as you lean and/or push into the client by pushing off with the back foot, there will be little or no loss of strength, and less muscular effort is necessary. However, when your upper extremity joints are not stacked (i.e., they are flexed), the force generated that must pass through the upper extremities will probably be lost to the client, because the joints of the upper extremity will tend to collapse further into flexion. Thus the force that was supposed to be delivered into the client's tissues is lost in creating movement of the therapist's body at the shoulder, elbow, wrist, and finger or thumb joints (Figures 4-8, B-C).

It is possible to transmit force through these unstacked, flexed upper extremity joints without loss of strength. However, it requires greater effort because muscles around the unstacked joints must be isometrically contracted to stabilize the joints, preventing them from collapsing. This results in greater effort and is less efficient for the therapist.

Category 3: Performing the Massage Stroke

Guideline #8: Generate Force Proximally
It has been stated that use of body weight via the external force of gravity is recommended whenever possible because it requires little or no effort. However, when it is necessary for you

4

Figure 4-8 Demonstration of force delivery through a therapist's upper extremities that are stacked and not stacked. **A** shows a therapist who has the elbow, wrist, and thumb joints of the upper extremities fully stacked. **B** shows the therapist with the elbow joints unstacked (i.e., flexed). As the force generated in the therapist's core is transmitted through the flexed elbow joints, these joints tend to collapse, and the therapist's trunk falls toward the client, as shown in **C**. Collapsing at unstacked upper extremity joints reduces the force delivered into the client.

BOX 4-10

Even perfectly stacked joints do not eliminate all effort and stress to the body. Although markedly less than with unstacked joints, there will still be some contraction effort on the part of the musculature to stabilize the stacked joints. Furthermore, because all of the therapist's force is efficiently transmitted through the joints, stacked joints are subjected to greater joint compression forces than are unstacked joints. However, by keeping the joints straight in line with the force being transmitted, all force from your trunk is transmitted without loss of strength to the client.

to use internal muscular effort to generate the therapeutic force for the treatment technique, there is a choice of which muscles to use.

When choosing between small and large muscles, it is always advantageous for you to generate the force using larger muscles of the body. A smaller muscle cannot generate the same maximal force that a larger muscle can. Furthermore, to the degree that a smaller muscle does generate the same force as a larger muscle, it requires a much greater effort to achieve this.

Looking at the muscles of the upper extremity from distal to proximal, it is evident that smaller muscles are located more distally and larger muscles are located more proximally. For example, the intrinsic finger joint muscles within the hand are smaller than the wrist joint muscles within the forearm, which are smaller than the elbow joint muscles within the arm, which are smaller than the shoulder joint muscles within the trunk. For this reason, whenever possible, it is recommended that a proximal generation of force from the trunk is done instead of a distal generation of force from the upper extremities.

In addition to the larger proximal core muscles of the trunk, large muscle groups of the lower extremities can also be engaged to create great force with little effort. By placing the feet appropriately, the therapist can push off the ground using powerful ankle joint plantarflexors and knee and hip joint extensors to generate strength of force that can be delivered into the client. (See Guideline #5 on page 35 for more information about proper positioning of your feet.) Furthermore, just as

BOX 4-11

Putting a number of the these guidelines together, it can be seen that the most efficient delivery of pressure into the client is a straight (stacked) line of force that travels unbroken from the therapist's lower extremities and core, into their upper extremities, and then into the client. This is true when generating force to press into the client. However, having a stacked line of force is just as important and efficient when the therapist is pulling on the client instead. Although pulling strokes are generally not employed as often as compression strokes, they are extremely valuable in certain instances and should be applied with the same efficiency of body mechanics.

the core of the body should be behind (in other words, in line with the force of the stroke that is transmitted through the upper extremities), the lower extremities should be oriented in the same line. The line of force through the therapist's body should travel in one straight line from the feet to the core and through the upper extremities into the client's body.

Guideline #9: Direct Force Perpendicular to the Contour of the Client's Body

When we discussed table height in Guideline #1, it was emphasized that the most efficient way to use gravity is to direct the force vertically downward. However, the body surface of the client that is being worked is not always horizontally flat. Therefore, although a vertically downward application of force is the most efficient way to use gravity, it is not always the most efficient direction to transmit force into the client's body. For example, when a client is prone, the client's back has contours created by the curves of the spinal column. Taking these contours into account, the therapist must change the direction of force so that it is perpendicular to the contour of the client's body at the point of contact. This means that the therapist will not always be pressing directly vertically downward; rather the therapist might have to direct the force diagonally so that it is perpendicular to the client's body surface.

There are even times when the therapist is working horizontally into the side of the client's body. For these cases it is important to realize that the most powerful and efficient delivery of force into the client's body is the force that is applied perpendicular to the body surface being worked. Any deviation from perpendicular will involve some loss of strength and efficiency, because some of the force will be transmitted into sliding along the tissue instead of pressing into it.

BOX 4-12

Trigonometric formulas (sine, cosine, and tangent) can be used to determine the exact amount of force that is lost when a massage stroke is not delivered perpendicular to the surface of the client's body.

To illustrate this idea, Figure 4-9 shows three different applications of force for a therapist working on a client's back. Note that in each case, the force is applied perpendicular to the contour of the region of the back that is being worked. If you try this in your practice, I believe that you will intuitively find it to be the easiest way to generate pressure with the least effort. A necessary addendum to this concept is that if a long stroke is being done—for example, one that covers the length of the spine—the contours encountered during that stroke will vary. For maximal efficiency, it is necessary for the therapist to adjust to these contours by changing the direction that pressure is applied; this necessitates changing the orientation of the core, and likely also necessitates changing the position of the feet.

BOX 4-13

The contact is defined as whatever surface of the therapist contacts and transmits force into the client.

Figure 4-9 Illustration of three applications of force into the back of a client. **A**, The thoracolumbar region is worked by applying the force diagonally in a cephalad direction (toward the head). **B**, The midthoracic region is worked by applying force vertically downward. **C**, The upper thoracic region is worked by applying the force diagonally in a caudal direction (toward the lower body). Note how the direction of the force of the stroke is different in each case, so that it is delivered perpendicular to the contour of the body surface that is being worked. Applying pressure perpendicular to the body surface contour is the most efficient delivery of force.

Guideline #10: Choose a Larger Contact Surface When Possible and Double-Support It

When deep pressure is being delivered, it must be transmitted into the client through whatever body part the therapist uses to contact the client. Apart from the occasional use of elbow, forearms, and feet, a bodyworker's contact is usually the hand. The danger is that over time, continually transmitting deep pressure through the hands will damage their relatively small joints. To protect the therapist's hands against injury, it is important for the contact surface of the hand to be as large as possible. For example, working with the palm of the hand instead of the fingers or thumb allows for deeper pressure to be given with less chance of injury to the therapist.

The disadvantage to using a larger contact instead of the fingers or thumb is that larger contacts tend to be less sensitive, making it more difficult for the therapist to assess both the quality of the client's tissues and the response of the client tissues to the pressure of the treatment as the massage is performed. The appropriate contact at any point during the massage can only be determined by the therapist. If you like to use fingers or thumbs a lot, I would recommend that you alternate between these contacts as often as possible. This distributes the stress load around the hand, giving each muscle and joint a chance to rest.

In addition to choosing a larger hand contact, it is important to double-support the contact. This means that the two hands are working on the client together instead of separately. One hand should be placed somewhat over the other so that the contact hand on the client is stabilized and reinforced by the other hand (Figure 4-10). Another benefit of double-supporting the contact is that it strengthens the therapist's contact, allowing for a stronger and more efficient delivery of force into the client. Protecting the contact area of the hand is particularly needed when working with smaller contacts, such as the fingers or thumbs. Although double-supporting the contact means that less surface area of the client can be covered during a stroke, the benefits when doing deep tissue work more than compensate for this. Figure 4-10 illustrates four double-supported contacts of the therapist's hands upon the client.

Figure 4-10 Four examples of a double-supported contact of a therapist's hands upon a client. **A,** Double-support of the thumb. **B,** Double-support of the fingers. **C,** Double-support of the ulnar side of the hand. **D,** Double-support of the palm of the hand.

 BOX 4-14

Stabilizing the contact upon the client by double-supporting it is often described as bracing the contact.

BOX 4-15

For a therapist with a hyperextendable interphalangeal joint of the thumb, double-supporting the thumb is critically important to prevent it from collapsing into hyperextension.

Summary

No matter what technique and style of delivery we have, doing massage is hard work and physically stresses the body; this reality cannot be avoided. However, if we learn to work more efficiently, we can decrease these stresses. The proposed guidelines of this chapter are meant to help increase the efficiency of our work and thereby minimize the stress to our body. As you practice them, keep in mind that any change made in body mechanics will most likely feel awkward at first, simply because it is different. However, with time, applying these guidelines should become more comfortable.

Although they are not comprehensive of all aspects of body mechanics for bodyworkers, these 10 guidelines are a solid foundation to build upon. Note that even though these guidelines were presented and discussed separately in this chapter, it is only by seamlessly weaving them into a cohesive whole that a fluid and efficient style for the delivery of bodywork can be achieved. Furthermore, by increasing the efficiency and decreasing the effort of our work, the quality of our work will likely improve as well. Increasing efficiency is learning to work smarter instead of working harder.

Chapter 5

Anatomy, Physiology, and Treatment of Trigger Points (TrPs)

Overview

This chapter defines a trigger point (TrP) and then covers the foundational anatomy, physiology, and pathology of myofascial TrPs. To understand the mechanism of how TrPs develop, sarcomere structure and the sliding filament mechanism are reviewed. Then the two major hypotheses, the *energy crisis hypothesis* and *dysfunctional endplate hypothesis,* for TrP genesis are discussed, including their fusion into what is called the *integrated trigger point hypothesis.* The relationship of the *pain–spasm–pain cycle* and the *contraction–ischemia cycle* are also related to the genesis of a TrP. Then the relationships between central and attachment TrPs, and key TrPs and satellite TrPs are examined, as well as the general factors that create TrPs. The effects of TrPs are discussed, including the concept and proposed mechanisms for how a TrP refers pain. The chapter concludes with an exploration of how TrPs can be located in clinical practice and a discussion of the major methods used by manual and movement therapists to treat TrPs, including the relative efficacy of the methods of sustained compression compared with deep-stroking massage. Note: Common patterns of TrPs in individual muscles with the typical corresponding referral zone(s) are given in Part III of this book.

Chapter Outline

Chapter Objectives

After completing this chapter, the student should be able to perform the following:

1. Define the key terms of this chapter.
2. List the different types of TrPs.
3. Discuss the similarities and differences between active and latent TrPs.
4. Describe the structure of a sarcomere and explain how the sliding filament mechanism works.
5. Discuss the relationship between the sliding filament mechanism, the energy crisis hypothesis, and the genesis of a TrP.
6. Describe how the pain–spasm–pain, contraction–ischemia, and pain–spasm–ischemia cycles relate to the genesis of a TrP.

7. Describe the dysfunctional endplate hypothesis.
8. Describe the relationship among the energy crisis, the dysfunctional endplate, and the integrated TrP hypotheses.
9. Discuss the relationship between central and attachment TrPs, including the role of enthesopathy.
10. List and discuss the general factors that tend to create TrPs.
11. Describe the effects of a TrP.
12. Discuss the relationship between a key TrP and a satellite TrP.

Continued

13. Discuss the two types of TrP referral patterns and the proposed mechanisms for how TrPs refer pain.

14. Discuss the methods and principles involved in locating a client's TrPs.

15. Discuss the various methods of TrP treatment, including the proposed mechanism for their validity and the possible benefit of one method versus the other.

Key Terms

active TrP
adaptively shorten
attachment TrP
central TrP
contraction–ischemia cycle
contracture
convergence–projection theory
cord spillover theory
deep-stroking massage
dysfunctional endplate hypothesis
energy crisis hypothesis
enthesopathy
essential referral zone

integrated TrP hypothesis
ischemia
ischemic compression
key TrP
latent TrP
motor point
myofascial TrP
pain–spasm–ischemia cycle
pain–spasm–pain cycle
pincer grip
primary referral zone
sarcomere
satellite TrP

sclerotogenous referred pain
secondary referral zone
shortened active insufficiency
sliding filament mechanism
spillover referral zone
stripping massage
sustained compression
taut band
trigger point (TrP)
TrP pressure release
twitch response
visceral referred pain

What is a Trigger Point?

A trigger point (TrP) is a focal area of hyperirritability that is locally sensitive to pressure and can refer symptoms (usually pain) to other areas of the body. TrPs are reported to exist in most every soft tissue of the body, including muscle, muscular fascia, periosteum, ligament, and skin. The term myofascial TrP is used to describe TrPs that exist within skeletal muscle tissue or skeletal muscular fascia (usually the tendon or aponeurosis of a muscle). This text will restrict its discussion to myofascial TrPs, which are the most common type of TrPs found in the body.

BOX 5-1

For simplicity of verbiage, unless the context is made otherwise clear, the term *TrP* will be used throughout this text to refer to a myofascial TrP.

Put simply, a skeletal muscle TrP is what the lay public refers to as a tight and painful muscle knot. More specifically, a skeletal muscle tissue TrP is a hyperirritable focal area of muscle hypertonicity (tightness) located within a taut band of skeletal muscle tissue. Furthermore, as with all TrPs, it is locally sensitive to palpatory pressure and can potentially refer pain or other symptoms to distant areas of the body.

All TrPs can be divided into two classifications, active TrPs and latent TrPs. Although the definitions are not fully consistent, it is generally agreed that latent TrPs do not cause local or referred pain unless they are first compressed, whereas active TrPs may produce local or referred pain even when they are not compressed. A latent TrP is essentially at a less severe stage than is an active TrP, and if left untreated, a latent TrP often develops into an active TrP.

Furthermore, myofascial TrPs are often divided into central TrPs and attachment TrPs. As their names imply, central TrPs are located in the center of a muscle (or more accurately, in the center of muscle fibers) and attachment TrPs are located at the attachment sites of a muscle.

BOX 5-2

If every muscle fiber of a muscle begins at one attachment of the muscle and ends at the other attachment of the muscle, then the center of a muscle would be the center of all its fibers. However, not all muscles have their fibers architecturally designed this way. For example, pennate muscles by definition do not have their fibers run from attachment to attachment. Furthermore, even fusiform muscles do not always have all their fibers run the entire length of a muscle. For this reason, the center of a muscle is not always synonymous with center of its fibers.

Effective clinical treatment of clients who present with myofascial pain syndromes requires an understanding of both why TrPs form in the first place and what the essential mechanism of a TrP is. This understanding is not possible unless sarcomere structure and the sliding filament mechanism of muscle contraction are first understood. For this reason, it is necessary to review these topics before continuing on with a discussion of TrPs.

Sarcomere Structure

A muscle is an organ that is made up of thousands of muscle fibers. Each muscle fiber is made up of thousands of myofibrils that run the length of the muscle fiber, and each myofibril is composed of thousands of sarcomeres laid end to end.

A sarcomere is bordered at both ends by a Z-line. Within a sarcomere, there are two types of filaments, actin and myo-

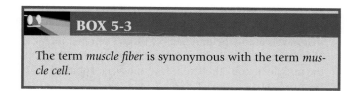

sin. The thin actin filaments are located on both sides of the sarcomere and are attached to the two Z-lines; the thick myosin filament is located at the center of the sarcomere. Furthermore, the myosin filament has projections called *heads* that can reach out and attach themselves to the actin filaments (Figure 5-1). Also important to note is that the sarcoplasmic reticulum of a muscle fiber has stored calcium ions within it.

When a muscle contracts, it does so because it has been ordered to contract by the nervous system. Given that a sarcomere is the basic structural unit and the basic functional unit of a muscle, to understand muscle contraction, it is necessary to first understand sarcomere function and its initiation by the

Figure 5-1 A sarcomere is bounded on both sides by Z-lines. The thin actin filaments attach to the Z-lines on both sides. The thick myosin filament is located in the center and contains projections called *heads.* A sarcomere is the basic structural and functional unit of muscle tissue. (From Muscolino JE: *Kinesiology: the skeletal system and muscle function,* enhanced edition, St Louis, 2007, Mosby.)

BOX 5-3

The term *muscle fiber* is synonymous with the term *muscle cell.*

---

nervous system. The process that describes sarcomere function is called the *sliding filament mechanism.*

Sliding Filament Mechanism

Following are the steps of the sliding filament mechanism:
1. When we will a contraction of a muscle, a message commanding this to occur originates in our brain. This message travels as an electrical impulse within our central nervous system.
2. This electrical impulse then travels out to the periphery in a motor neuron (nerve cell) of a peripheral nerve to go to the skeletal muscle. Where the motor neuron meets each individual muscle fiber is called the **motor point** and is usually located at approximately the midpoint (i.e., center) of the muscle fibers.
3. When the impulse gets to the end of the motor neuron, the motor neuron secretes its neurotransmitters (acetylcholine) into the synaptic cleft at the neuromuscular junction (Figure 5-2).
4. These neurotransmitters float across the synaptic cleft and bind to the motor endplate of the muscle fiber.

5

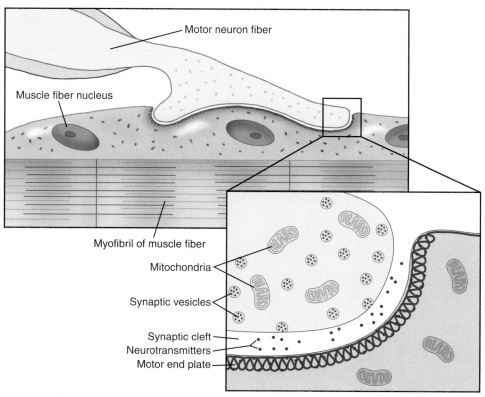

Figure 5-2 Neuromuscular junction. We see the synaptic vesicles containing the neurotransmitter molecules in the distal end of the motor neuron. These neurotransmitters are released into the synaptic cleft and then bind to the motor endplate of the muscle fiber's membrane. (Note: The inset box provides an enlargement.) (From Muscolino JE: *Kinesiology: the skeletal system and muscle function,* enhanced edition, St Louis, 2007, Mosby.)

5. The binding of these neurotransmitters onto the motor endplate causes an electrical impulse on the muscle fiber that travels along the muscle fiber's outer cell membrane. This electrical impulse is transmitted into the interior of the muscle fiber by the T tubules (transverse tubules) (Figure 5-3).

6. When this electrical impulse reaches the interior, it causes the sarcoplasmic reticulum of the muscle fiber to release stored calcium ions into the sarcoplasm (the cytoplasm of the muscle fiber).

7. These calcium ions then bind onto the actin filaments, causing a structural change that exposes the binding sites of actin filaments to the myosin heads.

8. Heads of the myosin filaments attach onto the binding sites of the actin filaments, creating myosin-actin cross-bridges.

9. These cross-bridges then bend, pulling the actin filaments in toward the center of the sarcomere (Figure 5-4).

10. If no ATP molecules are present, these cross-bridges will stay in place (hence the contraction is maintained) and no further sliding of the filaments will occur.

11. When ATP is present, the following sequence occurs: the cross-bridges between the myosin and actin filaments break because of the expenditure of energy of the ATP molecules, and the myosin heads attach to the next binding sites on the actin filaments, forming new cross-bridges. These new cross-bridges bend and pull the actin filaments further in toward the center of the sarcomere.

12. This process in Step 11 will repeat as long as ATP molecules are present to initiate the breakage, and calcium ions are present to keep the binding sites on the actin filaments exposed so that the next cross-bridges can be formed, which then pull the actin filaments further in toward the center of the sarcomere.

13. In this manner, sarcomeres of the innervated muscle fibers will contract to 100% of their ability.

14. When the nervous system message for contraction is no longer sent, neurotransmitters will no longer be released into the synapse. The neurotransmitters that were present are either broken down or reabsorbed by the motor neuron.

BOX 5-4

The steps listed here illustrate the sliding filament mechanism when the sarcomere (i.e., the entire muscle) is able to contract and shorten (concentrically contract). This only occurs if the force of the muscle's contraction is great enough to overcome whatever resistance force there is to shortening. Alternately, a muscle can contract and stay the same length (isometrically contract) or can contract and lengthen (eccentrically contract). Regardless of the type of contraction, the defining characteristic of a muscle contraction is the presence of the myosin-actin cross-bridges and the pulling force that they create.

BOX 5-5

ATP stands for "adenosine triphosphate." An ATP molecule can be likened to a battery because it stores energy in its bonds. Within a muscle fiber, its energy is used to provide the energy that is needed to both break myosin-actin cross-bridges and also reabsorb calcium ions back into the sarcoplasmic reticulum.

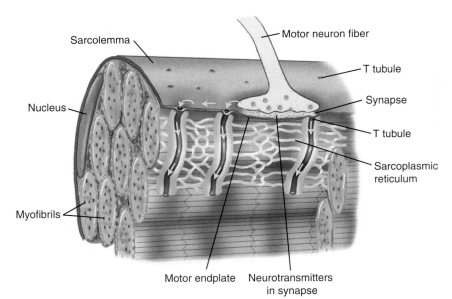

Figure 5-3 Binding of the neurotransmitters onto the motor endplate of the muscle fiber's membrane initiates an electrical impulse that travels along the outer membrane (sarcolemma) of the entire muscle fiber. This electrical impulse is then transmitted into the interior of the muscle fiber by the T tubules (transverse tubules) of the muscle fiber. (From Muscolino JE: *Kinesiology: the skeletal system and muscle function*, enhanced edition, St Louis, 2007, Mosby.)

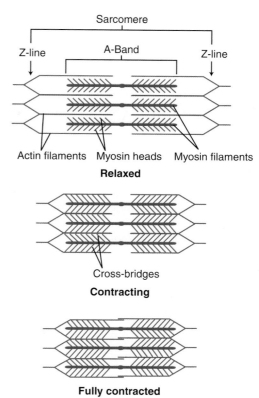

Figure 5-4 Steps of the sliding filament mechanism. **A,** Binding sites are exposed because of the presence of calcium ions (Ca++) that have been released by the sarcoplasmic reticulum. **B,** The myosin head forms a cross-bridge by attaching to one of the actin's binding sites. **C,** The myosin head bends, pulling the actin filament toward the center of the sarcomere. **D,** The myosin cross-bridge breaks. **E,** The process begins again when the myosin head attaches to another actin binding site. (From Muscolino JE: *Kinesiology: the skeletal system and muscle function,* enhanced edition, St Louis, 2007, Mosby.)

Figure 5-5 Illustration of how the sliding filament mechanism results in a change in length of a sarcomere. From the resting length of a sarcomere when it is relaxed, we see that as the sarcomere begins to contract, it begins to shorten toward its center. When the sarcomere is fully contracted, the sarcomere is at its shortest length. (From Muscolino JE: *Kinesiology: the skeletal system and muscle function,* enhanced edition, St Louis, 2007, Mosby.)

15. Without the presence of neurotransmitters in the synapse, no impulse is sent into the interior of the muscle fiber, and calcium ions are no longer released from the sarcoplasmic reticulum.
16. Calcium ions that were present in the sarcoplasm are reabsorbed by the sarcoplasmic reticulum by the expenditure of energy by ATP molecules.
17. Without the presence of calcium ions in the sarcoplasm, binding sites on actin filaments are no longer exposed, so it is no longer possible for new myosin-actin cross-bridges to form. Assuming that the old cross-bridges are released (because of the presence of ATP; see Step 11), the muscle contraction ceases.
18. The entire point of this process is that if actin filaments slide along the myosin filament toward the center of the sarcomere, then the Z-lines to which the actin filaments

are attached will be pulled in toward the center of the sarcomere and the sarcomere will shorten (Figure 5-5).
19. When the sarcomeres of a myofibril shorten, the myofibril shortens, pulling at its attachment ends.

Genesis of a TrP: Energy Crisis Hypothesis

Once normal muscle contraction is understood, it is not difficult to understand how a TrP can form. The most prominent theory for TrP genesis is called the energy crisis hypothesis. To understand the energy crisis hypothesis, it is necessary to understand the role that ATP molecules have within the sliding filament mechanism. ATP molecules provide the energy necessary to run the functions of a cell, including the sliding filament mechanism. Specifically, there are two steps within the sliding filament mechanism that require the input of energy from ATP molecules: ATP molecules are necessary to break the myosin-actin cross-bridges (Step 11), and they are necessary for reabsorption of calcium ions by the sarcoplasmic reticulum when the sarcomere contraction is complete (Step 16). If for any reason ATP molecules are not present during Step 11, the myosin-actin cross-bridges will not break and the affected sarcomeres will not be able to relax, thus forming a TrP. Furthermore, if ATP molecules are not present during

Step 16, the calcium ions cannot be reabsorbed into the sarcoplasmic reticulum. As long as calcium ions are present, active sites on actin molecules remain exposed and myosin-actin cross-bridges remain, continuing the contraction, thus forming a TrP.

BOX 5-6

The fact that a TrP is a local phenomenon is an important distinction, because when an entire muscle or a globally large portion of a muscle is tight, it is due to the pattern for tightness that is being directed from the gamma motor system of the central nervous system via muscle spindle reflex mediation. Therefore a globally tight muscle is tight because of central nervous system activity, whereas a TrP is a local phenomenon of muscle tightness. Some sources like to make this distinction by stating that a globally tight muscle occurs because of an excess of contraction, whereas a TrP occurs because of contracture. In this sense, the term *contracture* is used to emphasize that the mechanism of a TrP is not mediated and controlled by the central nervous system, whereas *contraction* denotes that the control is by the central nervous system.

Essentially, the energy crisis hypothesis is so named because if the sliding filament mechanism is deprived of ATP molecules, there will be a crisis due to insufficient energy, and the sarcomere contraction will continue, resulting in the formation of a TrP. The underlying cause of the lack of ATP molecules is ischemia (loss of arterial blood flow) to the region of sarcomeres affected due to the tightness of the muscle itself. When a muscle contracts, it becomes palpably harder and has the ability to constrict the blood vessels within it, restricting blood flow. A muscle contraction that is approximately 30% to 50% of its maximum is sufficient to close off arterial vessels located within it. When arterial blood vessels are closed off in this manner, the local muscle tissue loses its blood supply, resulting in a loss of nutrients including those needed to generate ATP molecules. Furthermore, this loss of ATP molecules occurs during a time of increased metabolic demand by the muscle, because its contraction requires ATP each time a cross-bridge breaks to then reform on a different active site of the actin filament. This initiates a vicious cycle called the contraction–ischemia cycle: muscle contraction causes ischemia, thereby creating a deficiency of ATP; without ATP, the muscle tissue cannot relax and therefore stays contracted; its contraction then continues to cut off the arterial blood supply furthering the ischemia, and so on (Figure 5-6, A). It is for this reason that once TrPs form, they tend to persist unless therapeutic intervention occurs.

Another exacerbating factor is that the venous vessels are also closed off due to the muscle contraction. Because it is the job of the venous vessels to remove waste products of metabolism, when veins are closed off, the waste products of metabolism remain in the tissues. Unfortunately these metabolic waste products are acidic and irritate the local muscle tissue, resulting in pain in the region, hence the tenderness that TrPs display. Ironically, the pain produced by these waste products tends to cause more spasming due to the pain–spasm–pain cycle (Figure 5-6, B), which only increases the ischemia.

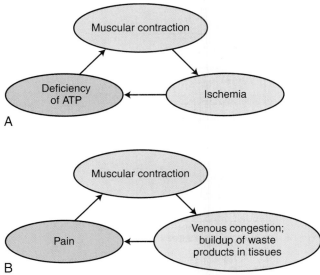

Figure 5-6 The contraction–ischemia and pain–spasm–pain cycles are illustrated. **A** shows the contraction–ischemia cycle. A strong muscular contraction closes off arterial blood supply, causing ischemia; this then results in a deficiency of ATP. Given that ATP is necessary to stop a muscle contraction, the muscle contraction continues, increasing the ischemia, and a vicious cycle ensues. **B** shows the pain–spasm–pain cycle. When muscle contraction closes off venous circulation, it causes a buildup (congestion) of noxious metabolic waste products that irritate the nerves in the area, resulting in pain. The pain triggers more muscular contraction, which then creates greater venous congestion of waste products and more pain, and a vicious cycle ensues.

Hence, we have a pain–spasm–ischemia cycle with TrPs that become entrenched in the muscle tissue.

With an understanding of the energy crisis hypothesis, we see that all that it takes to begin the process of TrP formation is for a part of a muscle to forcefully contract long enough to cause an *energy crisis* in the local muscle tissue. Given this, it is easy to see why TrPs are so prevalent in the body. In fact, it might be asked why TrPs do not form even more often than they do. The answer seems to be that the local muscle contraction must persist long enough to cause sufficient ischemia to create the energy crisis. Most of the time, we contract our muscles intermittently with periods of rest in between; these periods of rest allow a new flow of nutrients that can then be used for the production of ATP molecules in the muscle tissue. However, postural muscles very often contract isometrically for long periods of time without rest, such that ischemia and the resultant depletion of ATP is sufficient to create a TrP. This is one reason that TrPs are so often found in postural muscles; prominent examples include the trapezius and sternocleidomastoid.

Furthermore, irritation or injury to a region of a muscle is another factor often implicated in the formation of a TrP. When a region of a muscle is injured, highly irritating chemicals are released, which directly increases the sensitivity and tenderness of the area and also cause local swelling. This local swelling can press on nerves, causing more pain. It can also compress arterial blood vessels, causing ischemia. Furthermore, the pain caused by the irritating chemicals and the pressure from the swelling can initiate the pain–spasm–pain cycle.

Hence, TrPs tend to form within regions of a muscle that have contracted for long periods without rest, or within regions that have been irritated or injured. It is important to realize that once formed, a TrP is a local phenomenon. It does not continue because a person is directing the TrP to contract from the central nervous system; it is perpetuated because of the local factors in the muscle tissue at the TrP itself.

Central TrPs: Linking the Energy Crisis and Dysfunctional Endplate Hypotheses to Form the Integrated TrP Hypothesis

Interestingly, even though TrPs can form anywhere within a muscle, they most often form at the motor point of the muscle, usually located at the center of the muscle, where the motor neuron synapses with the muscle fibers. The proposed theory to explain why TrPs so often form at motor points is called the dysfunctional endplate hypothesis. This hypothesis posits that when a motor neuron continually carries the message for contraction to a muscle fiber, it secretes excessive amounts of acetylcholine into the synapse, causing the muscle fiber's motor endplate to produce excessive numbers of action potentials. This results in a sustained partial depolarization of the motor endplate, which then increases the local metabolic demand for ATP by the muscle fiber. This increased ATP usage by the motor endplate of the muscle fiber membrane further depletes the ATP available in the region of the motor endplate, which increases the energy crisis for the sarcomeres located closest to the motor endplate. Therefore sarcomeres located most closely to the motor endplate tend to form TrPs more easily than sarcomeres located in other regions of the muscle. Linking the energy crisis hypothesis with the dysfunctional endplate hypothesis is called the integrated TrP hypothesis. Because motor points of a muscle are usually located at the center of muscle fibers, most TrPs formed are central TrPs.

Central TrPs, Taut Bands, and Attachment TrPs

Once a central TrP has been created, its sarcomeres contract and shorten, pulling in toward their centers. This creates a constant pull upon the rest of the sarcomeres of the affected myofibril. This pull stretches these sarcomeres, creating a *taut band* of muscle tissue (Figure 5-7). For this reason, central TrPs are usually found within a taut band.

If the pulling force of the central TrP is sufficiently strong, the adjacent sarcomeres of the affected myofibril that lengthen will not be able to dissipate the entire pulling force of the central TrP, and its pull will be transferred to the ends of the myofibrils at their attachment into bone. Unfortunately, this pulling force irritates the ends of the myofibrils at or near the actual attachment into bone. The term enthesopathy is used to describe the condition that results from this constant irritation to the muscle's attachments, and can either cause a TrP to form in the sarcomeres of the skeletal muscle tissue near the attachment or cause a TrP to form within the muscle's tendon or the bone's periosteum at the muscle's attachment site. Whether formed within the skeletal tissue or its related fascial tissue, this TrP created by the enthesopathy due to the pull of the central TrP is called an *attachment TrP*. Hence, once central TrPs have formed, they create a taut band that tends to create an enthesopathy, which in turn can create an attachment TrP.

General Factors That Create TrPs

As stated, via the energy crisis hypothesis, TrPs tend to develop when a muscle is contracted for an excessive length of time. There are a number of circumstances that tend to create this scenario. Following is a list of these common circumstances that can lead to the formation of TrPs.
1. Excessive muscle contraction: Certainly this is the prime factor for TrP genesis. A muscle that contracts for an extended period, especially a long-held isometric contrac-

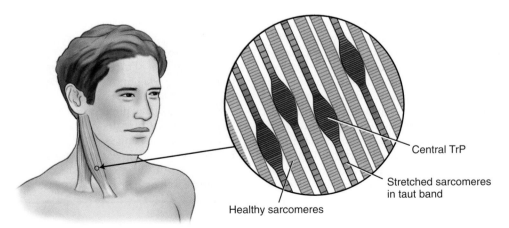

Figure 5-7 A central trigger point (TrP) located within a taut band. The sarcomeres of the TrPs can be seen to be shortened. This results in a pulling along the myofibrils in which the TrPs are located, causing a stretching of the remaining sarcomeres of the myofibrils. The pulling of these taut bands often causes an enthesopathy at the muscle's attachment, resulting in attachment TrPs. (Reprinted with permission by New Harbinger Publications, Inc. Modified from Davies C: *The trigger point therapy workbook: your self-treatment guide for pain relief*, ed 2, Oakland, Calif, 2004, New Harbinger. www.newharbinger.com)

Central TrP

Stretched sarcomeres in taut band

Healthy sarcomeres

5

tion, tends to close off the blood supply to the muscle tissue, resulting in ischemia and the formation of TrPs via the energy crisis hypothesis.

2. Irritation/injury/trauma: Whenever a muscle is physically irritated or injured, irritating chemicals are released into the local muscle tissue. These chemicals can create swelling in the muscle tissue, which compresses blood vessels, resulting in ischemia, thereby initiating TrP formation. These chemicals can also cause local pain and tenderness that can initiate the pain–spasm–pain and contraction–ischemia cycle, which can further lead to TrP formation.

3. Perceived pain: Any pain perceived to be in a muscle, even if the pain is referred from elsewhere in the body, can result in the tightening of that muscle via the pain–spasm–pain cycle. This tightening predisposes the muscle to TrP formation.

4. Muscle splinting: If there is any pain or damage to an adjacent tissue, especially a nearby joint, muscles in that region of the body tend to tighten up as a protective mechanism to splint the region. This splinting contraction of the muscle favors the formation of TrPs.

5. Prolonged shortening: Whenever a muscle remains in a shortened state for a prolonged period, it will tend to adaptively shorten. An adaptively shortened muscle tends to tighten (i.e., increased contraction), and this increased tension favors the development of TrPs.

6. Prolonged stretching: Even though stretching any soft tissue, including muscle, is theoretically good, if a muscle is excessively stretched and or stretched too quickly, the muscle spindle reflex will be initiated, causing the muscle to tighten. This will then predispose the muscle to the development of TrPs.

Effects of a TrP

The most obvious effect of having a TrP within a muscle is that the TrP is locally painful and may have a referral pattern of pain. Beyond that, TrPs tend to be located within taut bands that are also usually tender and painful upon palpation.

However, when a muscle harbors a TrP, there are other consequences that might affect the entire muscle. Given that a TrP creates a taut band in which it is located, the taut band of muscle tissue will resist stretching, and if stretching is attempted, pain will likely result. For this reason, a muscle with a TrP located within it very often results in decreased range of motion of the joint(s) crossed by that muscle. Furthermore, if a muscle is not stretched and is allowed to stay in a shortened state, the muscle tends to adapt to that shortened state. This adaptation can be both functional and structural. Functionally, the muscle can adaptively shorten because the nervous system, fearing possible pain or muscle tearing, tends to avoid motions of the body that would stretch that muscle. Structurally, the muscle can adaptively shorten because fibrous adhesions will tend to accumulate within the muscle, further decreasing its ability to lengthen and stretch. In addition, because of a principle known as the *length tension relationship curve*, muscles that are excessively tight and shortened become weaker.

Hence, when a muscle contains one or more TrPs, besides local or referred pain, muscle-wide effects often occur. Muscles harboring TrPs tend to become tighter and weaker. Of course,

BOX 5-7

The phenomenon of a tight and shortened muscle becoming weaker is known as shortened active insufficiency. When a sarcomere shortens, its actin filaments overlap, covering up and making inaccessible some of the active binding sites needed for myosin-actin cross-bridges to form. If fewer cross-bridges form, the strength of the contraction will be diminished, resulting in a weaker muscle.

whenever one muscle becomes functionally impaired, stresses occur within the body as other muscles try to compensate for this dysfunctional muscle. For this reason, it is often said that the presence of a first TrP, often called a key TrP, can cause the creation of other TrPs, called satellite TrPs.

BOX 5-8

Perhaps the easiest way to understand why adaptive shortening of a muscle occurs is to look at the example of hip joint flexor muscles. When we sit for prolonged periods of time, our hip flexors are shortened and slackened because sitting places our thigh into 90 degrees of flexion at the hip joint. The problem is that if in this position we want to further flex a thigh at the hip joint, the hip flexor muscles would not be immediately responsive to cause motion when they contract, because any contraction would have to first take out the slack that is present in the muscles. For this reason, the gamma motor system of the brain adaptively shortens these muscles by increasing their tension to match the shortened length that they are in when sitting. They are now no shorter than they were before, but the increased tension has removed the slack. If they are now ordered to contract, they will be more responsive and will be able to more quickly create further flexion of the thigh at the hip joint. For this reason, whenever we maintain postures for prolonged periods of time wherein a muscle or muscle group is shortened and slackened, the baseline resting tone of these muscles will gradually adapt to adjust to that shortened state, allowing them be more responsive when motion is needed.

It is this increased tension in the adaptively shortened muscle that predisposes it to the formation of TrPs. A further factor is that if a muscle is always held in a shortened state and is never stretched out, fascial adhesions will build up within the muscle. In time, these adhesions will make it that much more difficult for the muscle to lengthen and stretch out.

Key TrPs Creating Satellite TrPs

Once a key TrP has formed, it is common for its presence to create satellite TrPs, either in the same muscle or within other muscles of the body.

1. Central and attachment TrPs: Key central TrPs often create satellite attachment TrPs within the same taut band of muscle tissue. As previously explained, the attachment TrP

is caused by the enthesopathy (irritation) created by the pull of the central TrP's taut band.

2. Functional muscular mover group: Key TrPs within one muscle often create satellite TrPs in other muscles of the same functional group of movers. Given that a TrP often makes the muscle it is located in painful as well as tighter and weaker, the body tends to use other muscles that share the same joint action to engage and work instead. In time, these other muscles may be overworked and therefore become painful and contracted, and in turn develop satellite TrPs.

3. Antagonist muscles: Key TrPs within one muscle often create satellite TrPs in muscles of the antagonist group of muscles. Given that a muscle with TrPs tends to be tight, antagonist muscles often must contract more to even the pull across their shared joint so that the tight muscle with TrPs does not asymmetrically pull upon the joint, creating an asymmetric posture of the bones (and therefore body parts) at that joint.

4. Referral zones of pain: Key TrPs often cause satellite TrPs to form within the musculature located within the referral pain zone. Even though pain within the referral zone of a key TrP is not indicative of trauma or damage to the tissue of the referral zone, the nervous system interprets this pain as if the referral zone is experiencing trauma or damage. As a result, the pain–spasm–pain cycle kicks in, creating tightness of the musculature of the referral zone, which predisposes TrP formation in this area.

TrP Referral Patterns

Perhaps the most enigmatic aspect of a TrP is its referral pattern. Each muscular TrP, when tight enough or sufficiently compressed, tends to have a characteristic pattern of pain referral that may be felt locally or distant from the TrP itself. Usually the pain refers to what is known as the primary referral zone (also known as the essential referral zone). However, when more severe, a TrP may refer pain into what is called the secondary referral zone (also known as the spillover referral zone) in addition to the primary referral zone. In this textbook, the primary zone is indicated by a dark red color and the secondary zone is indicated by a lighter red color (Figure 5-8). It should be emphasized that even though typical TrP locations and referral patterns are mapped out for most muscles of the body, this does not mean that TrPs can only occur where shown in the illustrations in this book, or that the referral zones must always follow the patterns shown here. Although usual TrP locations and referral patterns are known, TrPs can occur anywhere within a muscle, and their referral patterns are not necessarily restricted to the patterns shown here.

TrP referral patterns of pain do not simply follow the course of a peripheral nerve as if the TrP entrapped a nerve and caused projection of pain along its course (similar to how a lumbar disc herniation can compress the sciatic nerve and cause pain along the course of the sciatic nerve). Rather, TrP referral is more similar to the type of referred pain that a heart attack is well known to cause. Only in the case of a TrP, instead of an internal visceral organ referring pain to the skin of the body (to the shoulder and chest region in the case of a heart attack), a TrP in a muscle usually refers pain to another region of the muscle, or just as commonly, to an entirely different muscle of the body.

Figure 5-8 Four TrPs, indicated by the Xs, are illustrated within the sternal head of the sternocleidomastoid (SCM) muscle. The primary (essential) referral zones of pain are indicated by the areas of dark red. When more severe, SCM sternal head TrPs may also refer pain into secondary (spillover) referral zones, indicated by the areas of light red.

The prevailing theory for how myofascial TrPs refer pain is called the convergence–projection theory. According to this theory, the sensory neurons that detect sensation and pain in one muscle converge with the sensory neurons that come from another muscle of the body (Figure 5-9). For example, if the sensory neurons from muscles A and B converge in the spinal cord, then when pain occurs due to a TrP in muscle A, these signals travel within sensory neurons that enter the spinal cord and converge with the sensory neurons that come from muscle B. When these signals of pain reach the brain along the common pathway from muscles A and B, the brain has no way of knowing if the pain originated in muscle A or muscle B. As a result, the pain may be projected (or it could be said to be mislocalized) to muscle B. In this way, the brain can perceive the pain that is caused by a TrP located in muscle A as coming from muscle B, even if there is no TrP located in muscle B.

If this theory were the only theory responsible for explaining TrP referral, then it would mean that all TrP referral pain patterns and the TrPs that caused them must be innervated by the same sensory neurons. This does not seem likely given the widespread referral patterns of some TrPs. Another proposed theory to explain the phenomenon of TrP referral patterns is called the cord spillover theory. It states that when excessive pain signals enter the spinal cord from a strongly active TrP, there is a "spillover" of these electrical signals in the cord from the sensory neurons coming from the muscle housing the TrP to interneurons that come from other muscles that do not have TrPs (Figure 5-10). This spillover causes these other interneurons to carry signals of pain to the brain, telling the brain that these other muscles have pain, even though they contain no pain-producing lesions. In effect, the pain has been referred from the muscle housing the TrP to other muscles that do not have TrPs.

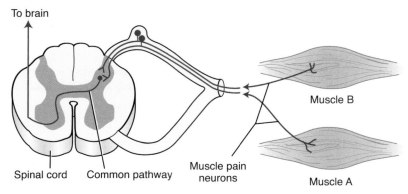

Figure 5-9 The convergence–projection theory for TrP referral. The convergence–projection theory posits that sensory pain neurons from different muscles converge in the spinal cord onto a common pathway that carries that information up to the brain. Therefore when pain signals enter the brain from the common pathway in the spinal cord, the brain cannot judge from which muscle the pain originated and therefore may refer (project) the pain to the muscle that does not have the TrP. (Modified from Mense S, Simons DG, Russell IJ: *Muscle pain: understanding its nature, diagnosis, and treatment*, Baltimore, 2000, Lippincott, Williams & Wilkins.)

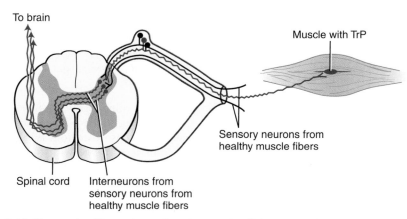

Figure 5-10 The cord spillover theory for trigger point (TrP) referral. The spillover theory posits that when strong pain signals enter the cord from the sensory neurons of a muscle with a TrP, the electrical activity can "spill over" and cause activity within adjacent interneurons that are part of the pathways of other muscles that do not have pain-producing TrPs.

BOX 5-10

There is one other explanation that is sometime offered to explain how TrP referral patterns occur. Similar to sclerotogenous referred pain (from ligaments and joint capsules) and visceral referred pain (from internal visceral organs), it appears that many TrP (myotogenous) referral pain patterns occur within aspects of the body that share the same embryologic origin as the location of the TrP itself. In other words, the location of the TrP and the location of the referral zone were derived from the same embryologic segment. Therefore it is proposed that given the common embryologic origins, the brain may have some mapping that continues to link these areas that may now be spread apart geographically within the body. Thus a TrP in one area of the body may refer pain to another, once embryologically related, area.

In all likelihood, both theories are probably true and combine to form the most common typical TrP referral patterns of pain that have been mapped. It is important to emphasize that TrP referral patterns do not always follow the most commonly mapped referral patterns that are shown in this and other books.

Locating and Treating TrPs

To treat a TrP, it must first be found. Although TrPs can be located anywhere within a muscle, they tend to occur in certain spots within certain muscles. Generally, TrPs are located at the center of a muscle fiber. If all muscles were fusiform with all their fibers running the full length of the muscle, then all central TrPs would be located at the center of the muscle. Unfortunately this is not always true. Pennate muscles and fusiform muscles that do not have fibers running the full length of the muscle can have their central TrPs in locations other than dead center within the muscle. For this reason, it is helpful to

---

BOX 5-11

Not all roundish nodules palpated within the client's soft tissues are TrPs. Be careful to discern TrPs from lipomas and lymph nodes. Lipomas are benign soft tissue tumors that generally feel soft and have the consistency of a gel caplet inserted under the skin; they may or may not be tender to compression. Lymph nodes/glands may mimic the feeling of a TrP if they are swollen, as they will be if the client has an active infection in that region of the body; swollen lymph nodes usually are tender to compression, but are usually not as hard as TrPs. However, long-standing swollen lymph nodes may calcify over time and eventually feel similar to a TrP on palpation. In addition to assessing palpatory quality, another way to distinguish a TrP from a lipomas or lymph node is to check for the presence of pain referral upon compression. Although not all TrPs refer pain to a distant site, many TrPs do. Lipomas and lymph nodes, however, do not refer pain when compressed.

---

know the fiber architecture of each muscle. In lieu of knowing this, there are commonly mapped-out TrP locations for each muscle of the body. These are shown in Muscle Palpation Tours located in Chapters 10 to 20 of Part III of this book.

Once your palpating fingers are in the correct location for a TrP, you should palpate for what likely feels like a small hard knot or marble embedded within the muscle tissue. Often, these TrPs are located within a taut band of fibers that can be strummed or twanged by running your fingers across (perpendicular to) them. Very often, if the taut band is sufficiently taut, a twitch response will occur in which the taut band involuntarily contracts when strummed. Of course, both TrPs and their associated taut bands are usually tender to palpation. Regarding methods of muscle palpation necessary to identify the location of a TrP, the reader is referred to Chapter 2, The Art and Science of Muscle Palpation.

Understanding the genesis of central and attachment TrPs and the mechanism of an actual TrP allows us to reason through the best treatment approach for clients with myofascial TrP syndromes.

For years, the recommended approach for treating TrPs has been the technique known as ischemic compression. Ischemic compression involves the application of deep pressure directly on the client's TrP and holding the pressure for a sustained length of time (approximately 10 seconds or more). The premise of ischemic compression (as its name implies) was to create ischemia in the TrP; then when the therapist removed the pressure, a surge of blood would rush in to the TrP. The problem with ischemic compression, besides the fact that it tended to be an extremely uncomfortable treatment for most clients due to the deep pressure that was recommended, is that given the fact that a TrP is already ischemic, why would therapy be aimed at creating ischemia? This has already been acknowledged by many authorities on TrPs. As a result, ischemic compression technique has been modified and renamed, and is now termed sustained compression or TrP pressure release. However, regardless of the new names, the essence of holding sustained compression upon the TrP is essentially unchanged (the only substantive

change is that less pressure is recommended, making it less painful for the client). The value to ischemic compression or any sustained compression or TrP pressure release technique is usually stated to create a surge of new blood into the TrP when the pressure is released. Using that logic, it would seem that a better treatment approach could be devised for working with TrPs.

Toward this end, the technique of deep-stroking massage (also known as stripping massage) has been recommended by many of the authorities on TrP theory and practice. David Simons states: "this method is probably the most effective way to inactivate central TrPs when using a direct manual approach, and it can be used to treat TrPs without producing excessive joint movement. The rationale is clear."[1] It is also the preferred method espoused in *The Trigger Point Therapy Workbook* by Clair Davies.[2]

Deep-stroking massage is done with short strokes that use moderately (but not excessively) deep pressure directly over the TrP. The deep stroking can be done in any direction, but at least some of the strokes should be done along the direction of the taut band containing the TrP. Approximately 30 to 60 short deep strokes should be done consecutively at a pace of 1 to 2 seconds per stroke, totaling a treatment session of approximately 1 minute per TrP.

BOX 5-12

The TrP treatment methods discussed in this chapter are hands-on myofascial approaches. Two other common methods used for the treatment of a TrP are spray and stretch, and TrP injections. Spray and stretch is done by applying a vapocoolant spray to the region of the TrP and then immediately stretching the muscle containing the TrP. TrP injections are injections of either saline solution or a local anesthetic directly into the TrP; this treatment is usually performed only by a licensed physician. Certainly other treatment options exist, including stretching, acupuncture, and physical therapy. Of these, stretching is certainly an option for most manual and movement therapists; and given that a TrP is, in effect, a tightening of a small region of a muscle; it stands to reason that stretching would be beneficial. There are many techniques that can be used when stretching a muscle. For a discussion of these techniques, see Chapter 6.

It can also be beneficial to continue the deep stroking along the taut band to the attachment of the muscle. The purpose of deep stroking is twofold. The primary purpose, as stated, is to create a flushing of blood into the TrP with each release of the pressure. This is the major advantage of doing deep-stroking massage 30 to 60 times in a row compared with 2 to 3 sustained pressures as recommended in the past. Given that the therapeutic aspect of this technique occurs with each release as new blood flushes in, more strokes mean more releases, which result in a better circulation of blood into the TrP. Given that the pathologic mechanism that creates a TrP is ischemia, the new circulation of blood allows nutrients to enter the TrP so that ATP molecules can be formed, eliminating the "energy crisis."

When done along the direction of the taut band, deep-stroking massage also has the advantage of helping to stretch the shortened sarcomeres within the TrP, breaking the myosin-actin cross-bridges with mechanical force. It is also recommended that the manual treatment be performed with the muscle on stretch to further aid in the stretching of shortened sarcomeres.

BOX 5-13

By the energy crisis hypothesis, any TrP treatment technique whose method depends upon mechanically deforming a TrP to break its cross-bridges would seem to be ultimately ineffective. If the local ischemia is not eliminated, then even if every myosin-actin cross-bridge of the TrP were broken, without the presence of the ATP molecules to reabsorb the calcium ions back into the sarcoplasmic reticulum, the continued presence of the calcium ions in the sarcoplasm would keep the active sites of the actin filaments exposed and new cross-bridges would immediately form, perpetuating the TrP.

If a TrP is long standing, the chance of fibrous adhesion formation increases. The microstretching of deep-stroking massage, especially if performed along the length of the muscle fibers, and with the muscle on stretch, helps to break up these patterns of adhesions before they form more fully and

---

BOX 5-14

Although most TrPs are treated with a flat pressure applied by the therapist's fingers, thumb, hand, or elbow, there are times when a pincer grip is recommended. A pincer grip involves grabbing the TrP between the thumb and another finger (usually the index or middle finger) and pinching or squeezing the TrP between them. This method is often employed when it is not desirable to transmit flat pressure deep to the TrP. For example, when working a TrP in the sternocleidomastoid muscle, flat pressure is often contraindicated because of the presence of the carotid artery immediately deep to portions of the muscle; in this region, a pincer grip can be safely used. A pincer grip also offers the ability to increase pressure on the TrP because it is trapped between the two treating fingers. The disadvantage is that pincer grip work is often less comfortable for the client.

---

become structurally entrenched. In addition, most types of deep tissue work have the advantage of helping to flush out toxins that have accumulated because of the venous congestion present in TrPs.

A special note regarding attachments TrPs: When central and attachment TrPs both exist within a muscle, the recommended course is to treat the central TrPs first. Given that attachment TrPs are usually caused by the pulling of the taut bands created by the central TrPs, if a central TrP is cleared up, its attachment TrP may clear up on its own. However, it is entirely possible for an attachment TrP in muscle tissue, once created, to now have its own vicious cycle of ischemia causing contraction, causing further ischemia, and so on. Furthermore, once this cycle has begun, the pain present as a result of the attachment TrP can trigger further contraction via the pain–spasm–pain cycle; and of course the pooling of toxins from venous congestion will also tend to perpetuate the presence of the TrP based on their irritating nature. For all these reasons, even though it is probably wisest and most efficient to first treat central TrPs, if central TrP treatment does not result in the easy dissolution of attachment TrPs, then it is advisable to directly treat the attachments TrPs as well.

BOX 5-15

The reasoning used for treating central TrPs before attachment TrPs can be applied to the treatment of any key TrPs before treating their satellite TrPs. Given that it is the presence of a key TrP that creates the satellite TrP, beginning with treatment of key TrPs may obviate the need to treat the satellite TrPs. The difficulty is knowing which TrPs are key TrPs and which ones are their satellite TrPs. Of course, even if it is determined which TrPs are key and which are satellite (e.g., central TrPs are often key and attachment TrPs are usually satellite), once formed, a satellite TrP may create its own vicious cycle and may not disappear unless treated directly.

References

1. Simons DG, Travell JG, Simons LS: *Myofascial pain and dysfunction: the trigger point manual,* vol 1, ed 2, Baltimore, 1999, Lippincott, Williams & Wilkins, p 41.
2. Davies C: *The trigger point therapy workbook: your self-treatment guide for pain relief,* Oakland, Calif, 2001, New Harbinger, p 33.

Chapter 6

Stretching

Overview

This chapter discusses the therapeutic tool of stretching. It begins with an explanation of some of the choices that are available to the therapist and trainer when stretching a client. Basic questions pertaining to stretching are then posed and answered so that the therapist can better understand how to incorporate stretching into therapeutic practice. The two basic stretching techniques, static stretching and dynamic stretching, are then described and contrasted, with an explanation of when each method is best applied. The chapter concludes with a discussion of the advanced stretching techniques: pin and stretch, contract relax (CR) stretching (often known as *PNF stretching*), and agonist contract (AC) stretching.

Chapter Outline

Chapter Objectives

After completing this chapter, the student should be able to perform the following:

1. Define the key terms of this chapter.
2. Describe the relationship between a line of tension and stretching.
3. Discuss the purpose and benefit of stretching and describe why stretching is done.
4. Explain how stretches can be reasoned out instead of memorized.
5. Describe the relationship between the pain–spasm–pain cycle and the muscle spindle reflex to the force exerted during a stretch.
6. Discuss when stretching should be done, especially with respect to an exercise workout routine.
7. Compare and contrast static stretching with dynamic stretching.
8. Discuss how and why the pin and stretch technique is done.
9. Describe how to perform the contract relax, agonist contract, and contract relax agonist contract stretching techniques.
10. Discuss the similarities and differences between contract relax stretching and agonist contract stretching.

Key Terms

active tension
agonist contract (AC) stretching
contract relax agonist contract (CRAC) stretching
contract relax (CR) stretching
dynamic stretching
Golgi tendon organ (GTO) reflex
good pain
line of tension

mobilization
muscle spindle reflex
myofibroblast
pain–spasm–pain cycle
passive tension
pin and stretch
postisometric relaxation (PIR) stretching

proprioceptive neuromuscular facilitation (PNF) stretching
reciprocal inhibition
static stretching
stretching
target muscle
target tissue
tension

Introduction

Stretching is a powerful therapeutic tool that is available to manual therapists and athletic trainers to improve the health of their clients. Although few people disagree about the benefits of stretching, there is a great deal of disagreement about how stretching should be done. There are many possible choices. Stretching can be performed statically or dynamically. Three repetitions (reps) can be done, each one held approximately 10 to 20 seconds, or 10 reps can be performed, each one held for approximately 2 to 3 seconds. A technique called *pin and stretching* can be done, or stretches that use neurologic reflexes to facilitate the stretch, such as contract relax (CR) and agonist contract (AC) stretching, can be performed. There are also choices regarding when stretching is best done: stretching can be done before or after strengthening exercise.

To best understand stretching so that we can apply it clinically for the optimal health of our clients, let's first look at the fundamental basis of stretching by posing and answering the following five questions: What is stretching? Why is stretching done? How do we figure out how to stretch muscles? How forcefully should we stretch? When should stretching be done? Then we can examine the types of stretching techniques that are available to the client and therapist/trainer.

1. What Is Stretching?

Simply defined, **stretching** is a method of physical bodywork that lengthens and elongates soft tissues. These soft tissues may be muscles and their tendons (collectively called *myofascial units*), ligaments, and/or joint capsules. When performing a stretch upon our client, we use the term **target tissue** to describe the tissue that we intend to stretch (or **target muscle** when we specifically want to stretch a muscle or muscle group). To create a stretch, the client's body is moved into a position that creates a **line of tension** that pulls on the target tissues, placing a stretch upon them (Figure 6-1). If the stretch is effective, the tissues will be lengthened.

2. Why Is Stretching Done?

Stretching is done because soft tissues may increase in tension and become shortened and contracted. Shortened and contracted soft tissues resist lengthening and limit mobility of the joint that they cross. The specific joint motion that is limited will be the motion of a body part (at the joint) that is in the opposite direction from the location of the tight tissues. For example, if the tight tissue is located on the posterior side of the joint, anterior motion of a body part at that joint will be limited, and if the tight tissue is located on the anterior side of the joint, posterior motion of a body part at that joint will be limited (Figure 6-2).

BOX 6-1

The tension of a tissue can be described as its resistance to stretch.

As stated, a shortened and contracted tissue can be described as having greater **tension**. Two types of tissue tension exist, passive tension and active tension. All soft tissues can exhibit increased passive tension. **Passive tension** results from increased fascial adhesions that build up over time in soft tissues.

Additionally, muscles may exhibit increased active tension. **Active tension** results when a muscle's contractile elements (actin and myosin filaments) contract via the sliding filament mechanism, creating a pulling force toward the center of the muscle. Whether a soft tissue has increased passive or active tension, this increased tension makes the tissue more resistant to lengthening. Therefore stretching is done to lengthen and elongate these tissues, hopefully restoring full range of motion and flexibility of the body.

BOX 6-2

Muscles have classically been considered to be the only tissue that can exhibit active tension. However, recent research has shown that fibrous connective tissues often contain cells called **myofibroblasts**, which evolve from fibroblasts normally found in the fibrous connective tissues. Myofibroblasts contain contractile proteins that can actively contract. Although not present in the same numbers that muscle tissue contains, connective tissue myofibroblasts may be present in sufficient number to be biomechanically significant when assessing the active tension of that connective tissue.

Figure 6-1 A client's right upper extremity is stretched. The line of tension created by this stretch is indicated by hatch marks and extends from the client's anterior forearm to the pectoral region. A stretch is exerted upon all tissues along the line of tension of the stretch.

Figure 6-2 When tissues located on one side of a joint are tight, motion of a body part at that joint to the opposite side will be limited. **A** shows a decreased flexion of the thigh at the hip joint due to taut tissues, tight hamstrings, at the posterior side of the hip joint. Similarly, tight hamstrings would also limit anterior tilt of the pelvis at the hip joint (anterior pelvic tilt is the reverse action of flexion of the thigh at the hip joint). If anterior hip joint tissues (especially hip joint flexor muscles, such as the tensor fasciae latae seen in this illustration) are tight, a decrease in range of motion of extension of the thigh at the hip joint will occur as seen in **B**. Similarly, tight anterior hip joint tissues also limit posterior tilt of the pelvis at the hip joint (posterior pelvic tilt is the reverse action of extension of the thigh at the hip joint).

3. How Do We Figure Out How to Stretch Muscles?

If our target tissue to be stretched is a muscle, the question is, How do we figure out what position the client's body must be put in to achieve an effective stretch of the target muscle or muscle group? Certainly there are many excellent books available for learning specific muscle stretches. Indeed, specific stretches for each of the muscles and muscle groups covered in Part III of this book are given. However, better than relying on a book or other authority to give us stretching routines that must be memorized, it is preferable to be able to figure out the stretches that our clients need.

Figuring out a stretch for a muscle is actually quite easy. Simply recall the actions that were learned for the target muscle, and then do the opposite of one or more of its actions. Because the actions of a muscle are what the muscle does when it shortens, then stretching and lengthening the muscle would be achieved by having the client do the opposite of the muscle's actions. Essentially, if a muscle flexes a joint, then extension of that joint would stretch it; if the muscle abducts a joint, then adduction of that joint would stretch it; if a muscle medially rotates a joint, then lateral rotation of that joint

would stretch it. If a muscle has more than one action, then the optimal stretch would consider all its actions.

For example, if the target muscle that is being stretched is the right upper trapezius, given that its actions are extension, right lateral flexion, and left rotation of the neck and head at the spinal joints, then stretching the right upper trapezius would require either flexion, left lateral flexion, and/or right rotation of the head and neck at the spinal joints.

When a muscle has many actions, it is not always necessary to do the opposite of all of them; however, at times it might be desired or needed. If the right upper trapezius is tight enough, simply doing flexion in the sagittal plane might be sufficient to stretch it. However, if further stretch is needed, then left lateral flexion in the frontal plane and/or right rotation in the transverse plane could be added as shown in Figure 6-3.

Even if not every plane of action is used for the stretch, it is still important to be aware of all the muscle's actions or a mistake might be made with the stretch. For example, if the right upper trapezius is being stretched by flexing and left laterally flexing the client's head and neck, it is important to not let the client's head and neck rotate to the left, because this will allow the right upper trapezius to be slackened and the tension of the stretch will be lost. Furthermore, given that the right upper trapezius also elevates the right scapula at the scapulocostal joint, it is also important to make sure that the right scapula is depressed or at least not allowed to elevate during the stretch, or the tension of the stretch will also be lost.

It can be very difficult to isolate a stretch so that only one target muscle is stretched. When a stretch is performed, usually an entire functional group of muscles is stretched at the same time.

For example, if a client's thigh is stretched into extension at the hip joint in the sagittal plane, the entire functional group of sagittal plane hip joint flexors will be stretched. To isolate one of the hip flexors usually requires fine tuning the stretch to achieve the desired result. If the stretch is done into extension in the sagittal plane and adduction in the frontal plane, then all hip flexor muscles that are also frontal plane adductors will be slackened and relaxed by the adduction, and the stretch will be focused on those hip flexor muscles that are also abductors,

Figure 6-3 The right upper trapezius is stretched in all three planes. The movements of a stretch of a target muscle are always antagonistic to the joint actions of that muscle. In this case, the right upper trapezius is an extensor in the sagittal plane, right lateral flexor in the frontal plane, and left rotator in the transverse plane of the head and neck at the spinal joints. Therefore, to stretch the right upper trapezius, the client's head and neck are flexed in the sagittal plane, left laterally flexed in the frontal plane, and right rotated in the transverse plane.

such as the tensor fasciae latae (TFL), the sartorius, and the anterior fibers of the gluteus medius and minimus.

If medial rotation of the thigh at the hip joint in the transverse plane is also added to the stretch so that the thigh is now being extended in the sagittal plane, adducted in the frontal plane, and medially rotated in the transverse plane, then all hip flexors and abductors that are also transverse plane medial rotators will be slackened and relaxed by medial rotation, and the stretch will now be focused on muscles that do flexion, abduction, and lateral rotation of the thigh at the hip joint. In this case, the sartorius will be the principal target muscle to be stretched because it is the only hip flexor and abductor muscle that also laterally rotates the thigh at the hip joint (the iliopsoas will also be stretched because it is a flexor and lateral rotator at the hip joint, and some sources state that it can also abduct). Of course, given that the sartorius is also a flexor of the leg at the knee joint, it is imperative that the knee joint is extended during the stretch, or the sartorius would be slackened by a flexed knee joint and the effectiveness of the stretch would be lost.

BOX 6-4

The functional group of flexors of the hip joint includes the tensor fasciae latae, anterior fibers of the gluteus medius and minimus, sartorius, rectus femoris, iliopsoas, pectineus, adductor longus, gracilis, and adductor brevis.

Had lateral rotation of the thigh at the hip joint been added as the third transverse plane component instead of medial rotation, then the sartorius, being a lateral rotator, would have been slackened and the TFL and anterior fibers of the gluteus medius and minimus, being medial rotators, would have been stretched instead. To then isolate the stretch to just the TFL or just the anterior fibers of the gluteus medius or minimus is difficult if not impossible, because these muscles all share the same actions in all three planes and therefore are stretched by the same joint position.

Therefore, whenever a client's body part is moved into a stretch in one direction, in other words in one plane, the entire functional group of muscles located on the other side of the joint is stretched. To then fine tune and isolate the stretch, to one or only a few of the muscles of this functional group requires adding other components to the stretch. These other components might involve adding other planes to the stretch, or they may involve adding a stretch to another joint if the target muscle crosses more than one joint (i.e., is a multijoint muscle).

Figuring out exactly how to fine tune a stretch to isolate a target muscle depends upon a solid foundation of knowledge of the joint actions of the muscles involved. Once this knowledge is attained, applying it can eliminate the need for memorizing tens or hundreds of stretches. In the place of memorization comes an ability to critically reason through the steps necessary to figure out whatever stretches are needed for the proper treatment of our clients!

4. How Forcefully Should We Stretch?

Stretching should never hurt. If stretching causes pain, it is likely that the target muscles or muscles in the vicinity of the target tissues will tighten in response to the pain via the pain–spasm–pain cycle. Furthermore, if the target muscle is either stretched too quickly or too forcefully, the muscle spindle reflex may be engaged, resulting in a tightening of the target muscle. ☺ Given that a stretch should relax and lengthen tissue, stretching that causes musculature to tighten defeats the purpose of the stretch.

For this reason, a stretch should never be done too quickly; stretching should always be done slowly and rhythmically. Furthermore, the therapist should be prudent and judicious regarding how far a client is stretched. And a stretch should never cause pain; theoretically, a stretch can be done as hard as possible, but always without pain. When in doubt, it is best to be conservative regarding the speed and forcefulness of a stretch. It is wiser to gently and slowly stretch a client over a number of sessions to safely achieve the goal of loosening the target tissues. It may take more sessions, but a positive outcome is essentially guaranteed. Imprudent stretching may not only set back the progress of the client's treatment program but may also cause damage that is difficult to reverse.

BOX 6-5

Clients often describe a stretch as being painful, but go on to say that the pain feels good. For this reason, a distinction should be made between what is often described by the client as good pain and true pain (or what might be called *bad pain*). Good pain is often the way that a client describes the sensation of the stretch; therefore causing good pain as a result of a stretch is fine. However, if a stretch causes true pain—in other words, the client winces and resists or fights the stretch—then the intensity of the stretch must be lessened. Otherwise, not only will the stretch not be effective, but the client is likely to be injured. A stretch should never be forced.

5. When Should Stretching Be Done?

Stretching should be done when the target tissues are most receptive to being stretched; this is when they are already warmed up. Not only do cold tissues resist stretching, resulting in little benefit, they are also more likely to be injured when stretched. For this reason, if stretching is linked to a physical exercise workout, the stretching should be done after the workout when the tissues are warmed up, not before the workout when the tissues are cold. This general principle is true if the type of stretching is the classic form, called *static stretching*. If dynamic stretching is done instead, then it is safe and appropriate to stretch before an exercise regimen when the tissues are cold, because dynamic stretching is a method of warming the tissues in addition to stretching them. For more on static versus dynamic stretching, see the next section.

BOX 6-6

Warming/heating the soft tissues of the body facilitates stretching them in two ways: first, heat is a central nervous system depressant helping the musculature relax; second, fascia is more easily stretched when warm.

BOX 6-7

Some sources state that static stretching done before strengthening exercise is actually deleterious to the performance of the exercise. Their reasoning is that when muscles are stretched, they are neurologically inhibited from contracting and consequently less able to contract quickly when needed to protect a joint from a possible sprain or strain during strenuous exercise.

If the client wants to stretch but does not have the opportunity to first engage in physical exercise to warm the target tissues, then the client may warm them by applying moist heat. There are a number of ways to do this. Taking a hot shower or bath, using a whirlpool, or placing a moist heating pad or hydrocollator pack upon the target tissues are all effective ways to warm target tissues before stretching them. Of all these choices, perhaps the most effective one is taking a hot shower, because it not only warms the tissues, but also the pressure of the water hitting the skin physically creates a massage that can help to relax the musculature of the region.

Basic Stretching Techniques: Static Stretching Versus Dynamic Stretching

Classically, stretching has been what is called static stretching, meaning that the position of the stretch is attained and then held statically for a period of time (Figure 6-4). The length of time recommended to statically hold a stretch has traditionally been between 10 and 30 seconds, and three reps have usually been recommended. However, the wisdom of this "classic" technique of stretching has recently been questioned.

The alternative to static stretching is called dynamic stretching, also known as mobilization. Dynamic stretching is done by moving the joints of the body through ranges of motion instead of holding the body in a static position of stretch. The idea is that whenever a joint is moved in a certain direction, the tissues on the other side of the joint are stretched. Following the example of Figure 6-2, if the hip joint is flexed (whether by the usual action of flexion of the thigh at the hip joint, or the reverse action of anterior tilt of the pelvis at the hip joint), then the tissues on the other side of the joint, the hip joint extensor muscles and other posterior soft tissues, will be stretched. Similarly, if the hip joint is extended (whether by extending the thigh at the hip joint or posteriorly tilting the pelvis at the hip joint), the hip joint flexor muscles and other anterior tissues, will be stretched.

By this concept, any joint motion of the body stretches some of the tissues of that joint. Of course, it is important when doing dynamic stretching that the joint motions are done in a careful, prudent, and graded manner, gradually increasing the intensity of the motions. For this reason, dynamic stretching begins with small ranges of motion carried out with little or no resistance. It then gradually builds up to full ranges

Figure 6-4 A client is performing a static stretch of her left arm and scapular region. Static stretches are done by bringing the body part to a position of stretch and then statically holding that position for a period of time. (From Muscolino JE: Stretch your way to better health, *Massage Ther J* 45[3]:167-171, 2006. Photo by Yanik Chauvin.)

of motion. If dynamic stretching is done before a physical workout, then the ranges of motion that are performed should be the same ranges of motion that will be asked of the body during the physical workout. And if the exercise entails some form of added resistance, then the added resistance of the exercise should gradually be added to the dynamic stretching after the full ranges of motion of the joints are done.

For example, before playing tennis, one would go through the motions of forehand, backhand, and serving strokes without a racquet in hand, beginning with small swings and building up to full range of motion swings. Then the same order of motions would be repeated, but this time with the added resistance of having the tennis racquet in hand (but not actually hitting a ball), starting with small swings and gradually working up to full range of motion swings. Finally, the person adds the full resistance of hitting the tennis ball while playing on the court, again, starting with gentle, short swings and gradually building up to full range of motion and powerful swings (Figure 6-5). The advantage of dynamic stretching as an exercise warmup is that not only is circulation increased, the tissues warmed up, the joints lubricated and brought through their ranges of motion, and the neural pathways that will be used during the exercise routine engaged, but with each motion that is done, soft tissues on the other side of the joint are stretched. Even though dynamic stretching is the ideal method to employ before engaging in physical exercise, it can certainly be done at any time.

Given the benefits of dynamic stretching, is there still a place for classic static stretching? Yes. As explained earlier, static stretching is beneficial if the tissues are first warmed up. This means that static stretching can be very effective after an exercise routine is done (or if the tissues are warmed up by applying moist heat). However, more and more sources are recommending that even static stretching should be performed in more of a movement-oriented "dynamic" manner. Whereas it was classically recommended to hold a stretch from 10 to 30 seconds, many sources now advocate that the stretch should be held for only 2 to 3 seconds. This then allows for approximately 8 to 10 reps to be done instead of the previously recommended 3. Something interesting to note is that as the method of static stretching is changed from a few long statically held stretches to more repetitions with the stretch being held for less time, static stretching increasingly resembles dynamic stretching.

Advanced Stretching Techniques: Pin and Stretch Technique

Beyond the choice of performing a stretch statically or dynamically, there are other, more advanced stretching options. One of these advanced options is pin and stretch technique. Pin and stretch technique is a stretching technique in which

A   B

Figure 6-5 Illustration showing the beginning stages of dynamic stretching for a forehand stroke in tennis. In **A**, a short forehand swing is done without holding a racquet. In **B**, a full range of motion swing is done without the racquet.

C

D

Figure 6-5, cont'd The person then progresses to holding a racquet to provide greater resistance, first with a short swing as seen in **C**, and then with a full range of motion swing as seen in **D**. After this, the person is ready to progress to the added resistance of playing tennis and hitting the ball. Note that with dynamic stretching, when the arm is brought posteriorly for the backswing, the muscles in front of the shoulder joint are stretched, and when the person swings forward with the forehand stroke, the muscles in back of the shoulder joint are stretched. (From Muscolino JE: Stretch your way to better health, *Massage Ther J* 45[3]:167-171, 2006. Photos by Yanik Chauvin.)

the therapist pins (stabilizes) one part of the client's body and then stretches the tissues up to that pinned spot.

The purpose of the pin and stretch is to direct a stretch to a more specific region of the client's body. As stated previously, when a body part is moved to create a stretch, a line of tension is created. Everything along the line of tension will be stretched. However, if we want only a certain region of the soft tissues along that line of tension to be stretched, then we can specifically direct the stretch to that region by using the pin and stretch technique.

For example, if a side-lying stretch is done on a client as demonstrated in Figure 6-6, A, the entire lateral side of the client's body from the therapist's right hand on the client's distal thigh to the therapist's left hand on the client's upper trunk will be stretched. The problem with allowing the line of tension of a stretch to spread over such a large region of the client's body is that if one region of soft tissue of the client's

body within that line of tension is very tight, it might stop the stretch from being felt in another area of the line of tension that we are specifically targeting to stretch.

Figure 6-6 A shows a side-lying stretch of a client. When done in this manner, the line of tension of the stretch is very broad, ranging from the therapist's right hand on the client's distal thigh to the therapist's left hand on the client's upper trunk. **B** and **C** demonstrate application of the pin and stretch technique to narrow the focus of the stretch. When the therapist pins the client's lower rib cage as shown in **B**, the focus of the stretch is narrowed to the client's lateral thigh and lateral lumbar region. And if the therapist pins the client's iliac crest as shown in **C**, the stretch is narrowed even further to just the tissues of the lateral thigh. Note: Hatch marks indicate the area that is stretched in all three figures. (Modified from Muscolino JE: Stretching the hip, *Massage Ther J* 46[4]:167-171, 2007. Photos by Yanik Chauvin.)

To focus the line of tension and direct the stretch to our target tissues, we can use the pin and stretch technique. If the therapist pins the client's lower rib cage, as seen in Figure 6-6, B, the stretch will no longer be felt in the client's lateral thoracic region; instead it will be specifically directed to the client's lateral pelvis and lateral lumbar region. If the therapist instead pins the client's iliac crest, as seen in Figure 6-6, C, the stretch will no longer be felt in the client's lateral lumbar region and will now be directed to only the lateral musculature and other soft tissues of the client's thigh. In effect, the pin and stretch technique pins and stabilizes a part of the client's body, thereby focusing and directing the force of the line of tension of the stretch to the specific target tissue(s).

Continuing with this example, if the target tissues are the gluteus medius and quadratus lumborum (as well as other muscles of the lateral pelvis and lateral lumber region), pinning the client at the lower rib cage, as seen in Figure 6-6, B, would be the ideal approach. If the target tissue is limited to the gluteus medius (and other muscles/soft tissues of the lateral pelvis), the ideal location to pin the client during this side-lying stretch is at the iliac crest, as seen in Figure 6-6, C. As can be seen here, pin and stretch is a powerful technique that allows for much greater specificity when stretching a client.

Advanced Stretching Techniques: Contract Relax and Agonist Contract Stretching Techniques

Two other advanced stretching techniques that are extremely effective are the contract relax (CR) stretching technique and the agonist contract (AC) stretching technique. Both advanced stretching techniques are similar in that they employ a neurologic reflex to facilitate the stretching of the target musculature. The CR technique uses the neurologic reflex called the Golgi tendon organ (GTO) reflex. The AC technique uses the neurologic reflex called *reciprocal inhibition*.

Contract relax (CR) stretching is perhaps better known as proprioceptive neuromuscular facilitation (PNF) stretching; it is also known as postisometric relaxation (PIR) stretching.

BOX 6-9

Regarding the contract relax stretching technique, the name *contract relax* is used because the target muscle is first *contracted*, and then it is *relaxed*. The name *proprioceptive neuromuscular facilitation* is used because a *proprioceptive neurologic* reflex (GTO reflex) is used to *facilitate* the stretch of the target muscle. The name *postisometric relaxation* is used because after (i.e., *post*) an *isometric* contraction, the target muscle is *relaxed* (because of the GTO reflex). In each case the name describes how the stretch is done.

CR stretching is done by first having the client isometrically contract the target muscle with moderate force against resistance provided by the therapist, then the therapist stretches the target muscle by lengthening it immediately afterward. The isometric contraction is usually held for approximately 5 to 10 seconds (although some sources recommend holding the

A   B

Figure 6-7 Contract relax (CR) stretching of the right lateral flexor musculature of the neck and head is shown. In **A**, the client is isometrically contracting the right lateral flexor musculature against resistance provided by the therapist. In **B**, the therapist is now stretching the right lateral flexor musculature by moving the client's neck and head into left lateral flexion. This procedure is usually repeated three times. (From Muscolino JE: Stretch your way to better health, *Massage Ther J* 45[3]:167-171, 2006. Photos by Yanik Chauvin.)

isometric contraction for as long as 30 seconds) and this procedure is usually repeated three times. Generally, the client is asked to hold in her breath while isometrically contracting against resistance, and then exhale and relax while the target muscle is being stretched.

BOX 6-10

Even though the contraction of a CR stretch is usually isometric, it can be done concentrically. In other words, when the client contracts against the resistance of the therapist, the therapist can allow the client to successfully shorten the muscle and move the joint. Whether the contraction is isometric or concentric, the GTO reflex will still be initiated, adding to the effectiveness of the stretch.

BOX 6-11

There are two choices for the client's breathing protocol when doing a CR stretch. The client can either hold in the breath when contracting the target muscle against the resistance of the therapist, or the client can exhale when contracting the target muscle (think *exertion* on *exhale*) against the therapist's resistance. Although contracting when exhaling is probably slightly preferred, if CR stretching will be combined with AC stretching to perform CRAC stretching, then it is necessary for the client to hold in the breath when contracting the target muscle.

The muscle group that is usually used to demonstrate CR stretching is the hamstring group; however this method of stretching can be used for any muscle of the body (Figure 6-7). The basis for CR stretching is the GTO reflex and works as follows: if the target muscle is forcefully contracted, the GTO reflex is engaged and results in inhibition of the target muscle (i.e., the muscle is inhibited or stopped from contracting). This is a protective reflex that prevents the forceful contraction from tearing the muscle and/or its tendon. As therapists, we can use this protective reflex to facilitate stretching our client's musculature, because muscles that are neurologically inhibited are more easily stretched.

BOX 6-12

It is customary for each rep of a CR stretch to begin where the previous rep ended. However, it is possible and sometimes desirable to take the client off stretch to some degree before beginning the next rep. Given that the mechanism of CR stretching is the GTO reflex, what is most important is that the client is able to generate a forceful enough contraction to stimulate this reflex. Sometimes this is not possible if the client is trying to contract when the target muscle is stretched extremely long.

Like CR stretching, agonist contract (AC) stretching also uses a neurologic reflex to "facilitate" the stretch of the target muscle; however, instead of the GTO reflex, AC stretching uses reciprocal inhibition. Reciprocal inhibition is a neurologic reflex that creates a more efficient joint action by preventing two muscles that have antagonistic actions from contracting at the same time. When a muscle is contracted, muscles that have antagonistic actions to the contracted muscle are inhibited from contracting (i.e., they are relaxed). Neurologically inhibited muscles are more easily stretched. For example, if the brachialis contracts to flex the forearm at the elbow joint, reciprocal inhibition would inhibit the triceps brachii from contracting and creating a force of elbow joint extension (that would oppose the action of elbow joint flexion by the brachialis).

To use reciprocal inhibition when stretching a client, have the client do a joint action that is antagonistic to the joint action of the target muscle. This will inhibit the target muscle, allowing for a greater stretch to be done at the end of this active movement (Figure 6-8). Generally, the position of stretch is only held for 1 to 3 seconds; this procedure is repeated approximately 10 times. The client is usually asked to breathe in before the movement, then exhale during the movement.

BOX 6-13

Regarding the agonist contract (AC) stretching technique, the name *agonist contract* is used because the *agonist* (mover) of a joint action is *contracted*, causing the antagonist (the target muscle that is to be stretched) on the other side of the joint to be relaxed (by reciprocal inhibition).

BOX 6-14

Agonist contract (AC) stretching that uses the neurologic reflex of reciprocal inhibition is the basis for Aaron Mattes' *Active Isolated Stretching (AIS)* technique.

The two methods of CR and AC stretching can be powerful additions to your repertoire of stretching techniques and may greatly benefit your clients. In fact, these two methods may be performed sequentially on the client, beginning with CR stretching followed by AC stretching; this protocol is called contract relax agonist contract (CRAC) stretching (Figure 6-9). CRAC stretching begins with the client isometrically contracting the target muscle against the therapist's resistance for approximately 5 to 8 seconds while holding in the breath (Figure 6-9, A); this is the CR aspect of the stretch. Next, the client actively contracts the antagonist muscles of the target muscle by moving the joint toward a stretch of the target muscle while breathing out (Figure 6-9, B); this is the AC aspect of the stretch. Then the client relaxes and the therapist moves the client into a further stretch of the target muscle while the client continues to breathe out or begins to breathe in (Figure 6-9, C). Combining CR with AC stretching can create an even greater stretch for the client's target musculature.

A

B

Figure 6-8 Agonist contract (AC) stretching for the right lateral flexor musculature of the neck is shown. **A** shows the client actively performing left lateral flexion of the neck, which both stretches the right lateral flexor musculature of the neck and results in reciprocal inhibition of the right lateral flexors. **B** shows that at the end of range of motion of left lateral flexion, the therapist then stretches the client's neck further into left lateral flexion, thereby further stretching the right lateral flexor musculature of the neck. This procedure is usually repeated 8 to 10 times. (Modified from Muscolino JE: Stretch your way to better health, *Massage Ther J* 45[3]:167-171, 2006. Photos by Yanik Chauvin.)

A

B

C

Figure 6-9 Contract relax agonist contract (CRAC) stretching is demonstrated for the right lateral flexion musculature of the neck. When these two stretching methods are both done, contract relax (CR) is usually done first, and then agonist contract (AC) is performed immediately afterward. **A** shows CR stretching technique with the client isometrically contracting the right lateral flexion musculature of her neck against the resistance of the therapist. At the end of this isometric contraction, instead of relaxing and having the therapist stretch her right lateral flexion muscles by moving her neck into left lateral flexion, the client actively moves her neck into left lateral flexion as seen in **B**. This active motion is part of the AC stretching technique. In **C**, the therapist now stretches the client's neck further into left lateral flexion. (Modified from Muscolino JE: Stretch your way to better health, *Massage Ther J* 45[3]:167-171, 2006. Photos by Yanik Chauvin.)

BOX 6-15

To simplify the difference between CR and AC stretching: with CR stretching, the client actively isometrically contracts the target muscle and then the therapist stretches it immediately afterward; with AC stretching, the client actively moves his or her body into the stretch of the target muscle and then the therapist further stretches the target muscle immediately afterward.

Conclusion

Stretching can be a very powerful treatment option. There are many choices when it comes to choosing the most effective stretching technique. Basic stretching techniques involve the choice between static and dynamic stretching. Although current research seems to favor dynamic over static stretching, the best choice likely depends upon the unique circumstances of each client. Beyond the choice of static versus dynamic stretching, advanced stretching techniques, such as pin and stretch, CR, AC, and CRAC stretching techniques, are extremely effective therapeutic tools when working clinically.

Upper Extremity Bone Palpation and Ligaments

Overview

Chapter 7 is one of three chapters of Part II of this book that addresses palpation of the skeleton. This chapter is a palpation tour of the bones, bony landmarks, and joints of the upper extremity. The tour begins with the shoulder girdle, then addresses the arm, forearm, and wrist region; and concludes with the hand. Although any one bone or bony landmark can be independently palpated, this chapter is set up sequentially to flow from one landmark to another, so it is recommended that the order presented here is followed. Muscle attachments for each of the palpated structures are also given (specific palpations for these muscles are covered in Part III of this book). The ligaments of the upper extremity are presented at the end of this chapter.

Chapter 8 presents the ligaments of the axial body and the palpation of the bones, bony landmarks, and joints of the axial body. Chapter 9 presents the ligaments of the lower extremity and the palpation of the bones, bony landmarks, and joints of the lower extremity.

Chapter Outline

The bones, bony landmarks, and joints of the following regions are covered:

Chapter Objectives

After completing this chapter, the student should be able to perform the following:

1. Define the key terms of this chapter.
2. Palpate each of the bones, bony landmarks, and joints of this chapter (listed in Key Terms).
3. State the muscle or muscles that attach to each of the bony landmarks of this chapter.
4. Describe the location of each of the ligaments of the upper extremity.

Key Terms

acromioclavicular (AC) joint
acromion process of the scapula
anatomic snuffbox
bicipital groove of the humerus
capitate
clavicle
coracoid process of the scapula
deltoid tuberosity of the humerus
distal interphalangeal (DIP) joint
dorsal tubercle of the radius
greater tubercle of the humerus

hamate
hook of the hamate
humeral shaft
inferior angle of the scapula
infraspinous fossa of the scapula
infraglenoid tubercle of the scapula
interphalangeal (IP) joint
lateral border of the scapula
lateral epicondyle of the humerus

lateral supracondylar ridge of the humerus
lesser tubercle of the humerus
Lister's tubercle of the radius
lunate
medial border of the scapula
medial epicondyle of the humerus
medial supracondylar ridge of the humerus
metacarpal base

Section 1: Shoulder Girdle

7

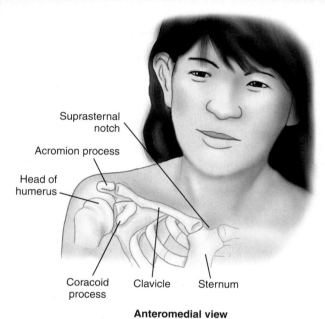

Suprasternal notch
Acromion process
Head of humerus
Coracoid process
Clavicle
Sternum

Anteromedial view

Figure 7-1 Anteromedial view of the shoulder girdle.

Anteromedial view

Figure 7-2 Sternoclavicular joint: Start by first locating the suprasternal notch of the manubrium of the sternum; then press laterally, feeling for the **sternoclavicular (SC) joint** between the sternum and the medial (proximal) end of the clavicle. To better palpate the SC joint, ask the client to actively move his or her arm in various ranges of motion while palpating the SC joint.

⊕ Go to http://evolve.elsevier.com/Muscolino/palpation for identification of bony landmark exercises.

Anteromedial view

Figure 7-3 Clavicle: From the SC joint, slide along the shaft of the **clavicle** from medial to lateral (proximal to distal) to feel its entire length. Notice that the medial end of the clavicle is convex anteriorly and the lateral end of the clavicle is concave anteriorly.

PLEASE NOTE: The sternocleidomastoid and upper trapezius muscles attach to the superior side of the clavicle. The pectoralis major, anterior deltoid, and subclavius muscles attach to the inferior side of the clavicle.

Anteromedial view

Figure 7-4 Coracoid process of the scapula: From the concavity at the lateral (distal) end of the clavicle, drop inferiorly off the clavicle to find the **coracoid process of the scapula** (which is located deep to the pectoralis major muscle). When palpating the coracoid process, notice that its apex (tip) points laterally. (If it is difficult to locate the coracoid process in this manner, then try to palpate it by first locating its apex. To do this, drop down from the far lateral end of the clavicle onto the head of the humerus and then press medially to find the apex of the coracoid process.)

PLEASE NOTE: Three muscles attach to the coracoid process: the short head of the biceps brachii, coracobrachialis, and the pectoralis minor.

Anteromedial view

Figure 7-5 Acromion process of the scapula: After palpating the coracoid process of the scapula, move back to the clavicle and continue palpating the clavicle laterally (distally) once again until you reach the **acromion process of the scapula**. The acromion process of the scapula is at the far lateral end (i.e., the tip of the shoulder).

PLEASE NOTE: The upper trapezius and deltoid muscles attach to the acromion process of the scapula.

Anteromedial view

Figure 7-6 Acromioclavicular joint: To best feel the **acromioclavicular (AC) joint**, palpate pressing medially from the acromion of the scapula toward the clavicle until you feel the AC joint. This is usually the easiest way to feel this joint line because the lateral end of the clavicle sticks up slightly superiorly above the acromion process.

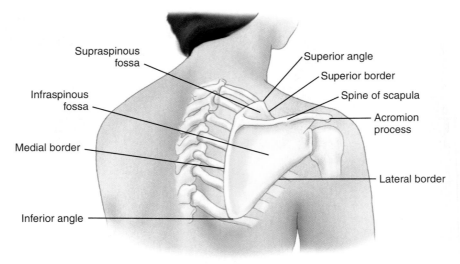

Posterolateral view

Figure 7-7 Posterolateral view of the scapula.

A   **Posterolateral view**   B   **Posterolateral view**

Figure 7-8 Acromion process and spine of the scapula: The **spine of the scapula** is the posterior continuation of the acromion process. To locate the spine of the scapula, begin on the acromion process **(A)** and continue palpating along it posteriorly. The spine of the scapula **(B)** can be palpated all the way to the medial border of the scapula. The spine of the scapula can be best palpated if you strum it perpendicularly by moving your palpating fingers up and down across it as you work your way posteriorly.

PLEASE NOTE: The posterior deltoid and trapezius muscles attach to the spine of the scapula. The rhomboid minor muscle attaches to the root of the spine of the scapula.

Posterolateral view

Figure 7-9 Supraspinous fossa: To palpate the **supraspinous fossa of the scapula**, locate the spine of the scapula and drop just off it superiorly. Palpate along the superior border of the spine of the scapula within the supraspinous fossa.
PLEASE NOTE: The supraspinous fossa is covered by the upper trapezius and the supraspinatus muscles. The supraspinatus muscle attaches to the supraspinous fossa.

Posterolateral view

Figure 7-10 Infraspinous fossa of the scapula: To palpate the **infraspinous fossa of the scapula**, locate the spine of the scapula and drop just off it inferiorly. The infraspinous fossa is larger than the supraspinous fossa.
PLEASE NOTE: The infraspinatus muscle attaches to the infraspinous fossa.

Posterolateral view

Figure 7-11 Medial border of the scapula (at the root of the spine of the scapula): Continue palpating along the spine of the scapula until you reach the **medial border of the scapula**. Where the spine of the scapula ends at the medial border is called the **root of the spine of the scapula**. It is helpful to have the client protract and retract the scapula (at the scapulocostal joint) to bring out the medial border of the scapula. Passively retracting the client's scapula makes it much easier to locate the medial border.
PLEASE NOTE: The levator scapulae and rhomboid muscles attach to the medial border of the scapula on the posterior side. The serratus anterior muscle attaches to the medial border on the anterior side.

Posterolateral view

Figure 7-12 Superior angle of the scapula: Once the medial border of the scapula has been located, palpate along it superiorly until you reach the **superior angle of the scapula**. It can be helpful to have the client elevate and depress the scapula as you palpate for its superior angle.
PLEASE NOTE: The levator scapulae muscle attaches to the superior angle of the scapula.

Posterolateral view

Figure 7-13 Inferior angle of the scapula: Palpate along the medial border of the scapula from the superior angle down to the **inferior angle of the scapula**.

PLEASE NOTE: The latissimus dorsi and teres major muscles attach onto or near the inferior angle of the scapula.

Posterolateral view

Figure 7-14 Lateral border of the scapula: Once you are at the inferior angle of the scapula, continue palpating superiorly along the **lateral border of the scapula**. It is easiest to feel the lateral border if your pressure is directed medially. The lateral border of the scapula can usually be palpated all the way to the **infraglenoid tubercle of the scapula**, just inferior to the glenoid fossa of the scapula. To confirm that you are on the infraglenoid tubercle, ask the client to extend his or her forearm at the elbow joint against resistance to bring out the infraglenoid attachment of the long head of the triceps brachii (you can provide the resistance to extension of the forearm at the elbow joint, or the resistance can be provided by the client pressing the forearm against his or her own thigh).

PLEASE NOTE: The teres major and teres minor muscles attach to the lateral border of the scapula; the long head of the triceps brachii attaches to the infraglenoid tubercle of the scapula. On the anterior side, the subscapularis muscle attaches onto or near the lateral border of the scapula.

Posterolateral view

Figure 7-15 Superior border of the scapula: The **superior border of the scapula** is more challenging to palpate than the medial and lateral borders. First, trace the medial border of the scapula up to the superior angle once again. Once the superior angle has been located, continue to palpate laterally along the superior border, with your pressure directed inferiorly against the superior border. Elevating the scapula (at the scapulocostal joint) may help to bring out the superior border a bit more. It is usually not possible to palpate the entire length of the superior border of the scapula.

PLEASE NOTE: The omohyoid muscle attaches to the superior border of the scapula. The levator scapulae muscle also attaches onto the superior border of the scapula at the superior angle.

Lateral view

Figure 7-16 Subscapular fossa of the scapula: The **subscapular fossa** is located on the anterior surface of the scapula and can be slightly challenging to palpate. With the client supine, grasp the medial border of the client's scapula with one hand and passively protract the scapula. With your other hand, palpate slowly but firmly against the anterior surface of the scapula.

PLEASE NOTE: The subscapularis muscle attaches to the subscapular fossa on the anterior side of the scapula; the serratus anterior muscle also attaches to the anterior side of the scapula, along the medial border.

7

Section 2: Arm and Forearm

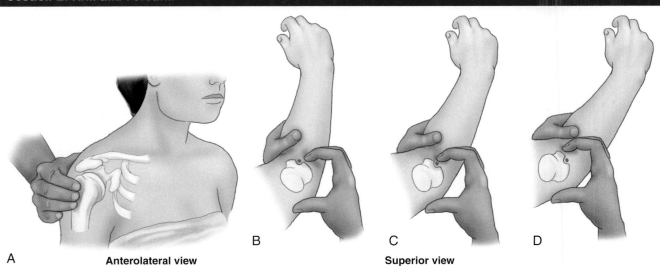

A

Anterolateral view

B   C   D

Superior view

Figure 7-17 Greater tubercle, bicipital groove, and lesser tubercle of the humerus: The **greater tubercle** is located on the lateral side of the **bicipital groove**; the **lesser tubercle** is located on the medial side. First locate the anterolateral margin of the acromion process of the scapula and then drop immediately off it onto the head of the humerus; you should be on the greater tubercle of the humerus **(A** and **B)**. Now, with a flat finger pad palpation across the anterior surface of the head of the humerus, passively move the client's arm into lateral rotation at the shoulder joint. You should be able to feel your palpating finger dropping into the bicipital groove as it passes under your finger pads **(C)**. As you continue to passively move the client's arm into lateral rotation, you will then feel the lesser tubercle under your fingers, just medial to the bicipital groove **(D)**. If you do not successfully feel the tubercles and bicipital groove, alternately move the client's arm through medial and lateral rotation, feeling for them.

PLEASE NOTE: The long head of the biceps brachii muscle runs through the bicipital groove; the supraspinatus, infraspinatus, and teres minor muscles attach onto the greater tubercle; the subscapularis muscle attaches onto the lesser tubercle.

Lateral view

Figure 7-18 Deltoid tuberosity: Feel for the **deltoid tuberosity**, which is approximately ⅓ of the way down the lateral side of the shaft of the humerus.

PLEASE NOTE: The deltoid attaches to the deltoid tuberosity of the humerus. Also attaching very close to the deltoid tuberosity is the proximal attachment of the brachialis.

A   B

Posterior view

Figure 7-19 Medial and lateral epicondyles of the humerus: To locate the **medial and lateral epicondyles of the humerus**, ask the client to flex the forearm at the elbow joint to approximately 90 degrees; place your palpating fingers on the medial and lateral sides of the client's arm **(A)** and move distally down the client's arm. Your palpating fingers will clearly run into the medial and lateral epicondyles of the humerus; they will prominently be the widest points along the sides of the humerus near the elbow joint **(B)**.

PLEASE NOTE: Five muscles attach onto the medial epicondyle of the humerus: pronator teres, flexor carpi radialis, palmaris longus, flexor carpi ulnaris, and flexor digitorum superficialis; the flexor pollicis longus also usually attaches onto the medial epicondyle. Six muscles attach to the lateral epicondyle of the humerus: the extensor carpi radialis brevis, extensor digitorum, extensor digiti minimi, extensor carpi ulnaris, anconeus, and supinator.

7

Posterior view

Figure 7-20 Olecranon process of the ulna: The **olecranon process of the ulna** is extremely easy to locate. With the thumb and middle finger on the medial and lateral epicondyles of the humerus, place your index finger on the olecranon process, located halfway between the two epicondyles. Note: If the client's elbow joint is flexed, the olecranon process will be located farther distally than the two epicondyles of the humerus. Be careful with palpatory pressure between the medial epicondyle of the humerus and the olecranon process of the ulna due to the presence of the ulnar nerve, known in lay terms as the "funny bone."
PLEASE NOTE: The triceps brachii and anconeus muscles attach onto the olecranon process.

Posterior view

Figure 7-21 Olecranon fossa of the humerus: Once the olecranon process of the ulna has been located, the **olecranon fossa of the humerus** is fairly easy to locate. The client's forearm must be partially flexed at the elbow joint so that the olecranon fossa of the humerus is exposed (in full extension, the olecranon process of the ulna is located in and obstructs palpation of the olecranon fossa of the humerus). Find the most proximal midline point of the olecranon process of the ulna and drop off it just proximally and you will feel the olecranon fossa of the humerus.
PLEASE NOTE: The distal tendon of the triceps brachii muscle overlies the olecranon fossa of the humerus.

A   B

Lateral view

Figure 7-22 Lateral supracondylar ridge of the humerus: From the lateral epicondyle of the humerus **(A)**, palpate just proximally onto the **lateral supracondylar ridge of the humerus** with your pressure directed medially against it **(B)**.
PLEASE NOTE: The brachioradialis and extensor carpi radialis longus muscles attach onto the lateral supracondylar ridge of the humerus.

7

Lateral view

Figure 7-23 Lateral humeral shaft: The majority of the **humeral shaft** is deep to musculature and difficult to directly palpate. However, the anterolateral shaft may be palpated. From the lateral supracondylar ridge, continue palpating the lateral shaft of the humerus proximally with your pressure directed medially against the shaft between the brachialis and triceps brachii muscles.

PLEASE NOTE: Attaching onto or near the lateral shaft of the humerus are the brachialis and triceps brachii muscles.

Lateral view

Figure 7-24 Radial head: The **radial head** lies at the proximal end of the radius. To palpate it, begin at the lateral epicondyle of the humerus and drop immediately distal to it. It is possible to feel the joint space between the head of the radius and the humerus (the capitulum is the landmark of the humerus that is directly next to the head of the radius and is also palpable here). To bring out the radial head, place two fingers on either side (proximal and distal) of it and ask the client to alternately pronate and supinate the forearm at the radioulnar joints; the spinning of the head of the radius can be felt under your fingers.

A

B

Medial view

Figure 7-25 Medial supracondylar ridge of the humerus: From the medial epicondyle of the humerus **(A)**, palpate just proximally onto the **medial supracondylar ridge of the humerus** with your pressure directed laterally against it **(B)**.

PLEASE NOTE: The pronator teres attaches to the most distal end of the medial supracondylar ridge of the humerus (as well as to the medial epicondyle).

Medial view

Figure 7-26 Medial shaft of the humerus: The majority of the medial shaft of the humerus is also palpable. However, you must be careful with your palpatory pressure here because of the presence of a number of nerves and arteries. To palpate the medial shaft of the humerus, continue palpating proximally from the medial supracondylar ridge of the humerus with your pressure directed laterally against the medial shaft.

PLEASE NOTE: Attaching onto or near the medial shaft of the humerus are the brachialis, coracobrachialis, and triceps brachii muscles. Farther proximally, the latissimus dorsi and teres major muscles also attach near the medial shaft of the humerus.

Medial view

Figure 7-27 Ulnar shaft: The entire medial border of the **ulnar shaft** is easily palpable. Begin on the medial side of the olecranon process and continue palpating distally with your pressure directed laterally against the medial border of the ulna until you reach the distal end of the ulna.

PLEASE NOTE: Three muscles attach onto the medial border of the shaft of the ulna: the ulnar head of the flexor carpi ulnaris, the ulnar head of the extensor carpi ulnaris, and the flexor digitorum profundus.

Lateral view

Figure 7-28 Lateral shaft of the radius: The majority of the lateral **radial shaft** is palpable. Begin approximately midshaft and palpate into the lateral radius with your pressure directed medially against the lateral shaft of the radius. Asking the client to alternately pronate and supinate the forearm at the radioulnar joints will help bring out the shaft of the radius. Continue palpating the lateral shaft of the radius proximally until you reach the head of the radius (there is a part of the proximal, lateral radial shaft that is difficult to palpate because it is deep to the supinator muscle).

PLEASE NOTE: The supinator, pronator teres, and flexor pollicis longus muscles attach onto the lateral shaft of the radius.

7

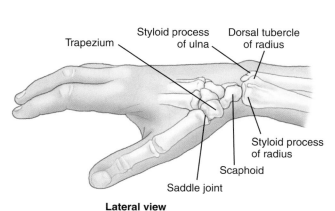

Lateral view

Figure 7-29 Lateral view of the wrist/hand.

Trapezium — Styloid process of ulna — Dorsal tubercle of radius — Styloid process of radius — Scaphoid — Saddle joint

Lateral view

Figure 7-30 Styloid process of the radius: Now that the lateral shaft of the radius has been located, continue palpating it distally until you reach the **styloid process of the radius** located at the distal end of the lateral radial shaft. (Note: There is a small portion of the distal lateral radial shaft that is not directly palpable because it is deep to three deep thumb muscles of the posterior forearm.)

PLEASE NOTE: The brachioradialis muscle attaches onto the styloid process of the radius.

YOU ARE HERE

7

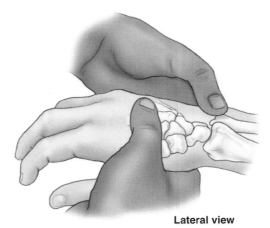

Lateral view

Figure 7-31 Dorsal (Lister's) tubercle: The **dorsal tubercle** (also known as **Lister's tubercle**) is located on the posterior side of the distal end of the radius. From the radial styloid, palpate posteriorly onto the radius; the dorsal tubercle will be a prominence located in the middle of the distal posterior radial shaft.
PLEASE NOTE: The dorsal tubercle separates the distal tendons of the extensors carpi radialis longus and brevis muscles from the distal tendon of the extensor pollicis longus muscle.

Lateral view

Figure 7-32 Styloid process of the ulna: The **styloid process of the ulna** is located at the distal end of the ulna on the posterior side. From the dorsal tubercle of the radius, move medially onto the posterior surface of the distal ulna and feel for the prominence of the ulnar styloid.

Section 3: Radial Side of the Wrist (Scaphoid and Trapezium)

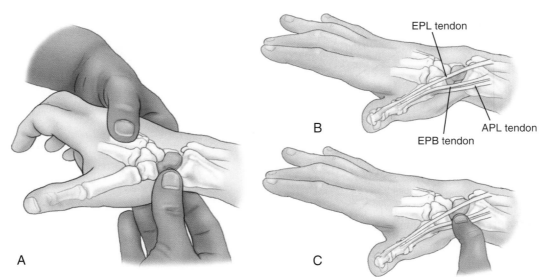

Lateral (radial) view

Figure 7-33 Scaphoid: The **scaphoid** is the carpal bone located in the proximal row of carpals on the lateral (radial) side, directly distal to the lateral side of the radius. It can be palpated dorsally, laterally, and anteriorly. Begin palpating the scaphoid laterally by dropping distally onto it from the radial styloid **(A)**. To bring out the scaphoid, ask the client to alternately do active radial and ulnar deviation of the hand at the wrist joint; the scaphoid will alternately press into your palpating finger with ulnar deviation and then disappear with radial deviation. To palpate the scaphoid on the dorsal side, ask the client to extend and abduct the thumb; this brings out the **anatomic snuffbox**, a depression bordered by the distal tendons of three thumb muscles (abductor pollicis longus [APL], extensor pollicis brevis [EPB], and extensor pollicis longus [EPL]) **(B)**. The scaphoid forms the floor of the anatomic snuffbox. Palpate the scaphoid by palpating between the tendons that border the anatomic snuffbox **(C)**. Asking the client to alternately do active ulnar and radial deviation of the hand at the wrist joint will also help bring out the scaphoid here. (Note: To palpate the scaphoid anteriorly, see Figure 7-37, A.)
PLEASE NOTE: The three muscles whose distal tendons border and define the anatomic snuffbox are the abductor pollicis longus and extensor pollicis brevis on the lateral side, and the extensor pollicis longus on the medial side.

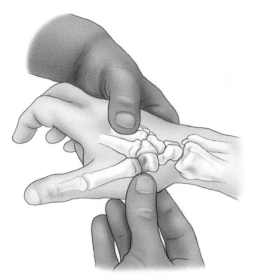

Lateral (radial) view

Figure 7-34 Saddle joint of the thumb: The **saddle joint of the thumb** is the carpometacarpal joint of the thumb and is located between the trapezium and the base of the metacarpal of the thumb. To palpate it, begin proximally from the palpation of the lateral side of the scaphoid (see Figure 7-33, A) and palpate distally until you feel the joint line between the trapezium and the metacarpal of the thumb. Perhaps even easier is to begin distally by first locating the lateral shaft of the metacarpal of the thumb and then palpating proximally until you feel the joint line between the metacarpal of the thumb and the trapezium. If you are unsure whether you are on this joint, ask the client to actively move the thumb and feel for the movement of the metacarpal of the thumb relative to the trapezium at the joint line.

Lateral (radial) view

Figure 7-35 Trapezium: Once the saddle joint of the thumb has been located, palpate just proximally to it and you will be directly on the lateral surface of the **trapezium**. The tubercle of the trapezium can also be palpated anteriorly (see Figure 7-37, B).

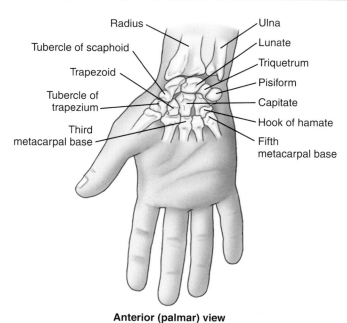

Radius — Ulna
Tubercle of scaphoid — Lunate
Trapezoid — Triquetrum
Tubercle of trapezium — Pisiform
Third metacarpal base — Capitate
— Hook of hamate
Fifth metacarpal base

Anterior (palmar) view

Figure 7-36 Anterior (palmar) view of the wrist.

7

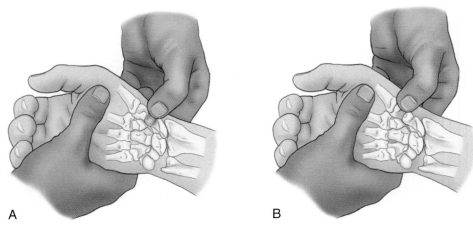

A   B

Anterior (palmar) view

Figure 7-37 Tubercles of scaphoid and trapezium: The tubercles of the scaphoid and trapezium are prominent and palpable anteriorly. To locate the **tubercle of the scaphoid**, begin on the lateral surface of the scaphoid (see Figure 7-33, A) and move approximately ¼ to ½ inch (.5 to 1 cm) anteriorly until you feel the tubercle of the scaphoid **(A)**. To locate the **tubercle of the trapezium**, begin on the lateral surface of the trapezium (see Figure 7-35) and move approximately ½ inch (1 cm) anteriorly until you feel the tubercle of the trapezium **(B)**. Note: The tubercle of the trapezium is located approximately ½ inch (1 cm) distal to the tubercle of the scaphoid.

PLEASE NOTE: The opponens pollicis muscle attaches onto the tubercle of the trapezium. The abductor pollicis brevis muscle attaches onto both the tubercle of the scaphoid and the tubercle of the trapezium. The flexor pollicis brevis muscle attaches onto the anterior surface of the trapezium. The transverse carpal ligament (flexor retinaculum) that forms the roof of the carpal tunnel also attaches to the tubercles of the scaphoid and trapezium.

Section 4: Central Carpal Bones of the Wrist (Capitate, Lunate, and Trapezoid)

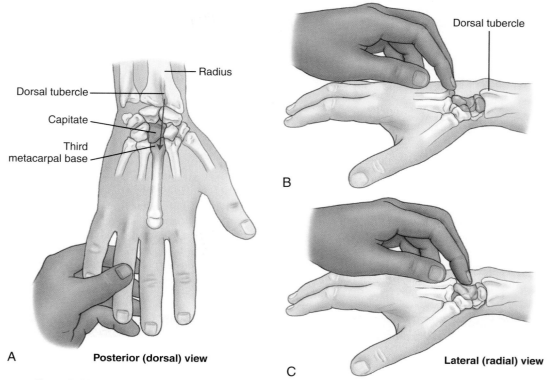

A **Posterior (dorsal) view**

B

C **Lateral (radial) view**

Figure 7-38 Third metacarpal base and the capitate: The dorsal (Lister's) tubercle of the radius, base of the third metacarpal, and **capitate** (of the distal row of carpal bones) are all located in a straight line on the dorsal side of the wrist/hand region **(A)**. First locate the dorsal tubercle of the radius (see Figure 7-31); from there, palpate distally for the base of the third metacarpal **(B)**. A **metacarpal base** is the expanded proximal end of a metacarpal (the base of the third metacarpal is the largest and most prominent of the metacarpal bases and is located directly medial to the base of the head of the second metacarpal). Once the base of the third metacarpal has been located, drop just off it proximally onto the capitate **(C)**. To bring out the capitate, ask the client to do active flexion and ulnar deviation of the hand at the wrist joint, and the capitate can be felt pressing up into your palpating finger.

PLEASE NOTE: The adductor pollicis muscle attaches onto the anterior side of the capitate.

Lateral (radial) view

Figure 7-39 Lunate: The **lunate** is the carpal bone located in the proximal row of carpals between the scaphoid and the triquetrum. The best place to palpate the lunate is posteriorly. To find the lunate, move proximally from the capitate and slightly in the ulnar direction. This area will feel like a depression. Now ask the client to alternately do active flexion and extension of the hand at the wrist joint. Upon wrist joint flexion, the lunate can be felt pressing up into your palpating finger; upon wrist joint extension, the lunate disappears from palpation.

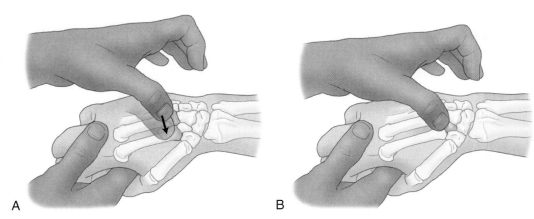

Posterolateral (dorsoradial) view

Figure 7-40 Second metacarpal base and the trapezoid: The **trapezoid** is the carpal bone that is located in the distal row of carpals, directly next to the trapezium and just proximal to the base of the second metacarpal. The best place to palpate the trapezoid is posteriorly. First locate the base of the third metacarpal (see Figure 7-38, B) and drop off it in the radial direction onto the base of the second metacarpal **(A)**. Once the base of the second metacarpal has been found, drop off it proximally and you will be on the trapezoid **(B)**. To bring out the trapezoid, ask the client to do active flexion and ulnar deviation of the hand at the wrist joint and the trapezoid can be felt to press up against your palpating finger.

Section 5: Ulnar Side of the Wrist (Triquetrum, Hamate, and Pisiform)

Medial (ulnar) view

Figure 7-41 Triquetrum: The **triquetrum** is a carpal bone located in the proximal row of carpals on the medial (ulnar) side, directly distal to the styloid process of the ulna on the posterior side of the wrist. The easiest way to palpate the triquetrum is to locate the medial border of the styloid process of the ulna, then drop distally off the ulnar styloid and you will be directly on the triquetrum. To bring out the borders of the triquetrum, ask the client to alternately do active radial and ulnar deviation of the hand at the wrist joint; the triquetrum will press against your palpating finger with radial deviation and will disappear from palpation with ulnar deviation.

Medial (ulnar) view

Figure 7-42 Fifth metacarpal base and the hamate: It is challenging, but the **hamate** can often be palpated on the ulnar side of the wrist. After locating the triquetrum on the ulnar side, palate farther distal for the base of the fifth metacarpal **(A)**. From the base of the fifth metacarpal, drop immediately proximal into a little depression that is located between the base of the fifth metacarpal and the triquetrum; the ulnar surface of the hamate can often be palpated there **(B)**.

A   B

C   D

Posteromedial (dorsoulnar) view

Figure 7-43 Fourth metacarpal base and hamate and triquetrum dorsally: From the dorsal side of the base of the fifth metacarpal **(A)**, move radially onto the base of the fourth metacarpal **(B)**. From there, drop proximally onto the dorsal surface of the hamate **(C)**. From the dorsal surface of the hamate, drop proximally (and stay toward the ulnar side) onto the dorsal surface of the triquetrum **(D)**.

Section 6: Anterior Wrist

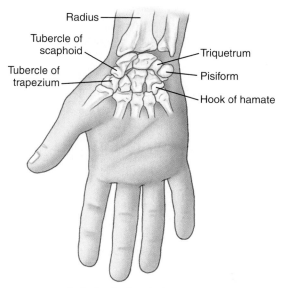

Radius

Tubercle of scaphoid

Tubercle of trapezium

Triquetrum

Pisiform

Hook of hamate

Anterior (palmar) view

Figure 7-44 Anterior (palmar) view of the wrist.

7

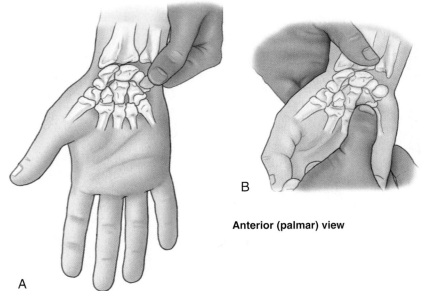

B

Anterior (palmar) view

A

Figure 7-45 Pisiform and hook of the hamate: The **pisiform** is a carpal bone located anteriorly on top of the triquetrum, in the proximal row of carpals on the ulnar side. The pisiform is prominent and easily palpated on the anterior side of the wrist, just distal to the ulna **(A)**. The hamate is also easily palpated anteriorly in the palm. Specifically, the **hook of the hamate** is palpable here. Begin by locating the pisiform; then palpate approximately ½ to ¾ inch (1 to 1.5 cm) distal and lateral (i.e., toward the midline of the hand) from the pisiform **(B)**. Note: The hook of the hamate is fairly pointy and can be somewhat tender to palpation.

PLEASE NOTE: The flexor carpi ulnaris and abductor digiti minimi manus muscles attach onto the pisiform. The flexor carpi ulnaris, flexor digiti minimi manus, and opponens digiti minimi muscles attach onto the hook of the hamate.

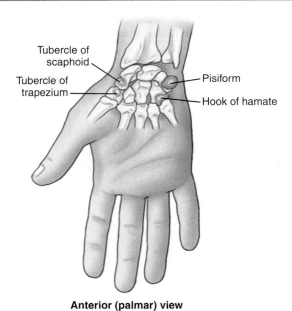

Tubercle of scaphoid

Tubercle of trapezium

Pisiform

Hook of hamate

Anterior (palmar) view

Figure 7-46 Review of four prominent anterior carpal landmarks: There are four carpal landmarks that are prominent and fairly easy to palpate in the anterior wrist. They are the pisiform and hook of the hamate on the ulnar side, and the tubercle of the scaphoid and tubercle of the trapezium on the radial side.

Section 7: Hand

Lateral (radial) view

Figure 7-47 Metacarpals and metacarpophalangeal joints: There are five **metacarpals**, located distal to the carpal bones and proximal to the phalanges of the fingers. All five metacarpals are easily palpable on the dorsal, ulnar, and radial sides. For each metacarpal, first locate its dorsal side anywhere along the middle of the **metacarpal shaft** (Note: The second metacarpal and the second **metacarpophalangeal [MCP] joint** are illustrated being palpated.) Once the shaft has been located, follow the metacarpal shaft proximally until you feel the expanded base (the base of the third metacarpal is the largest of the five). If you palpate just proximal to each base, the carpometacarpal joint for each individual metacarpal bone can be palpated (the palpation of all five metacarpal bases has already been covered in this chapter). Now palpate each metacarpal shaft on either its dorsal or radial side distally until you feel the expanded **metacarpal head**. Palpating just distal to the head of each metacarpal, the metacarpophalangeal joints can be discerned.

PLEASE NOTE: The flexor carpi radialis, flexor carpi ulnaris, extensor carpi radialis longus, extensor carpi radialis brevis, extensor carpi ulnaris, opponens digiti minimi, adductor pollicis, palmar interossei, and dorsal interossei manus muscles attach onto the second through fourth metacarpals. The abductor pollicis longus, flexor pollicis brevis, opponens pollicis, adductor pollicis, and dorsal interossei manus muscles attach onto the first metacarpal.

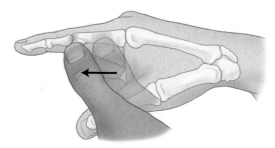

Lateral (radial) view

Figure 7-48 Phalanges and interphalangeal joints of the hand: There are three **phalanges** for each of the fingers except the thumb, which has only two phalanges. Furthermore, each phalanx has a proximal expanded **base**, a **shaft**, and a distal expanded **head**. The bases, shafts, and heads of each of the phalanges are easily palpable on the dorsal, ulnar, and radial sides (Note: Because of the presence of the fingernail, the distal phalanx is moderately more difficult to palpate). Between the proximal and middle phalanges of each finger is the **proximal interphalangeal (PIP) joint**. Between the middle and distal phalanges of each finger is the **distal interphalangeal (DIP) joint**. Between the proximal and distal phalanges of the thumb is the **interphalangeal (IP) joint**.

This figure illustrates palpation of the radial (lateral) side of the shaft of the proximal phalanx and the PIP joint of the index finger.

PLEASE NOTE: The abductor digiti minimi manus, flexor digiti minimi manus, palmar interossei, and dorsal interossei manus muscles attach onto the proximal phalanges of the second through fourth fingers.

Lateral (radial) view

Figure 7-49 This figure illustrates palpation of the radial (lateral) side of the shaft of the middle phalanx and the DIP joint of the index finger.

PLEASE NOTE: The flexor digitorum superficialis, extensor digitorum, extensor digiti minimi, and extensor indicis muscles attach onto the middle phalanges of the second through fourth fingers.

Lateral (radial) view

Figure 7-50 This figure illustrates palpation of the radial (lateral) side of the shaft of the distal phalanx of the index finger.

PLEASE NOTE: The flexor digitorum profundus, extensor digitorum, extensor digiti minimi, and extensor indicis muscles attach onto the distal phalanges of the second through fourth fingers.

7

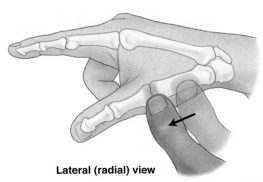

Lateral (radial) view

Figure 7-51 This figure illustrates palpation of the radial (lateral) side of the shaft of the metacarpal and the metacarpophalangeal (MCP) joint of the thumb.

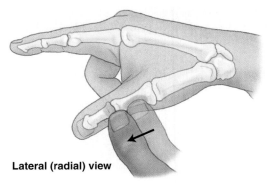

Lateral (radial) view

Figure 7-52 This figure illustrates palpation of the radial (lateral) side of the shaft of the proximal phalanx and the interphalangeal (IP) joint of the thumb.
PLEASE NOTE: The abductor pollicis brevis, flexor pollicis brevis, adductor pollicis, and extensor pollicis brevis muscles attach onto the proximal phalanx of the thumb.

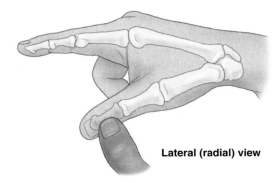

Lateral (radial) view

Figure 7-53 This figure illustrates palpation of the radial (lateral) side of the shaft of the distal phalanx of the thumb.
PLEASE NOTE: The flexor pollicis longus and extensor pollicis longus muscles attach onto the distal phalanx of the thumb.

Section 8: Ligaments of the Upper Extremity

Figure 7-54 Anterior view of the ligaments of the right upper extremity.

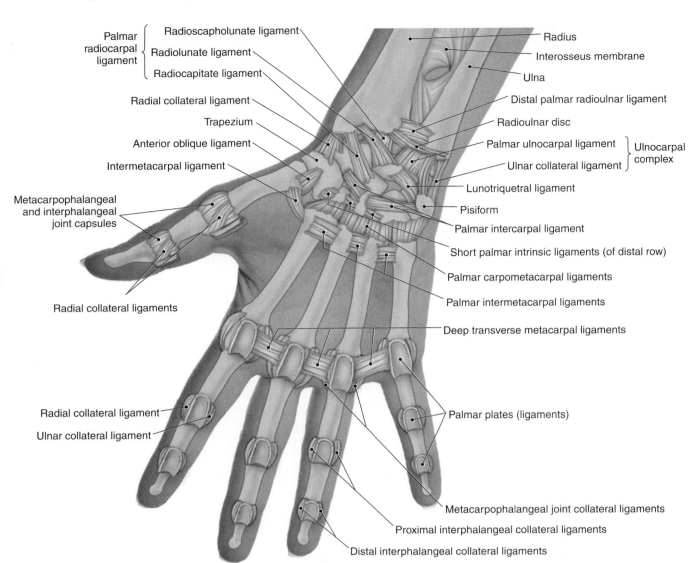

Palmar
radiocarpal
ligament
{
Radioscapholunate ligament
Radiolunate ligament
Radiocapitate ligament

Radial collateral ligament
Trapezium
Anterior oblique ligament
Intermetacarpal ligament

Metacarpophalangeal
and interphalangeal
joint capsules

Radial collateral ligaments

Radial collateral ligament
Ulnar collateral ligament

Radius
Interosseus membrane
Ulna
Distal palmar radioulnar ligament
Radioulnar disc
Palmar ulnocarpal ligament } Ulnocarpal
Ulnar collateral ligament } complex
Lunotriquetral ligament
Pisiform
Palmar intercarpal ligament
Short palmar intrinsic ligaments (of distal row)
Palmar carpometacarpal ligaments
Palmar intermetacarpal ligaments
Deep transverse metacarpal ligaments

Palmar plates (ligaments)

Metacarpophalangeal joint collateral ligaments
Proximal interphalangeal collateral ligaments
Distal interphalangeal collateral ligaments

Figure 7-55 Anterior view of the ligaments of the right wrist and hand.

Clavicle

Superior transverse scapular ligament

Acromioclavicular ligament

Glenohumeral joint capsule

Humerus

Elbow joint capsule

Radial collateral ligament

Radius

Interosseus membrane

Ulnar collateral ligament

Olecranon process of ulna

Styloid process of radius

Radial collateral ligament

Extensor retinaculum

Distal dorsal radioulnar ligament

Ulnar collateral ligament

Radial collateral ligaments

Ulnar collateral ligaments

Metacarpophalangeal
and interphalangeal
joint capsules

Figure 7-56 Posterior view of the ligaments of the right upper extremity.

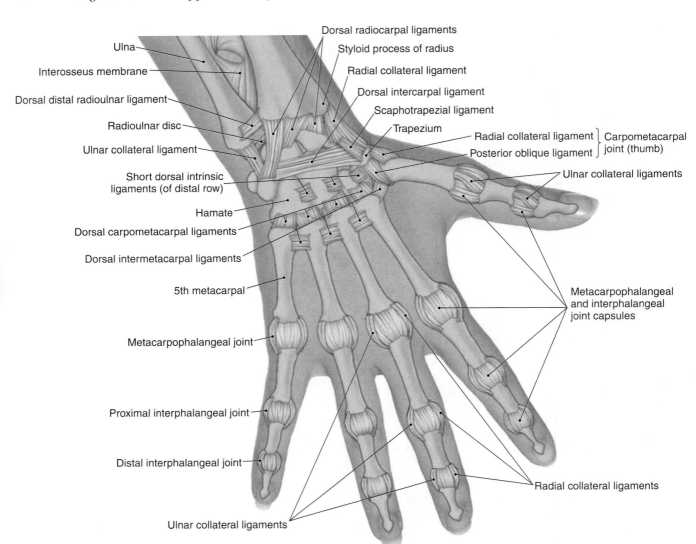

Figure 7-57 Posterior view of the ligaments of the right wrist and hand.

Axial Body Bone Palpation and Ligaments

Overview

Chapter 8 is one of three chapters of Part II of this book that addresses palpation of the skeleton. This chapter is a palpation tour of the bones, bony landmarks, and joints of the axial body. The tour begins with the face, then addresses the cranium and anterior and posterior neck, and concludes with the anterior and posterior trunk. Although any one bone or bony landmark can be independently palpated, this chapter is set up sequentially to flow from one landmark to another, so it is recommended that the order presented here is followed. Muscle attachments for each of the palpated structures are also given (specific palpations for these muscles are covered in Part III of this book). The ligaments of the axial body are presented at the end of this chapter.

Chapter 7 presents the ligaments of the upper extremity and the palpation of the bones, bony landmarks, and joints of the upper extremity. Chapter 9 presents the ligaments of the lower extremity and the palpation of the bones, bony landmarks, and joints of the lower extremity.

Chapter Outline

The bones, bony landmarks, and joints of the following regions are covered:

Section 1: Face, 94
Section 2: Cranium, 96

Chapter Objectives

After completing this chapter, the student should be able to perform the following:

1. Define the key terms of this chapter.
2. Palpate each of the bones, bony landmarks, and joints of this chapter (listed in Key Terms).
3. State the muscle or muscles that attach to each of the bony landmarks of this chapter.
4. Describe the location of each of the ligaments of the axial body.

Key Terms

angle of Louis
angle of the mandible
anterior tubercles (of cervical transverse processes)
articular pillar
articular processes
body of the mandible
carotid tubercle (of C6)
cervical pillar
condyle (of the ramus) of the mandible
coronoid process (of the ramus) of the mandible
costal cartilages
cricoid cartilages

external occipital protuberance (EOP)
facet joints (of the spine)
frontal bone
hyoid bone
inferior nuchal line of the occiput
intercostal spaces
interscapular region
interspinous space
frontal bone
jugular notch
laminar groove (of the spine)
mastoid process of the temporal bone
maxilla

nasal bone
occipital bone
parietal bone
posterior tubercle of C1
posterior tubercles (of cervical transverse processes)
ramus of the mandible
rib cage
ribs
spinous processes (SPs)
sternomanubrial joint
superior nuchal line of the occiput
suprasternal notch of the manubrium of the sternum

temporal bone
temporomandibular joint (TMJ)
thyroid cartilage

transverse process (TP) of C1
transverse processes (TPs)
vertebra prominens (of C7)

xiphoid process of the sternum
zygomatic arch of the temporal bone
zygomatic bone

Section 1: Face

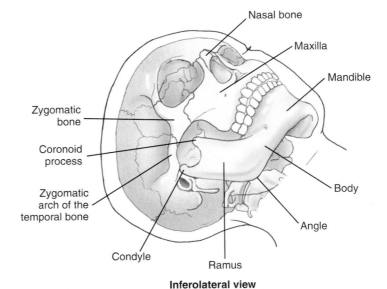

Figure 8-1 An oblique (inferolateral) view of the face.

Nasal bone

Maxilla

Mandible

Zygomatic bone

Coronoid process

Zygomatic arch of the temporal bone

Body

Angle

Condyle

Ramus

Inferolateral view

Inferolateral view

Figure 8-2 Body and angle of the mandible: The **body of the mandible** is subcutaneous and easily palpable. Begin palpating the inferior border of the body of the mandible anteriorly and continue palpating it laterally and posteriorly until the **angle of the mandible** is reached. The angle of the mandible is the transition area where the body of the mandible becomes the ramus of the mandible.

PLEASE NOTE: The following muscles attach onto the external surface of the body of the mandible: depressor anguli oris, depressor labii inferioris, mentalis, and platysma. The digastric, mylohyoid, and geniohyoid muscles attach onto the internal surface of the body of the mandible. The masseter and medial pterygoid muscles attach onto the angle of the mandible.

Go to http://evolve.elsevier.com/Muscolino/palpation for identification of bony landmark exercises.

Inferolateral view

Figure 8-3 Ramus (posterior border) and condyle of the mandible: The **ramus of the mandible** branches off from the body of the mandible at the angle of the mandible. The posterior border of the ramus is fairly easily palpable for its entire course and gives rise to the **condyle (of the ramus) of the mandible**. To palpate the ramus, begin at the angle of the mandible and palpate superiorly along the posterior border until the condyle is reached, anterior to the ear. To bring out the condyle, ask the client to alternately open and close the mouth. This allows one to feel the movement of the condyle of the mandible at the **temporomandibular joint (TMJ)**. (Note: The condyle can also be palpated from within the ear. Wearing a finger cot or glove, gently place your palpating finger inside the client's ear, press anteromedially, and ask the client to alternately open and close the mouth. The movement of the condyle of the mandible at the TMJ will be clearly palpable.)

PLEASE NOTE: The lateral pterygoid muscle attaches onto the condyle of the mandible.

Inferolateral view

Figure 8-4 Coronoid process of the mandible: The anterior border of the ramus of the mandible gives rise to the **coronoid process (of the ramus) of the mandible**. From outside the mouth, the coronoid process is difficult to palpate but can be felt if the mandible is depressed (i.e., the mouth is opened). Find the zygomatic bone and palpate directly inferior to it while asking the client to slightly move the mandible up and down, maintaining a position of the mouth that is nearly fully open.

PLEASE NOTE: The temporalis and masseter muscles attach onto the coronoid process of the mandible.

Inferolateral view

Figure 8-5 Ramus and coronoid process from inside the mouth: The anterior border of the ramus is easily palpable from the inside. To palpate the anterior border of the mandible inside the mouth, use a finger cot or glove and gently press posterolaterally. To palpate the coronoid process from inside the mouth, simply continue palpating along the anterior border of the ramus superiorly to the coronoid process.

Inferolateral view

Figure 8-6 Maxilla: The **maxilla**, also known as the *upper jaw*, is subcutaneous and easily palpated. First locate the maxilla superior to the mouth and then continue exploring all aspects of the maxilla.

PLEASE NOTE: The orbicularis oris, nasalis, depressor septi nasi, levator labii superioris alaeque nasi, levator labii superioris, and levator anguli oris muscles attach onto the maxilla.

Inferolateral view

Figure 8-7 Zygomatic bone: The **zygomatic bone**, commonly referred to as the *cheek bone*, is easily palpated inferolateral to the eye. Once located, explore the zygomatic bone to its borders with the maxilla, frontal bone, and temporal bone.

PLEASE NOTE: The masseter, zygomaticus minor, and zygomaticus major muscles attach onto the zygomatic bone.

8

Figure 8-8 Nasal bone: The **nasal bone** is easily palpable at the superior end of the nose. Note: The inferior end of the nose, which is composed of cartilage, is softer and more pliable.
PLEASE NOTE: The procerus muscle overlies the nasal bone.

Inferolateral view

Section 2: Cranium

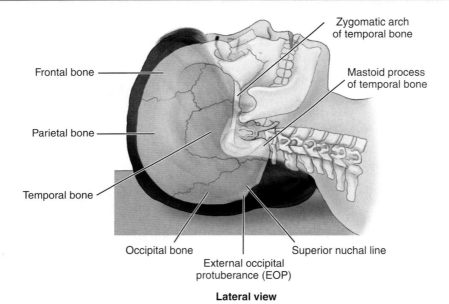

Zygomatic arch
of temporal bone

Frontal bone

Mastoid process
of temporal bone

Parietal bone

Temporal bone

Occipital bone   Superior nuchal line

External occipital
protuberance (EOP)

Lateral view
Figure 8-9 A lateral view of the head.

Figure 8-10 Frontal and parietal bones: The frontal and parietal bones are subcutaneous and easily palpable. First locate the **frontal bone** superior to the eye and then continue to palpate posteriorly onto the **parietal bone**, which is located at the top of the head.
PLEASE NOTE: The orbicularis oculi and corrugator supercilii muscles attach onto the frontal bone; the frontalis muscle overlies the frontal bone. The temporalis muscle attaches onto the parietal bone. The temporoparietalis muscle and the galea aponeurotica of the occipitofrontalis muscle overlie the parietal bone.

Lateral view

A

B

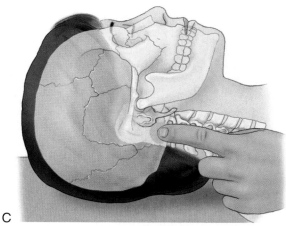

C

Lateral view

Figure 8-11 Temporal bone: The **temporal bone** is located on the side of the head (inferior to the parietal bone) **(A)**.

PLEASE NOTE: The temporalis muscle attaches to the majority of the temporal bone, making it more difficult to palpate this bone directly. Also, the temporoparietalis muscle overlies the temporal bone.

To palpate the zygomatic arch of the temporal bone, first find the zygomatic bone (see Figure 8-7). Once located, continue palpating the zygomatic bone posteriorly until you reach the **zygomatic arch of the temporal bone (B)**. It can be helpful to strum your fingers vertically over the zygomatic arch. The entire length of the zygomatic arch of the temporal bone can be palpated.

To palpate the **mastoid process of the temporal bone**, palpate just posterior to the earlobe, then press medially and strum over the mastoid process by moving your palpating finger anteriorly and posteriorly **(C)**.

PLEASE NOTE: The masseter muscle attaches onto the zygomatic arch of the temporal bone. The sternocleidomastoid, splenius capitis, and longissimus capitis muscles attach onto the mastoid process of the temporal bone.

8

A

B

C

Lateral view

Figure 8-12 Occipital bone: The **occipital bone** is located at the back of the skull; it is subcuta-neous and easily palpable **(A)**.

The **external occipital protuberance (EOP)** is a midline bump on the superior nuchal line of the occiput at the back of the head. The EOP is usually fairly large and prominent and therefore readily palpable **(B)**.

To palpate the **superior nuchal line of the occiput**, begin by locating the EOP at the center of the superior nuchal line; then palpate laterally for the superior nuchal line. It should feel like a raised ridge of bone running horizontally. It can be helpful to strum your fingers vertically over the superior nuchal line **(C)**. The superior nuchal line is fairly prominent and easily palpable on some people and much more challenging to palpate on others. Note: The **inferior nuchal line of the occiput** runs parallel and is located inferiorly to the superior nuchal line. It is usually difficult to palpate. If its palpation is attempted, first locate the superior nuchal line and then palpate inferior to it for the inferior nuchal line.

PLEASE NOTE: The occipitalis muscle attaches to the occipital bone. The upper trapezius mus-cle attaches to the external occipital protuberance and the superior nuchal line. The splenius capitis and sternocleidomastoid muscles also attach to the superior nuchal line of the occiput.

Section 3: Anterior Neck

Note: With all palpations in the anterior neck, a careful and sensitive touch is necessary and palpatory pressure must be applied gradually. There are many structures in the anterior neck that are very sensitive and can be tender. Furthermore, the carotid arteries are found in the anterior neck and pressure upon them can not only potentially restrict blood flow within them to the anterior brain, but can also trigger a neurologic reflex (the carotid reflex) that can lower blood pressure. For

this reason, it is best to palpate the anterior neck unilaterally (i.e., one side at a time). If you feel that your palpating fingers are on the carotid artery, either move slightly off it, or gently displace it from your palpating fingers. Generally, palpation of the structures of the anterior neck is best accomplished if the client's neck is relaxed and either in a neutral position or a position of slight passive flexion. Note: Some of the following palpations are cartilage structures, not bony landmarks.

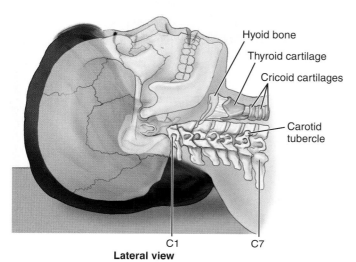

Lateral view

Figure 8-13 A lateral view of the neck.

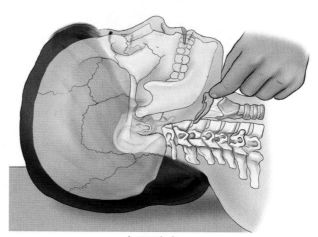

Lateral view

Figure 8-14 Hyoid bone: The **hyoid bone** is found in the anterior neck, inferior to the mandible (located at the level of the third cervical vertebra). To find the hyoid bone, begin at the mandible and move inferiorly in the anterior neck until you feel hard bony tissue. Once on the hyoid bone, ask the client to swallow, and movement of the hyoid bone will be felt. The hyoid bone is very mobile and it is possible to passively move it from left to right. A note of trivia: The hyoid bone is the only bone in the human body that does not articulate (form a joint) with another bone.
PLEASE NOTE: All four suprahyoid muscles and all four infrahyoid muscles (except the sternothyroid) attach onto the hyoid bone.

Lateral view

Figure 8-15 Thyroid cartilage: The **thyroid cartilage** is located in the anterior neck, inferior to the hyoid bone (the thyroid cartilage is located at the level of the fourth and fifth cervical vertebrae). Once the hyoid bone has been located, drop off it inferiorly; you will feel a joint space and then the thyroid cartilage will be felt. Palpate the small midline superior notch **(A)**; then gently palpate both sides of the thyroid cartilage **(B)**. Movement of the thyroid cartilage will be clearly felt if the client is asked to swallow. Palpation of the thyroid cartilage must be done gently and carefully because the thyroid gland often overlies part of the thyroid cartilage.

PLEASE NOTE: The sternothyroid and thyrohyoid muscles attach onto the thyroid cartilage.

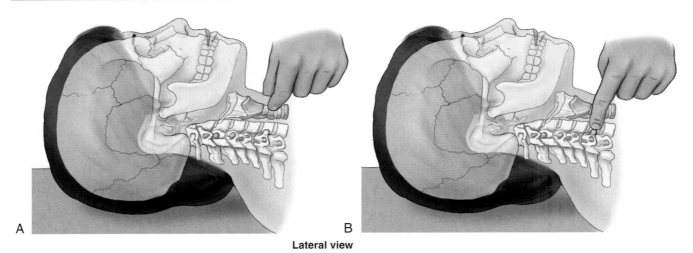

Lateral view

Figure 8-16 First cricoid cartilage and the carotid tubercle of C6: Directly inferior to the thyroid cartilage in the anterior neck is the first cricoid ring of cartilage at the sixth cervical vertebral level. To palpate the first cricoid cartilage, first locate the thyroid cartilage and continue to palpate along it inferiorly until a small joint line is felt. Immediately inferior to this joint line is the first cricoid cartilage **(A)**. Subsequent **cricoid cartilages** are located inferior to the first cricoid cartilage and may be palpated until their palpation is no longer possible at the level of the suprasternal notch of the manubrium of the sternum. Palpation of the cricoid cartilages must be done gently and carefully because the thyroid gland overlies them.

The **carotid tubercle** is the anterior tubercle of the transverse process of the sixth cervical vertebra. It is the largest anterior tubercle and is palpable in the anterior neck. To palpate the carotid tubercle, find the first cricoid cartilage and then drop off it laterally approximately ½ inch (1 cm); the carotid tubercle will be felt by pressing firmly but gently in a posterior direction **(B)**.

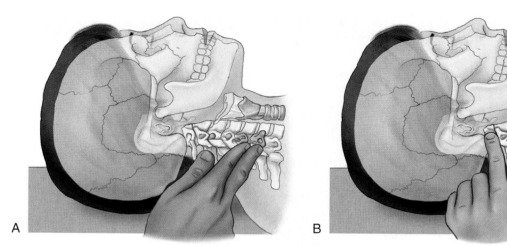

Lateral view

Figure 8-17 Transverse processes of C1 through C7: The **transverse processes (TPs)** of C2 through C7 are bifid and have **anterior tubercles** and **posterior tubercles**. These TPs may be palpated, but must be palpated with gentle pressure because their tubercles are pointy, and pressing the overlying musculature into them can be tender for the client. Begin by finding the carotid tubercle (anterior tubercle of the TP of C6); then palpate inferiorly and superiorly to find the other TPs. The direction of your pressure should be posterior and/or posteromedial **(A)**.

The **transverse process (TP) of C1** (the atlas) has the widest transverse process of the cervical spine. The TP of C1 can be palpated at a point that is directly posterior to the posterior border of the ramus of the mandible, directly anterior to the mastoid process of the temporal bone, and directly inferior to the ear. In this depression of surrounding soft tissue, the hard transverse process of C1 will be readily palpable **(B)**. Pressure should be gentle because this landmark is often sensitive and tender to pressure, and the facial nerve (CN VII) is located nearby.

PLEASE NOTE: The following muscles attach onto the TPs of C2 through C7: the levator scapulae, scalene group, longus colli, longus capitis, erector spinae group, transversospinalis group, intertransversarii, and levatores costarum. The following muscles attach onto the TP of C1: the levator scapulae, splenius cervicis, obliquus capitis inferior, obliquus capitis superior, rectus capitis anterior, rectus capitis lateralis, and intertransversarii.

8

8

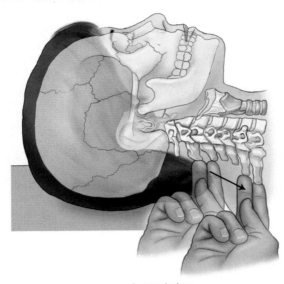

Lateral view

Figure 8-18 Spinous processes of C2 through C7: The **spinous processes (SPs)** of the cervical spine are palpated in the midline of the posterior neck. There are seven cervical vertebrae; however, not all of the cervical SPs are always palpable. Because of the lordotic curve of the spine of the neck (concave posteriorly), the SPs are often deep in the concavity and therefore difficult to palpate. The exact number of cervical SPs that can be palpated is primarily determined by the degree of the cervical curve of the client. The most prominent cervical SPs are those of C2 and C7; these two are always palpable. Begin by finding the external occipital protuberance in the midline of the occiput. From there, drop inferiorly off the occiput onto the cervical spine; the first cervical SP that will be palpable will be the SP of C2. As with most cervical SPs, the C2 SP is bifid (i.e., it has two points instead of one). It should be noted that these bifid points are not always symmetrical; one may be larger than the other. From C2, continue palpating inferiorly, feeling for additional cervical SPs. In some individuals, the next SP that will be readily palpable will be the one on C7 at the inferior end of the cervical spine.

The SP of C7 is clearly larger than the other lower cervical SPs, giving C7 the name **vertebra prominens**. In other individuals who have a decreased cervical spinal curve, it may be possible to palpate and count all the SPs from C2 to C7. Note: C1 (the atlas) does not have an SP; it has what is called a *posterior tubercle*. To palpate the **posterior tubercle of C1**, palpate between the SP of C2 and the occiput, pressing anteriorly into the soft tissue.

PLEASE NOTE: The following muscles either attach directly onto the SPs of the cervical spine, or attach into the nuchal ligament that overlies the SPs of the cervical spine: the upper trapezius, splenius capitis, splenius cervicis, interspinales, erector spinae group, and transversospinalis group. Furthermore, the rhomboid minor and serratus posterior superior muscles attach onto the spinous process of C7, the rectus capitis posterior major and obliquus capitis inferior muscles attach onto the SP of C2, and the rectus capitis posterior minor muscle attaches onto the posterior tubercle of C1.

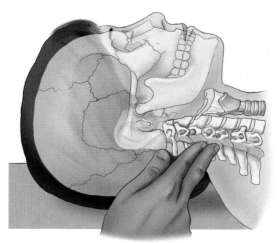

Lateral view

Figure 8-19 Articular processes (facet joints) of the cervical spine: The inferior and superior **articular processes** that create the **facet joints** of the cervical spine also create what is called the **articular pillar** or the **cervical pillar** because of the way they are stacked. They are easily palpable at the lateral side of the laminar groove (approximately one inch [2.5 cm] lateral to the SPs). The client must be supine and relaxed for palpation to be successful. Begin palpation at the spinous process of C2 and palpate laterally for the articular process of C2. Continue to palpate inferiorly until you reach the bottom of the neck. Note: The articular processes of the cervical spine are an excellent contact point when performing specific joint mobilizations to the cervical spine.

PLEASE NOTE: Muscles of the erector spinae group and the transversospinalis group attach onto the articular processes of the cervical spine.

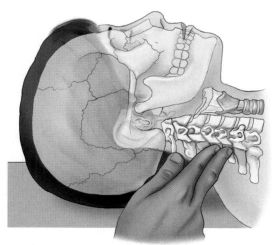

Lateral view

Figure 8-20 Laminar groove of the cervical spine: The **laminar groove** of the cervical spine is the groove that is found between the spinous processes medially and the articular processes laterally (i.e., the laminar groove overlies the laminae of the vertebrae). A number of muscles lie in the laminar groove, so direct palpation of the laminae at the floor of the laminar groove is difficult. Palpate just lateral to the SPs and you will be in the laminar groove.

PLEASE NOTE: The transversospinalis group attaches into the laminar groove of the neck. Many other muscles overlie the laminar groove.

Section 5: Anterior Trunk

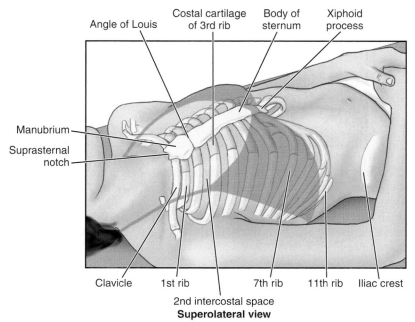

Figure 8-21 Superolateral view of the anterior trunk.

8

Superolateral view

Figure 8-22 Suprasternal notch of the sternum: The **suprasternal notch of the manubrium of the sternum** is subcutaneous and easily palpable. Simply palpate at the superior border of the sternum, and the depression of the suprasternal notch will be readily felt between the medial ends of the two clavicles. Note: The suprasternal notch is also known as the **jugular notch**.

Superolateral view

Figure 8-23 Angle of Louis: The **angle of Louis** is a horizontal prominence of bone on the sternum, formed by the **sternomanubrial joint**, which is the junction between the manubrium and the body of the sternum. (Note: The second sternocostal joint—in other words, where the second rib meets the sternum—is at the level of the angle of Louis.) To locate the angle of Louis, begin at the suprasternal notch of the manubrium and palpate inferiorly along the anterior surface of the manubrium until you feel a slight horizontal prominence of bone. It can be helpful to feel the angle of Louis by strumming vertically across it.

Superolateral view

Figure 8-24 Xiphoid process of the sternum: The **xiphoid process of the sternum** is at the inferior end of the sternum. The xiphoid process is cartilaginous but may calcify into bone as a person ages. To locate the xiphoid process, continue palpating inferiorly along the anterior surface of the sternum from the angle of Louis until you feel the small, pointy xiphoid process at the inferior end. Because the xiphoid process is made of cartilage, it is usually possible to exert mild pressure upon it and feel it move. Note: The xiphoid process is a landmark often used to find the proper hand position to administer CPR.

PLEASE NOTE: The rectus abdominis muscle attaches to the external surface of the xiphoid process; the transversus thoracis and diaphragm muscles attach to its internal surface.

Superolateral view

Anterolateral view

Figure 8-25 Anterior rib cage: The anterior side of the **rib cage** is composed of 12 **ribs**, seven **costal cartilages** that join the ribs to the sternum, and the 11 **intercostal spaces** located between the adjacent ribs and/or costal cartilages. All ribs, costal cartilages, and intercostal spaces can be palpated anteriorly and anterolaterally (except where the breast tissue of female clients interferes with palpation). The ribs and/or costal cartilages will be sensed as hard bony/cartilaginous tissue located subcutaneously, and the intercostal spaces will be sensed as depressions of soft tissue located between the ribs and/or the costal cartilages. Once each rib has been successfully palpated, try to follow it medially and laterally for its entire course, as far as possible.

To palpate ribs two through ten: Palpate the anterior rib cage lateral to the sternum. Generally, for ribs two through ten, it is easiest to identify them by strumming across them in a superior to inferior manner. Inferior to the medial end of the clavicle is the first intercostal space. The second rib is located at the level of the angle of Louis. From there, palpate inferiorly and count the intercostal spaces and ribs until you find the seventh costal cartilage **(A)**. Because of the contour of the rib cage, it is best to continue palpating ribs seven through ten and their costal cartilages more laterally in the anterior trunk **(B)**.

To palpate ribs eleven and twelve: Ribs eleven and twelve are called *floating ribs* because they do not articulate with the sternum. They must be palpated at the bottom of the rib cage, superior to the iliac crest, in the lateral and/or posterolateral trunk. It is often easiest to palpate the eleventh and twelfth ribs by pressing directly into and feeling for their pointy ends. (Note: This pressure should be firm but gentle because you are pressing soft tissue into the hard pointy end of a bone.)

To palpate the first rib: The first rib is probably the most challenging to palpate, but it can be felt. To palpate the first rib, find the superior border of the upper trapezius muscle and then drop off it anteriorly and direct your palpatory pressure inferiorly against the first rib **(C)**. Asking the client to take in a deep breath will elevate the first rib up against your palpating fingers and make palpation easier.

PLEASE NOTE: Many muscles attach to and/or overlie the anterior rib cage, including the serratus anterior, pectoralis major, pectoralis minor, subclavius, external intercostals, internal intercostals, rectus abdominis, external abdominal oblique, internal abdominal oblique, and transversus abdominis. The transversus thoracis and diaphragm attach to the internal surface of the anterior rib cage.

Section 6: Posterior Trunk

Note: Palpation of the scapula is covered in Chapter 7.

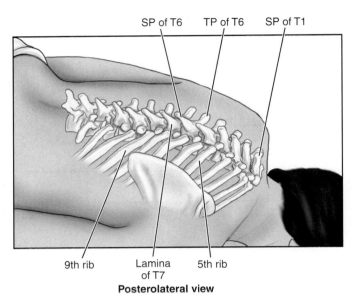

Posterolateral view

SP of T6   TP of T6   SP of T1

9th rib   Lamina of T7   5th rib

Figure 8-26 Superolateral view of the posterior trunk.

Posterolateral view

Figure 8-27 Spinous processes of the trunk: The spinous processes (SPs) of the twelve thoracic and five lumbar vertebrae are all palpable. Begin by locating the SP of C7 (also known as the *vertebra prominens*). It will usually be the first very prominent SP inferior to the SP of C2.

When the client is prone, if there is confusion as to which SP is C7, the following is a method to determine it. Palpate the SPs of the lower cervical spine with fingers on two or three of the prominent ones. Then passively flex and extend the client's head and neck. The SP of C6 will disappear from palpation with extension; the SP of C7 will not (i.e., the SP of C7 will be the highest SP palpable during flexion and extension).

Once the SP of C7 has been located, palpate each vertebral SP by placing your middle finger on the SP of that vertebra and your index finger in the **interspinous space** between that vertebra and the vertebra below. Continue palpating down the spine in this manner. It is usually possible to count the SPs from C7 to L5. Note: The SPs of the thoracic region are usually easily palpable because of the kyphotic thoracic spinal curve. However, palpating the lumbar SPs is a bit more challenging because of the lordotic lumbar spinal curve; to accomplish this, deeper pressure may be needed in the lumbar region.

PLEASE NOTE: The following muscles attach onto SPs of the trunk (thoracic and/or lumbar spine): the trapezius, splenius capitis, splenius cervicis, latissimus dorsi, rhomboids major and minor, serratus posterior superior, serratus posterior inferior, erector spinae group, transversospinalis group, and interspinales.

Posterolateral view

Figure 8-28 Transverse processes (TPs) of the trunk: The TPs of the trunk can be challenging to discern, but many of them can be palpated. Usually the TPs of the thoracic region can be felt approximately 1 inch (2.5 cm) lateral to the spinous processes (SPs). However, to determine the exact vertebral level of a TP can be difficult, because it is not located at the same level as the SP of the same vertebra. To determine the level of the TP that is being palpated, use the following method. Place one palpating finger on an SP, then press down onto the TPs nearby one at a time until you feel the pressure upon a TP move the SP that is under the palpating finger. The vertebral level of that TP will be the same as that of the SP that moved. This method is usually successful for the thoracic spine; palpation of the TPs of the lumbar spine is much more challenging.

PLEASE NOTE: The following muscles attach onto TPs of the trunk (thoracic and/or lumbar spine): the erector spinae group, transversospinalis group, quadratus lumborum, intertransversarii, levatores costarum, and psoas major.

Posterolateral view

Figure 8-29 Laminar groove of the trunk: The laminar groove of the thoracic and lumbar regions is the groove that is found between the SPs medially and the TPs laterally (i.e., the laminar groove overlies the laminae of the vertebrae). Palpate just lateral to the SPs and you will be in the laminar groove.

PLEASE NOTE: The transversospinalis group attaches into the laminar groove of the trunk. Many other muscles overlie the laminar groove.

Posterolateral view

Figure 8-30 Posterior rib cage: The ribs and intercostal spaces of the rib cage can be palpated in the posterior trunk in the **interscapular region** (between the scapulae) of the upper thoracic spine and in the region of the lower thoracic spine as well. Begin palpating in the interscapular region of the posterior trunk by vertically strumming across the ribs (up and down). Once you have gotten the feel of the ribs and intercostal spaces in this region, palpate each rib by simultaneously placing one finger pad on it and another finger pad on the adjacent intercostal space. Palpate all 12 ribs (above and below your starting point) in this manner. Depending upon the musculature of the client, it may be easy or somewhat difficult to discern all the ribs. Where the scapulae are not in the way, follow the ribs and intercostal spaces as far lateral as possible.

PLEASE NOTE: The following muscles attach onto the rib cage posteriorly: the latissimus dorsi, serratus posterior superior, serratus posterior inferior, erector spinae group, quadratus lumborum, levatores costarum, external intercostals, and internal intercostals. The subcostales and the diaphragm attach to the internal side of the posterior rib cage. Although primarily anterior, the external abdominal oblique, internal abdominal oblique, and transversus abdominis are located somewhat posteriorly on the rib cage as well.

8

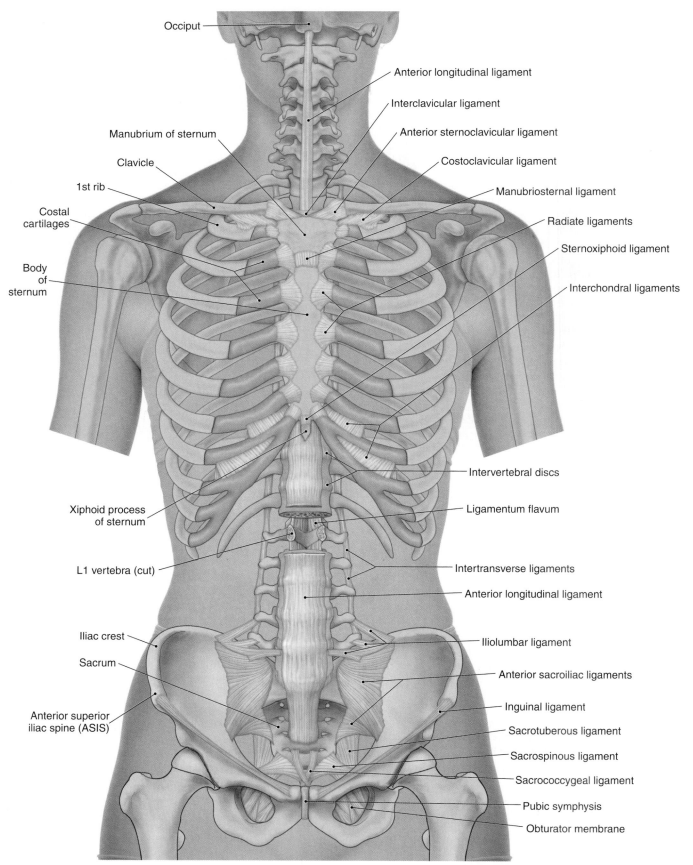

Occiput

Anterior longitudinal ligament

Interclavicular ligament

Manubrium of sternum

Anterior sternoclavicular ligament

Clavicle

Costoclavicular ligament

1st rib

Manubriosternal ligament

Costal cartilages

Radiate ligaments

Sternoxiphoid ligament

Body of sternum

Interchondral ligaments

Intervertebral discs

Xiphoid process of sternum

Ligamentum flavum

L1 vertebra (cut)

Intertransverse ligaments

Anterior longitudinal ligament

Iliac crest

Iliolumbar ligament

Sacrum

Anterior sacroiliac ligaments

Inguinal ligament

Anterior superior iliac spine (ASIS)

Sacrotuberous ligament

Sacrospinous ligament

Sacrococcygeal ligament

Pubic symphysis

Obturator membrane

Figure 8-31 Anterior view of the ligaments of the axial skeleton. One vertebral body has been removed.

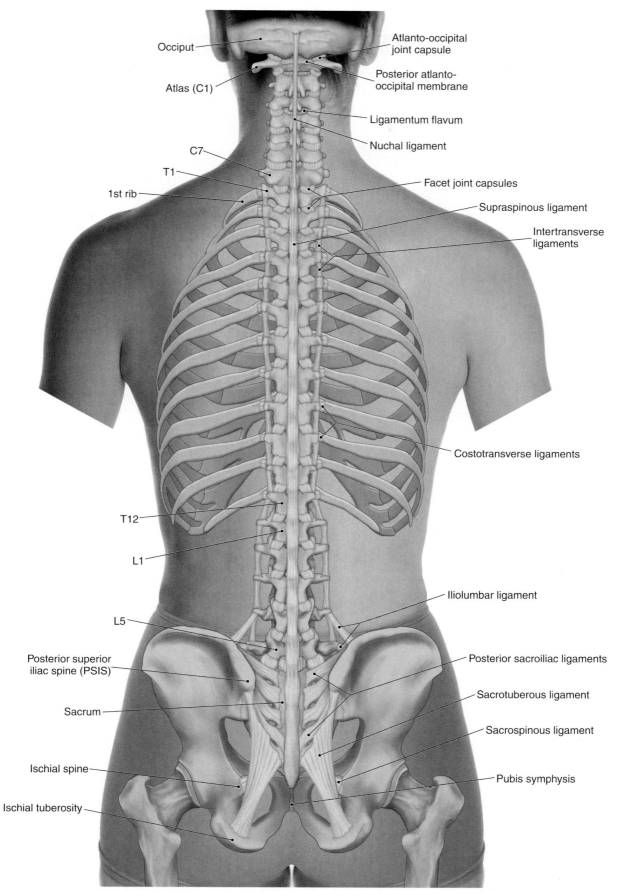

Figure 8-32 Posterior view of the ligaments of the axial skeleton. Note: The posterior atlanto-occipital membrane is the superior continuation of the ligamentum flavum.

Alar ligament

Occiput

Posterior atlanto-occipital membrane

Atlas (C1) (cut)

Accessory atlanto-axial ligament

Axis (C2) (cut)

Ligamentum flavum (cut)

Interspinous ligament

Occiput (cut)

Tectorial membrane (cut)

Cruciate ligament of dens

Posterior longitudinal ligament (cut)

Ligamenta flava

Figure 8-33 Posterior view of the ligaments of the upper cervical region. The atlas and axis have been cut. Notes: 1) The posterior atlanto-occipital membrane is the superior continuation of the ligamentum flavum. 2) The tectorial membrane is the superior continuation of the posterior longitudinal ligament. 3) The occiput has been cut on the right side to expose the tectorial membrane. 4) The tectorial membrane has been cut to expose the cruciate ligament of the dens, alar, and accessory atlantoaxial ligaments.

Anterior atlanto-occipital membrane

Anterior arch of atlas (C1)

Cruciate ligament of dens

Axis (C2)

Posterior longitudinal ligament

Anterior longitudinal ligament

Facet joint capsules

Body of C4

Intervertebral discs

Tectorial membrane

Occiput

Posterior atlanto-occipital ligament

Posterior tuberale of atlas (C1)

Supraspinous ligament

Nuchal ligament

Ligamenta flava

C7 spinous process

Interspinous ligament

A

8

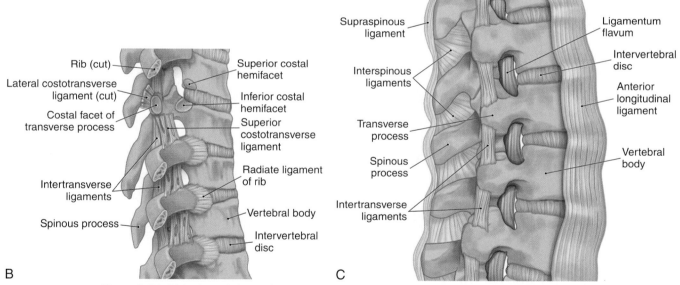

Rib (cut)

Lateral costotransverse ligament (cut)

Costal facet of transverse process

Intertransverse ligaments

Spinous process

Superior costal hemifacet

Inferior costal hemifacet

Superior costotransverse ligament

Radiate ligament of rib

Vertebral body

Intervertebral disc

B

Supraspinous ligament

Interspinous ligaments

Transverse process

Spinous process

Intertransverse ligaments

Ligamentum flavum

Intervertebral disc

Anterior longitudinal ligament

Vertebral body

C

Figure 8-34 Right lateral views of the ligaments of the spine. **A** is a sagittal section that shows the ligaments of the cervical spine. Note: The tectorial membrane is the superior continuation of the posterior longitudinal ligament. **B** shows ligaments of the thoracic spine. The ribs have been cut; one rib has been entirely removed to show the transverse process attachment of a superior costotransverse ligament; the facets for the rib are also seen. **C** shows the ligaments of the lumbar spine.

Lower Extremity Bone Palpation and Ligaments

Chapter 9 is one of three chapters of Part II of this book, which addresses palpation of the skeleton. This chapter is a palpation tour of the bones, bony landmarks, and joints of the lower extremity. The tour begins with the pelvis, then addresses the thigh and leg, and concludes with the foot. Although any one bone or bony landmark can be independently palpated, this chapter is set up sequentially to flow from one landmark to another, so it is recommended that you follow the order presented here. Muscle attachments for each of the palpated structures are also given (specific palpations for these muscles are covered in Part III of this book). The ligaments of the lower extremity are presented at the end of this chapter.

Chapter 7 presents the ligaments of the upper extremity and the palpation of the bones, bony landmarks, and joints of the upper extremity. Chapter 8 presents the ligaments of the axial body and the palpation of the bones, bony landmarks, and joints of the axial body.

Chapter Outline

The bones, bony landmarks, and joints of the following regions are covered:

Chapter Objectives

After completing this chapter, the student should be able to perform the following:

1. Define the key terms of this chapter.
2. Palpate each of the bones, bony landmarks, and joints of this chapter (listed in Key Terms)
3. State the muscle or muscles that attach to each of the bony landmarks of this chapter.
4. Describe the location of each of the ligaments of the lower extremity.

Key Terms

anterior inferior iliac spine (AIIS)
anterior superior iliac spine (ASIS)
calcaneal tuberosity
calcaneus
coccyx
cuboid
distal interphalangeal (DIP) joint
distal phalanx
femoral condyles
fibular shaft
fibular tubercle of the calcaneus
first cuneiform
gluteal fold

greater trochanter of the femur
head of the fibula
head of the talus
iliac crest
interphalangeal (IP) joint
ischial tuberosity
knee joint
lateral femoral condyle
lateral malleolus of the fibula
lateral tibial condyle
lesser trochanter of the femur
medial femoral condyle
medial malleolus of the tibia
medial tibial condyle

medial tubercle of the talus
metatarsal
metatarsal base
metatarsal head
metatarsophalangeal (MTP) joint
middle phalanx
navicular tuberosity
patella
phalanges (singular: phalanx)
posterior superior iliac spine (PSIS)
proximal interphalangeal (PIP) joint
proximal phalanx

Section 1: Pelvis

9

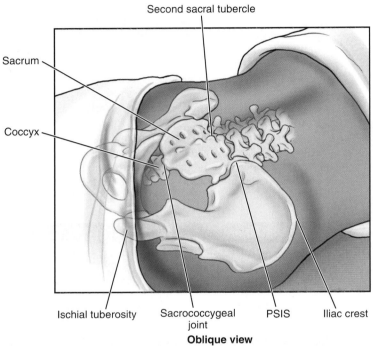

Second sacral tubercle

Sacrum

Coccyx

Ischial tuberosity   Sacrococcygeal joint   PSIS   Iliac crest

Oblique view

Figure 9-1 An inferolateral oblique view of the posterior pelvis. *PSIS,* Posterior superior iliac spine.

Go to http://evolve.elsevier.com/Muscolino/palpation for identification of bony landmark exercises.

Superolateral view

Figure 9-2 Iliac crest: The **iliac crest** is subcutaneous and easily palpable. With the client prone, place your palpating fingers on the iliac crest and follow it as far anterior as possible. It ends at the anterior superior iliac spine (ASIS). Then follow the iliac crest posteriorly to the posterior superior iliac spine (PSIS).
PLEASE NOTE: The following muscles attach onto the iliac crest: the latissimus dorsi, erector spinae group, quadratus lumborum, external abdominal oblique, internal abdominal oblique, transversus abdominis, gluteus maximus, and tensor fasciae latae.

Superolateral view

Figure 9-3 The posterior superior iliac spine: The **posterior superior iliac spine (PSIS)** is the most posterior aspect of the iliac crest and is usually visually prominent as well as easily palpable. It is located approximately 2 inches (5 cm) from the midline of the superior aspect (the base) of the sacrum. The PSIS is easily located because the skin drops in around the medial side of it, forming a dimple in most individuals. First visually locate the dimple; then palpate into it, pressing slightly laterally against the PSIS.
PLEASE NOTE: The latissimus dorsi and gluteus maximus muscles attach onto the PSIS.

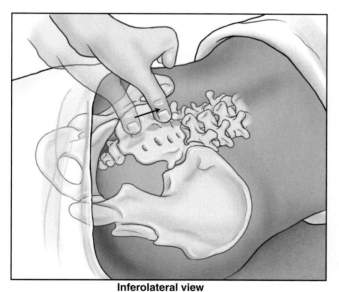

Inferolateral view

Figure 9-4 Sacrum: From the PSIS, palpate the midline of the **sacrum**, feeling for the **sacral tubercles**. Once a sacral tubercle is located, continue palpating superiorly and inferiorly for the other sacral tubercles. The second sacral tubercle is usually at the level of the PSISs. Note: The **sacroiliac (SI) joint**, located between the sacrum and ilium on each side, is not directly palpable because of the overhang of the PSIS and the presence of the joint ligaments.
PLEASE NOTE: The following muscles attach onto the posterior sacrum: the latissimus dorsi, erector spinae group, transversospinalis group, and gluteus maximus. The piriformis and iliacus attach onto the anterior sacrum.

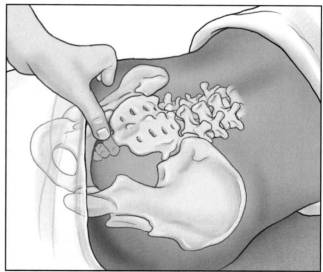

Inferolateral view

Figure 9-5 Coccyx: The **coccyx** is located directly inferior to the sacrum. It is subcutaneous and usually easily palpable. At the most superior aspect of the coccyx, the **sacrococcygeal joint** can usually be palpated.
PLEASE NOTE: The gluteus maximus muscle attaches onto the coccyx.

9

Inferolateral view

Figure 9-6 Ischial tuberosity: The **ischial tuberosity** is located deep to the **gluteal fold**, slightly medial to the midpoint of the buttock. It is best to palpate it from the inferior perspective so that the palpating fingers do not have to palpate through the gluteus maximus. Moderate to deep pressure is necessary to palpate the ischial tuberosity; however, it is not difficult to feel and is usually not tender for the client. Once located, strum across the ischial tuberosity both horizontally and vertically to palpate it in its entirety.

PLEASE NOTE: The adductor magnus, inferior gemellus, quadratus femoris, and hamstring muscles attach onto the ischial tuberosity.

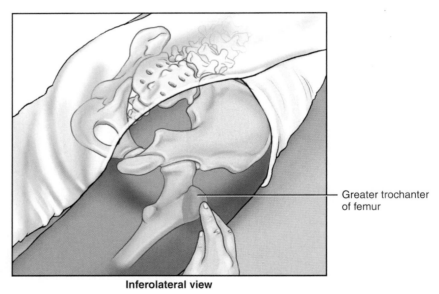

Inferolateral view

Figure 9-7 Greater trochanter of the femur: The **greater trochanter of the femur** is valuable to palpate along with the bony landmarks of the posterior pelvis because the majority of the muscles of the posterior pelvis attach distally onto the greater trochanter. It is fairly large (approximately 1.5 × 1.5 inches [4 × 4 cm]) and subcutaneous, hence it is fairly easy to palpate. From the ischial tuberosity, palpate at the same level (or slightly superior) on the lateral proximal thigh and the greater trochanter can be found; strum along it vertically and horizontally to feel the entire greater trochanter.

PLEASE NOTE: The following muscles attach onto the greater trochanter: the gluteus medius, gluteus minimus, piriformis, superior gemellus, obturator internus, inferior gemellus, and vastus lateralis.

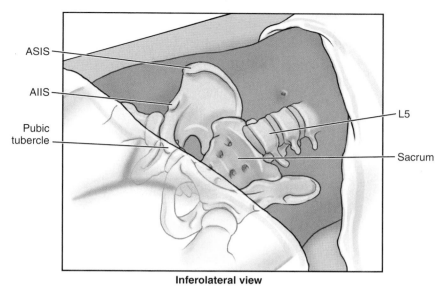

Inferolateral view

Figure 9-8 An inferolateral oblique view of the anterior pelvis. *AIIS,* Anterior inferior iliac spine; *ASIS,* anterior superior iliac spine.

Inferolateral view

Figure 9-9 Anterior superior iliac spine: The **anterior superior iliac spine (ASIS)** is the most anterior aspect of the iliac crest. It is usually visually prominent as well as easily palpable. From the iliac crest (see Figure 9-2), continue palpating anteriorly until you reach the ASIS.
PLEASE NOTE: The tensor fasciae latae and sartorius muscles attach onto the ASIS.

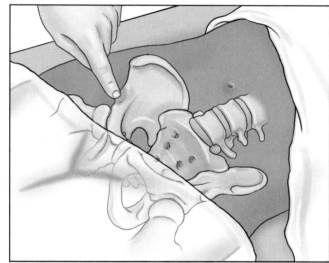

Inferolateral view

Figure 9-10 Anterior inferior iliac spine: Because of the thickness of musculature that overlies the **anterior inferior iliac spine (AIIS)**, it can be difficult to palpate. One method to locate it is to drop inferiorly from the ASIS and feel for the AIIS deeper into the tissue. However, the best method is to first locate the rectus femoris muscle of the quadriceps femoris group and then follow it proximally to its attachment onto the AIIS with the client's hip joint passively flexed. Note: this requires comfort and familiarity with muscle palpation of the rectus femoris (see page 433).
PLEASE NOTE: The rectus femoris muscle attaches onto the AIIS.

Inferolateral view

Figure 9-11 Pubic bone and pubic tubercle: The **pubic bone** is located at the most inferior aspect of the anterior abdomen. The **pubic tubercle** is on the anterior surface of the body of the pubic bone near the pubic symphysis joint and is at approximately the same level as the superior aspect of the greater trochanter of the femur. To locate the pubic bone, begin by palpating more superiorly on the anterior abdominal wall, then carefully and gradually palpate farther inferiorly, pressing gently into the abdominal wall until the pubic bone is felt. It helps to use the ulnar side of the hand and direct the pressure posteriorly and inferiorly. It is important that the abdominal wall muscles are relaxed so that when the pubic bone is reached, it will be readily felt.

PLEASE NOTE: The following muscles attach onto the superior ramus of the pubis and/or the body of the pubis: the rectus abdominis, pectineus, adductor longus, gracilis, and adductor brevis.

Section 2: Thigh and Leg

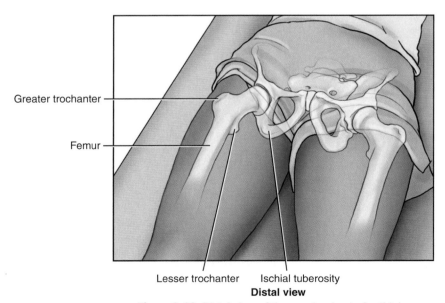

Greater trochanter

Femur

Lesser trochanter   Ischial tuberosity
Distal view

Figure 9-12 Distal view of the proximal anterior thigh.

Distal view

Figure 9-13 Greater trochanter: Begin palpation of the thigh by locating again the **greater trochanter of the femur**. The greater trochanter is located in the proximal lateral thigh, at approximately the same level as the public tubercle. It is fairly large (approximately 1.5 × 1.5 inches [4 × 4 cm]) and subcutaneous, hence it is fairly easy to palpate; strum along it vertically and horizontally to feel the entire greater trochanter.

PLEASE NOTE: The following muscles attach onto the greater trochanter: the gluteus medius, gluteus minimus, piriformis, superior gemellus, obturator internus, inferior gemellus, and vastus lateralis.

Distal and medial view

Figure 9-14 Lesser trochanter: The **lesser trochanter of the femur** is located in the proximal medial thigh. It is a palpable landmark, but is appreciably more challenging to discern, so palpating it with certainty requires more advanced palpation skills and knowledge of the psoas major muscle. To locate the lesser trochanter of the femur, the distal aspect of the psoas major muscle must be located (see page 387). Once located, follow the psoas major distally as far as possible. Then have the client relax their thigh in a position of flexion and lateral rotation of the thigh at the hip joint to relax and slacken the psoas major; then press in against the femur, feeling for the lesser trochanter.

PLEASE NOTE: The psoas major and iliacus muscles (iliopsoas muscle) attach onto the lesser trochanter.

Patella

Distal and anterior view

Figure 9-15 Patella: The **patella** (kneecap) is a prominent sesamoid bone located anterior to the distal femur. To best palpate the patella, have the client supine with the lower extremity relaxed. Palpate the entire patella, gently gliding along the patella horizontally and vertically.

PLEASE NOTE: The quadriceps femoris group attaches onto the patella.

Trochlear groove

Patella

Femur

Knee joint

Femoral
condyles

Tibial condyles

Head of fibula

Tibial
tuberosity

Lateral
malleolus

Medial
malleolus

Anterolateral view

Figure 9-16 Anterolateral view of the leg with the knee joint flexed to 90 degrees.

Anterolateral view

Figure 9-17 Trochlear groove of the femur: To palpate the **trochlear groove of the femur**, the knee joint should be flexed approximately 90 degrees (when the knee joint is fully extended, the patella moves proximally within the trochlear groove and obstructs its palpation) and the quadriceps femoris musculature relaxed. Now palpate immediately proximal to the patella in the midline of the anterior femur and the trochlear groove will be evident. (Note: The patella is not shown in this figure.)

Anterolateral view

Figure 9-18 Knee joint: With the client's **knee joint** flexed to approximately 90 degrees, drop off the inferior aspect of the patella and the joint line of the knee will be palpable both medially and laterally. Palpate within the joint space as well as superiorly against the femur and inferiorly against the tibia as you continue to palpate the knee joint toward the posterior side medially and laterally.
PLEASE NOTE: The medial and lateral menisci are palpable against the anterior tibia within the joint line of the knee.

Anterolateral view

Figure 9-19 Femoral condyles: The inferior margins of the **medial femoral condyle** and **lateral femoral condyle** are palpable by pressing proximally up against the femur from the joint line of the knee on both sides of the patella. Once located, palpate farther proximally onto the medial and lateral **femoral condyles**.
PLEASE NOTE: The following muscles attach onto the femoral condyles: the adductor magnus, gastrocnemius, plantaris, and popliteus.

Anterolateral view

Figure 9-20 Tibial condyles: The superior margins of the **medial tibial condyle** and **lateral tibial condyle** are palpable by pressing distally down against the tibia from the joint line of the knee on both sides of the patella. Once located, palpate farther distally onto the medial and lateral **tibial condyles**.
PLEASE NOTE: The biceps femoris and semimembranosus muscles attach onto the posterior surface of the tibial condyles. The gluteus maximus and tensor fasciae latae attach onto the lateral tibial condyle via the iliotibial band.

Anterolateral view

Figure 9-21 Head of the fibula: As you continue palpating along the superior margin of the lateral condyle of the tibia, you will reach the head of the fibula. The **head of the fibula** is the most proximal landmark of the fibula, located on the posterolateral side of the knee, and can be palpated anteriorly, laterally, and posteriorly. Note: The common fibular nerve is superficial near the head of the fibula, so care should be taken when palpating here.
PLEASE NOTE: The biceps femoris, fibularis longus, soleus, and extensor digitorum longus muscles attach onto the head of the fibula.

Anterolateral view

Figure 9-22 Tibial tuberosity: The **tibial tuberosity** is a prominent landmark located at the center of the proximal shaft of the anterior tibia, approximately 1 to 2 inches (2.5 - 5 cm) distal to the inferior margin of the patella. The quadriceps femoris muscle group attaches onto the tibial tuberosity.

9

9

Anterolateral view

Figure 9-23 Tibial shaft: From the tibial tuberosity, the entire anteromedial **tibial shaft** is subcutaneous and easily palpable. Begin palpating at the tibial tuberosity and continue palpating distally until you reach the medial malleolus at the end of the anteromedial tibial shaft.

PLEASE NOTE: The tibialis anterior, pes anserine group (sartorius, gracilis, semitendinosus), and quadriceps femoris group of muscles attach onto the anterior tibial shaft. The popliteus, soleus, tibialis posterior, and flexor digitorum longus muscles attach onto the posterior tibial shaft.

Anterolateral view

Figure 9-24 Medial malleolus: The **medial malleolus of the tibia** is the very prominent bony landmark at the ankle region that is located on the medial side. As you palpate down the anteromedial shaft of the tibia, you will reach the medial malleolus. Palpate the circumference of this large bony landmark.

Anterolateral view

Figure 9-25 Lateral malleolus: The **lateral malleolus of the fibula** is the very prominent bony landmark that is located at the lateral side of the ankle region. The lateral malleolus is the distal expanded end of the fibula. Notice that the lateral malleolus of the fibula is located somewhat farther distal than is the medial malleolus of the tibia.

Anterolateral view

Figure 9-26 Fibular shaft: The distal **fibular shaft** is palpable in the distal leg. Begin palpating the fibula at the lateral malleolus, and continue palpating the lateral shaft of the fibula proximally until you can no longer feel it deep to the overlying musculature. **PLEASE NOTE:** The fibularis longus and brevis muscles attach to the lateral fibular shaft. The extensor digitorum longus, extensor hallucis longus, and fibularis tertius muscles attach to the anterior fibular shaft. The soleus, tibialis posterior, and flexor hallucis longus muscles attach to the posterior fibular shaft.

9

Section 3: Medial Foot

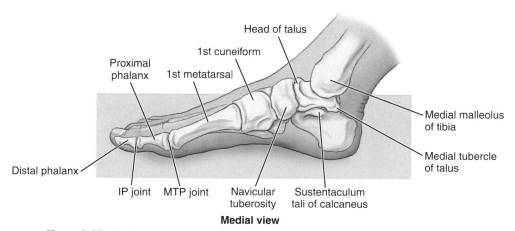

Head of talus

1st cuneiform

Proximal phalanx   1st metatarsal

Medial malleolus of tibia

Distal phalanx

Medial tubercle of talus

IP joint   MTP joint   Navicular tuberosity   Sustentaculum tali of calcaneus

Medial view

Figure 9-27 Medial view of the foot. *IP,* Interphalangeal; *MTP,* metatarsophalangeal.

Medial view

Medial view

Figure 9-28 Phalanges and interphalangeal joint of the big toe: Begin palpating the medial side of the foot distally at the proximal and distal phalanges of the big toe **(A)**. The interphalangeal (IP) joint between them can be palpated as well **(B)**.
PLEASE NOTE: The extensor hallucis longus and extensor hallucis brevis muscles attach onto the dorsal side of the phalanges of the big toe; the flexor hallucis longus, flexor hallucis brevis, adductor hallucis, and abductor hallucis muscles attach onto the plantar side of the phalanges of the big toe.

Figure 9-29 First metatarsophalangeal joint: From the proximal phalanx of the big toe, continue palpating proximally along the medial surface of the foot and you will feel the joint line of the first metatarsophalangeal (MTP) joint.

Medial view

Medial view

Figure 9-30 First metatarsal: The dorsal and medial surfaces of the first metatarsal are subcutaneous and easily palpable. As with the metacarpals of the hand, the expanded distal head and expanded proximal base of the metatarsals are palpable. (Note: The distal head of the first metatarsal is palpable on the dorsal, medial, and planter sides of the foot.)
PLEASE NOTE: The tibialis anterior, fibularis longus, and first dorsal interosseus muscles attach to the first metatarsal.

Figure 9-31 First cuneiform: Just proximal to the base of the first metatarsal on the medial and dorsal sides, the joint line between the first metatarsal and first cuneiform is palpable. Move just proximal to the joint line and the first cuneiform is palpable.
PLEASE NOTE: The tibialis anterior, fibularis longus, and tibialis posterior muscles attach to the first cuneiform.

Medial view

Figure 9-32 Navicular tuberosity: Continuing proximal from the first cuneiform, the **navicular tuberosity** is quite prominent and palpable.
PLEASE NOTE: The tibialis posterior muscle attaches to the navicular tuberosity.

Medial view

Figure 9-33 Head of the talus: The **head of the talus** is immediately posterior to the navicular. The **talonavicular joint** between these two bones is most evident if you have the client invert and evert the foot.
PLEASE NOTE: The talus is the only tarsal bone that has no muscle attachments.

Medial view

Figure 9-34 Sustentaculum tali of the calcaneus: From the navicular tuberosity (see Figure 9-32), move your palpating finger approximately 1 inch (2.5 cm) directly posterior and the **sustentaculum tali of the calcaneus** should be palpable (or from the head of the talus, drop slightly posterior and in the plantar direction). The sustentaculum tali forms a shelf upon which the talus sits. The joint line between the sustentaculum tali and the talus above is often palpable. As a point of reference, the medial malleolus of the tibia is located approximately 1 inch (2.5 cm) directly above (proximal to) the sustentaculum tali.

Medial view

Figure 9-35 Medial tubercle of the talus: Slightly posterior to the sustentaculum tali (posterior and plantar to the medial malleolus) the **medial tubercle of the talus** can be palpated.

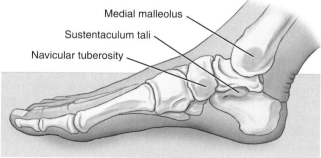

Medial malleolus
Sustentaculum tali
Navicular tuberosity

Medial view

Figure 9-36 Most prominent landmarks of the medial foot: The three most prominent landmarks of the medial foot are the medial malleolus of the tibia, sustentaculum tali of the calcaneus, and the navicular tuberosity.

Medial view

Figure 9-37 Posterior surface of the calcaneus: The posterior surface of the **calcaneus** is palpable as you continue palpating along the medial side to the posterior side of the foot.
PLEASE NOTE: The gastrocnemius, soleus, and plantaris muscles attach to the posterior surface of the calcaneus.

Section 4: Lateral Foot

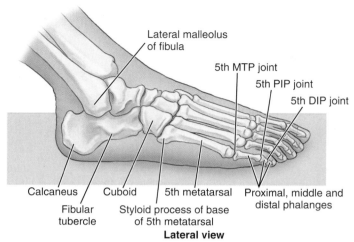

Lateral malleolus
of fibula

5th MTP joint

5th PIP joint

5th DIP joint

Calcaneus   Cuboid   5th metatarsal   Proximal, middle and
distal phalanges

Fibular
tubercle

Styloid process of base
of 5th metatarsal

Lateral view

Figure 9-38 Lateral view of the foot. *DIP,* Distal interphalangeal; *MTP,* metatarsophalangeal; *PIP,* proximal interphalangeal.

A

B

Lateral view

Figure 9-39 Phalanges and interphalangeal (IP) joints of the little toe: Begin palpating the lateral side of the foot distally at the proximal, middle, and distal phalanges of the little toe **(A)**. The **proximal interphalangeal (PIP) joint** and **distal interphalangeal (DIP) joint** between the phalanges can be palpated as well **(B)**.
PLEASE NOTE: The extensor digitorum brevis and extensor digitorum longus muscles attach to the dorsal surface of the phalanges of the little toe. The flexor digitorum brevis, flexor digitorum longus, flexor digiti minimi pedis, abductor digiti minimi pedis, and third plantar interosseus muscles attach to the plantar surface of the phalanges of the little toe.

Lateral view

Figure 9-40 Fifth metatarsophalangeal (MTP) joint: From the proximal phalanx of the little toe, continue palpating proximally along the lateral surface of the foot and you will feel the joint line of the fifth MTP joint. Note: The proximal phalanx of the little toe extends quite a bit more proximally than do the other proximal phalanges of the foot; therefore the fifth MTP joint is found more proximally than are the other MTP joints of the foot.

A

B

Lateral view

Figure 9-41 Fifth metatarsal: Proximally from the fifth metatarsophalangeal joint is the fifth metatarsal. The dorsal and lateral surfaces of the fifth metatarsal are readily palpable. Palpate from the expanded distal head to the middle of the shaft of the fifth metatarsal **(A)**. Continue palpating proximally until you reach the large expanded proximal base **(B)**. The base of the fifth metatarsal flares out and is called the **styloid process of the fifth metatarsal**.

PLEASE NOTE: The dorsal surface of the base of the fifth metatarsal is the attachment site of the fibularis brevis and fibularis tertius muscles. The flexor digiti minimi pedis muscle attaches to the plantar surface of the base of the fifth metatarsal.

Lateral view

Figure 9-42 Cuboid: Just proximal to the fifth metatarsal along the lateral side of the foot is a depression where the **cuboid** lies. The depression is created by a combination of the flaring of the base of the fifth metatarsal (the styloid process of the fifth metatarsal) and the concave shape of the lateral border of the cuboid. Palpate with firm pressure medially into this depression and the cuboid can be felt.

PLEASE NOTE: The tibialis posterior and flexor hallucis brevis muscles attach to the plantar surface of the cuboid. A groove in the lateral border of the cuboid is created by the passage of the distal tendon of the fibularis longus muscle from the dorsal to the plantar surface of the foot.

Lateral view

Figure 9-43 Lateral calcaneus: From the cuboid, continue palpating proximally along the lateral surface of the foot and the lateral surface of the calcaneus will be evident; it is subcutaneous and easily palpable. The **fibular tubercle of the calcaneus** is palpable distal to the lateral malleolus of the fibula.

PLEASE NOTE: The extensor digitorum brevis and extensor hallucis brevis muscles attach to the lateral surface of the calcaneus. The fibular tubercle is a valuable landmark because it separates the distal tendons of the fibularis longus and fibularis brevis muscles.

9

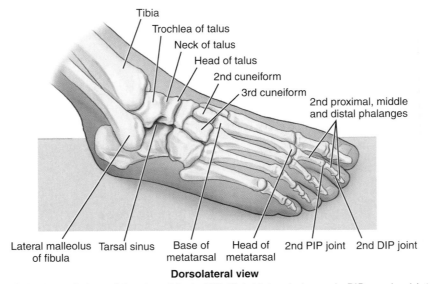

Tibia
Trochlea of talus
Neck of talus
Head of talus
2nd cuneiform
3rd cuneiform
2nd proximal, middle and distal phalanges

Lateral malleolus of fibula | Tarsal sinus | Base of metatarsal | Head of metatarsal | 2nd PIP joint | 2nd DIP joint

Dorsolateral view

Figure 9-44 Lateral view of the dorsal foot. *DIP*, Distal interphalangeal; *PIP*, proximal interphalangeal.

Dorsolateral view

Figure 9-45 Anterior talus: The anterior aspect of the talus, especially on the lateral side, can be palpated distal to the tibia. The anterior aspect of the **trochlea of the talus** is fairly easily palpated directly medial to the distal end of the lateral malleolus of the fibula. A greater portion of the anterior talus becomes palpable if the client's foot is passively inverted and plantarflexed.

Dorsolateral view

Figure 9-46 Tarsal sinus: If you palpate directly distal and anteromedial to the lateral malleolus of the fibula, you will feel a depression. This depression overlies the **tarsal sinus**, which is the space that leads into the **subtalar joint** cavity between the talus and the calcaneus. To best palpate the tarsal sinus, direct your palpatory pressure medially and inferiorly.

PLEASE NOTE: The extensor digitorum brevis and extensor hallucis brevis muscles overlie the tarsal sinus.

A

B

Dorsolateral view

Figure 9-47 Phalanges (singular: phalanx) of toes two through four: The **phalanges** and metatarsals of toes two through four are easily palpable on the dorsum of the foot. Start distally and palpate the **distal phalanx**, **middle phalanx**, and **proximal phalanx** of each toe **(A)**, and the joint lines between these phalanges, the proximal interphalangeal (PIP) and distal interphalangeal (DIP) joints **(B)**.

PLEASE NOTE: The extensor digitorum brevis, extensor digitorum longus, and dorsal interossei pedis muscles attach to the dorsal surfaces of the phalanges of toes two through four. The flexor digitorum brevis, flexor digitorum longus, and first and second plantar interossei muscles attach to the plantar surfaces of the phalanges of toes two through four.

Dorsolateral view

Figure 9-48 Metatarsophalangeal (MTP) joints of toes two through four: From the proximal phalanx of each of toes two through four, continue palpating the dorsal side of the foot proximally and you will feel the MTP joint line between the proximal phalanx and the metatarsal of each of these toes.

Dorsolateral view

Figure 9-49 Metatarsals of toes two through four: Proximally from the metatarsophalangeal joint line of each toe, the metatarsal can be palpated. The distal expanded **metatarsal head**, shaft, and proximal expanded **metatarsal base** are all subcutaneous and easily palpable.

PLEASE NOTE: The dorsal interossei pedis, plantar interossei, adductor hallucis, and tibialis posterior muscles attach to the metatarsals of toes two through four.

Dorsolateral view

Figure 9-50 Second and third cuneiforms: The second and third cuneiforms can be palpated on the dorsal side of the foot. The **second cuneiform** is directly proximal to the second metatarsal; the **third cuneiform** is directly proximal to the third metatarsal. From the base of the second and third metatarsals, palpate directly proximally and you will feel the **tarsometatarsal joint** line between the metatarsal and the cuneiform; proximal to the joint line, the cuneiform itself is palpable.

PLEASE NOTE: The tibialis posterior muscle attaches to the plantar surfaces of the second and third cuneiforms.

Section 6: Plantar Foot

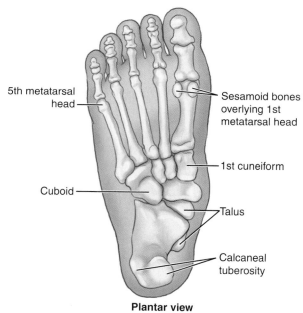

5th metatarsal head

Sesamoid bones overlying 1st metatarsal head

1st cuneiform

Cuboid

Talus

Calcaneal tuberosity

Plantar view

Figure 9-51 Plantar view of the foot.

Plantar view

Figure 9-52 Metatarsal heads of toes one through five: The heads of all five metatarsals are palpable on the plantar surface of the foot. Although all five metatarsals are palpable, because of the concavity of the transverse arch of the foot, the heads of the first and fifth metatarsals are most prominent. Begin by palpating the head of the fifth metatarsal and then continue medially, palpating each of the other four metatarsal heads. Overlying the plantar surface of the head of the first metatarsal are two small **sesamoid bones**. When palpating the head of the first metatarsal on the plantar side, it is actually the two sesamoids that are felt.

PLEASE NOTE: The flexor hallucis brevis attaches into the sesamoid bones that overlie the head of the first metatarsal.

Plantar view

Figure 9-53 Calcaneal tuberosity: The **calcaneal tuberosity** can often be palpated on the plantar side of the foot. With the client's foot relaxed, palpate with firm pressure on either side of the midline of the plantar side of the calcaneus. The medial aspect of the calcaneal tuberosity is often more prominent than the lateral aspect.

PLEASE NOTE: The abductor hallucis, abductor digiti minimi pedis, and flexor digitorum brevis muscles attach to the calcaneal tuberosity on the plantar surface of the calcaneus. The quadratus plantae and tibialis posterior muscles also attach onto the plantar surface of the calcaneus (but not the calcaneal tuberosity).

9

9

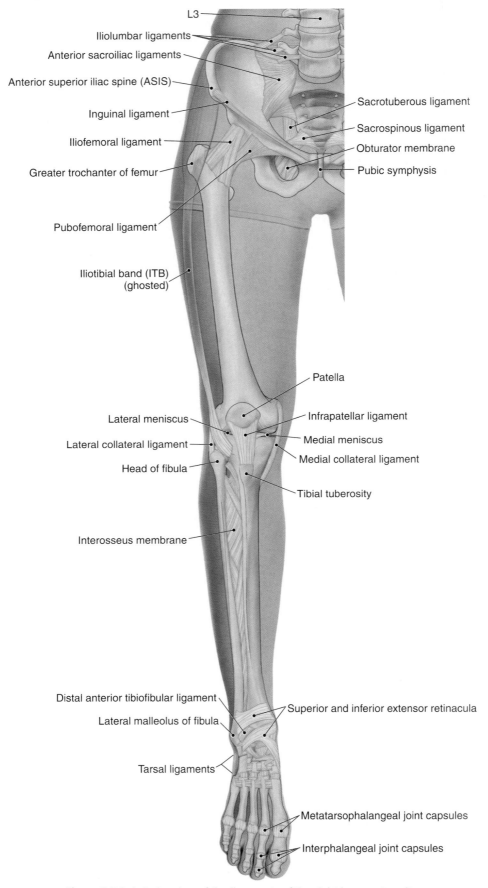

- L3
- Iliolumbar ligaments
- Anterior sacroiliac ligaments
- Anterior superior iliac spine (ASIS)
- Inguinal ligament
- Iliofemoral ligament
- Greater trochanter of femur
- Pubofemoral ligament
- Iliotibial band (ITB) (ghosted)
- Lateral meniscus
- Lateral collateral ligament
- Head of fibula
- Interosseus membrane
- Distal anterior tibiofibular ligament
- Lateral malleolus of fibula
- Tarsal ligaments

- Sacrotuberous ligament
- Sacrospinous ligament
- Obturator membrane
- Pubic symphysis
- Patella
- Infrapatellar ligament
- Medial meniscus
- Medial collateral ligament
- Tibial tuberosity
- Superior and inferior extensor retinacula
- Metatarsophalangeal joint capsules
- Interphalangeal joint capsules

Figure 9-54 Anterior view of the ligaments of the right lower extremity.

Figure 9-55 Posterior view of the ligaments of the right lower extremity.

9

Interphalangeal joint
capsules

Metatarsophalangeal joint
capsules and plantar plates

Plantar intermetatarsal
ligaments

5th metatarsal

1st cuneiform

2nd cuneiform

Plantar cuneonavicular
ligaments

Cuboid

Navicular tuberosity

Long plantar
ligament

Spring ligament

Short plantar
ligament

Talus

Sustentaculum tali
of calcaneus

Figure 9-56 Plantar view of the ligaments of the right foot.

Figure 9-57 Medial view of the ligaments of the right foot.

Figure 9-58 Lateral view of the ligaments of the right foot.

Chapter 10

Tour #1—Palpation of the Muscles of the Shoulder Girdle

Overview

This chapter is a palpation tour of the muscles of the shoulder girdle. The tour begins with muscles on the posterior side and then addresses the muscles on the anterior side. Palpation for the posterior shoulder girdle muscles is shown in the prone position, and palpation of the anterior shoulder girdle muscles is shown in the supine position. Alternate palpation positions are also described. The major muscles or muscle groups of the region are each given a separate layout, and there are also a few detours to other muscles of the region. Trigger point (TrP) information and stretching are given for each of the muscles covered in this chapter. The chapter closes with an advanced *Whirlwind Tour* that explains the sequential palpation of all of the muscles of the chapter.

Chapter Outline

Chapter Objectives

After completing this chapter, the student should be able to perform the following for each of the muscles covered in this chapter:

1. State the attachments.
2. State the actions.
3. Describe the starting position for palpation.
4. Describe and explain the purpose of each of the palpation steps.
5. Palpate each muscle.
6. State the "Palpation Key."
7. Describe alternate palpation positions.
8. State the locations of the most common TrP(s).
9. Describe the TrP referral zones.
10. State the most common factors that create and/or perpetuate TrPs.
11. State the symptoms most commonly caused by TrPs.
12. Describe and perform a stretch.

Video demonstrations of the muscle palpations in this chapter are presented in Chapter 10 on DVD 1.

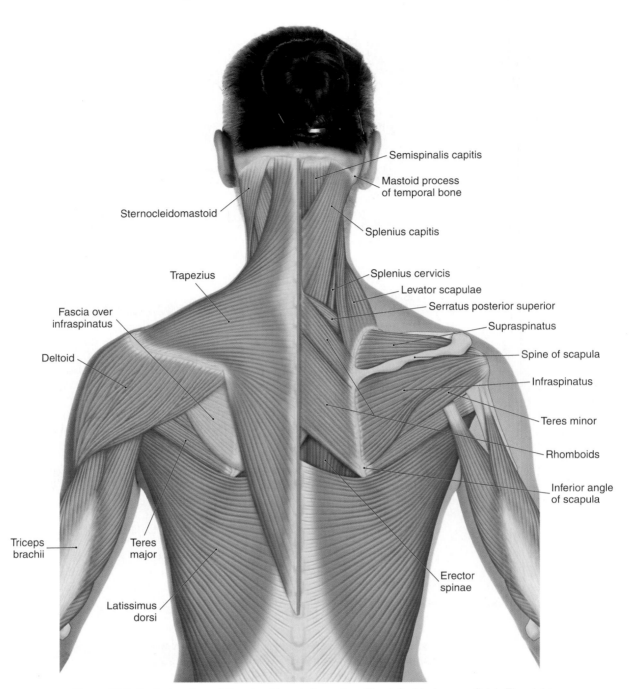

Figure 10-1 Posterior view of the shoulder girdle region. The left side is superficial. The right side is deep (the deltoid, trapezius, sternocleidomastoid, and infraspinatus fascia have been removed).

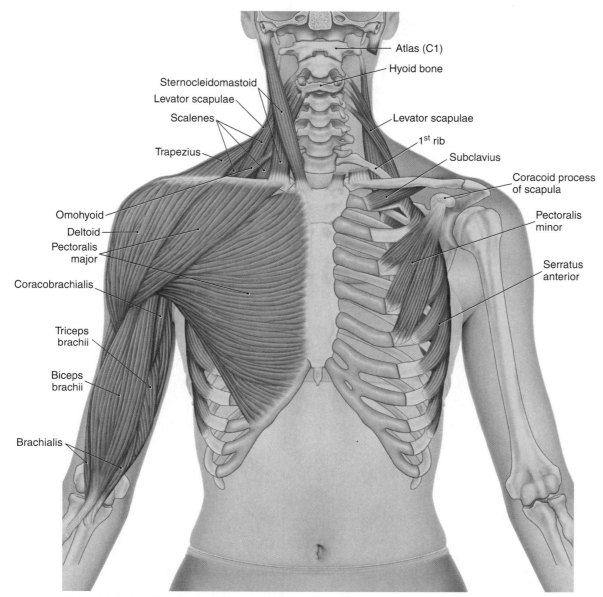

Atlas (C1)

Hyoid bone

Sternocleidomastoid

Levator scapulae

Scalenes

Trapezius

Levator scapulae

1st rib

Subclavius

Coracoid process of scapula

Omohyoid

Deltoid

Pectoralis major

Coracobrachialis

Pectoralis minor

Serratus anterior

Triceps brachii

Biceps brachii

Brachialis

10

Figure 10-2 Anterior view of the shoulder girdle region. The right side is superficial. The left side is deep (the deltoid, pectoralis major, trapezius, scalenes, omohyoid, and muscles of the arm have been removed; the sternocleidomastoid has been cut).

10

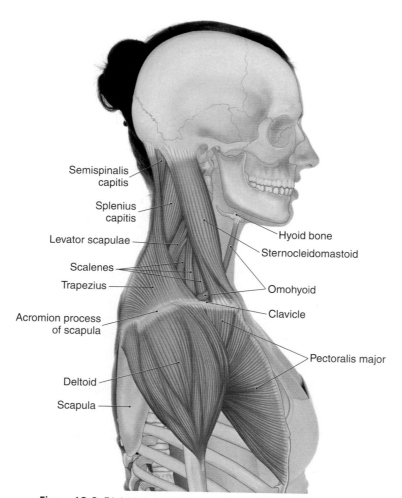

Semispinalis
capitis

Splenius
capitis

Levator scapulae

Scalenes

Trapezius

Acromion process
of scapula

Deltoid

Scapula

Hyoid bone

Sternocleidomastoid

Omohyoid

Clavicle

Pectoralis major

Figure 10-3 Right lateral view of the shoulder girdle and neck region.

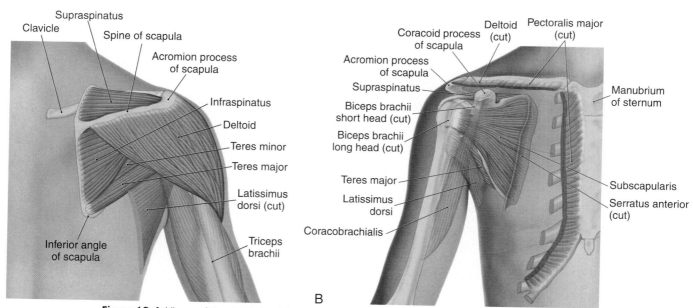

Clavicle

Supraspinatus

Spine of scapula

Acromion process
of scapula

Infraspinatus

Deltoid

Teres minor

Teres major

Latissimus
dorsi (cut)

Inferior angle
of scapula

Triceps
brachii

A

Coracoid process
of scapula

Deltoid
(cut)

Pectoralis major
(cut)

Acromion process
of scapula

Supraspinatus

Biceps brachii
short head (cut)

Biceps brachii
long head (cut)

Teres major

Latissimus
dorsi

Coracobrachialis

Manubrium
of sternum

Subscapularis

Serratus anterior
(cut)

B

Figure 10-4 Views of the right shoulder girdle region. **A** is a posterior view. **B** is an anterior view;
the majority of the deltoid and pectoralis major have been cut and removed.

Figure 10-5 Right lateral view of the shoulder girdle and trunk region.

❏ **ATTACHMENTS:**

o External occipital protuberance, medial ⅓ of the superior nuchal line, nuchal ligament, and the spinous processes of C7 through T12 *to the* lateral ⅓ of the clavicle, acromion process, and spine of the scapula

❏ **ACTIONS:**

o Upper trapezius: elevates, retracts, and upwardly rotates the scapula at the scapulocostal joint; extends, laterally flexes, and contralaterally rotates the head and neck at the spinal joints
o Middle trapezius: retracts the scapula at the scapulocostal joint
o Lower trapezius: depresses, retracts, and upwardly rotates the scapula at the scapulocostal joint

Starting position (Figure 10-7):

o Client prone with arm resting on the table at the side of the body
o Therapist standing to the side of the client
o Palpating hand placed just lateral to the lower thoracic spine (on the lower trapezius)

Palpation steps:

1. Ask the client to abduct the arm at the shoulder joint to 90 degrees with the elbow joint extended, and to slightly retract the scapula at the scapulocostal joint by pinching the shoulder blade toward the spine (Figure 10-8). Adding gentle resistance to the client's arm abduction with your support hand might be helpful.
2. Palpate the lower trapezius. To locate the lateral border, palpate perpendicular to it (Figure 10-9, A). Once located, palpate the entire lower trapezius.
3. Repeat for the middle trapezius between the scapula and the spine. Strum perpendicular to the direction of the fibers (i.e., strum vertically) (Figure 10-9, B).
4. Repeat for the upper trapezius.
5. To further engage the upper trapezius, ask the client to do slight extension of the head and neck at the

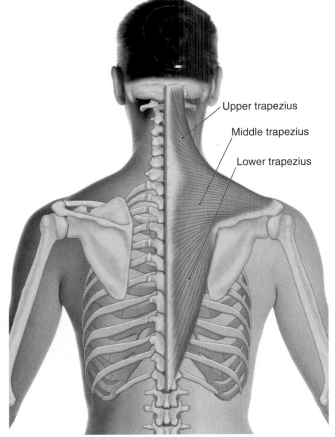

Figure 10-6 Posterior view of the right trapezius. The sternocleidomastoid, levator scapulae, and splenius capitis are ghosted in.

spinal joints. Then palpate the entire upper trapezius (Figure 10-9, C).

6. Once the trapezius has been located, have the client relax it and palpate to assess its baseline tone.

Figure 10-7 Starting position for prone palpation of the right trapezius.

Figure 10-8 To engage the entire right trapezius, the client abducts the arm at the shoulder joint (resistance can be added as shown) and slightly retracts the scapula at the scapulocostal joint.

TRAPEZIUS—PRONE—cont'd

Figure 10-9 Palpation of the right trapezius. **A** shows palpation of the lower trapezius. **B** shows palpation of the middle trapezius. **C** shows palpation of the upper trapezius. Palpation of the upper trapezius is facilitated by asking the client to slightly extend the head and neck at the spinal joints. For all three parts of the trapezius, palpate by strumming perpendicular to the fiber direction as shown.

Palpation Notes:

1. Abducting the arm at the shoulder joint requires an upward rotation force by the upper and lower trapezius to stabilize the scapula. Retracting the scapula engages the entire trapezius, especially the middle trapezius.
2. Clients will often lift the arm up into the air when asked to retract the scapula. Emphasize that the client should "pinch the shoulder blade back." However, the client should not retract the scapula excessively, or the scapula will move too close to the spine, and the retractor musculature in the interscapular region will bunch up, making it difficult to palpate the middle trapezius.
3. When asking the client to extend the head and neck to further engage the upper trapezius, do not have the client extend very far or it will be difficult to palpate into the neck.
4. The lateral border of the lower trapezius is often visible; look for it before placing your palpating hands on the client.

Palpation Key:

Fly like an airplane: If both trapezius muscles are palpated at the same time, both arms out to the sides make the client appear to be flying like an airplane.

TRAPEZIUS—PRONE—cont'd

TRIGGER POINTS

1. Trigger points (TrPs) in the upper trapezius often result from or are perpetuated by acute or chronic overuse of the muscle. Examples include chronic postures of elevation of the shoulder girdle; anteriorly held head; any chronic posture due to poor ergonomics, especially while sitting at the computer or crimping the phone between the shoulder and ear; resisting depression of the shoulder girdle when the upper extremity is hanging, especially when the upper extremity is carrying a weight; trauma (e.g., whiplash); compression forces (e.g., carrying a heavy purse or backpack on the shoulder, having a tight bra strap); or chronic stress/tension (holding the shoulder girdles uptight). Middle trapezius TrPs are activated/perpetuated by a chronic rounded shoulder posture, or when driving and holding the top of the steering wheel. Lower trapezius TrPs are activated/perpetuated by chronically pressing the shoulder girdles down (e.g., supporting the chin in the hand, pressing the hands down on the sitting surface when seated).

2. TrPs in the upper trapezius tend to produce a classic stiff neck with restricted contralateral lateral flexion and ipsilateral rotation of the neck at the spinal joints, a posture of an elevated shoulder girdle, pain at the end of contralateral rotation of the neck, and tension headaches. Middle trapezius TrPs tend to produce inhibition and weakness of the middle trapezius resulting in chronically protracted shoulder girdles (rounder shoulders), and goose bumps on the arm (and sometimes on the thigh). Lower trapezius TrPs tend to produce burning pain, and inhibition and weakness of the lower trapezius resulting in elevated shoulders. TrPs in all parts of the trapezius may produce spinal joint dysfunction of the vertebrae to which they are attached.

3. The referral patterns of upper trapezius TrPs must be distinguished from the referral patterns of TrPs in the sternocleidomastoid, masseter, temporalis, occipitalis, splenius cervicis, levator scapulae, semispinalis capitis, cervical multifidus, and lower trapezius. Middle trapezius referral patterns must be distinguished from the levator scapulae, erector spinae and transversospinalis of the trunk, and lower trapezius. Lower trapezius referral patterns must be distinguished from the cervical multifidus, levator scapulae, rhomboids, scalenes, infraspinatus, latissimus dorsi, serratus anterior, erector spinae and transversospinalis of the trunk, intercostals, and upper trapezius.

4. TrPs in the trapezius are often incorrectly assessed as cervical disc syndrome, temporomandibular joint (TMJ) syndrome, or occipital neuralgia.

5. Associated TrPs of the upper trapezius often occur in the scalenes, splenius capitis and cervicis, levator scapulae, rhomboids, semispinalis capitis, temporalis, masseter, and the contralateral upper trapezius. Associated TrPs of the middle trapezius often occur in the pectoralis major and minor, and the erector spinae and transversospinalis muscles of the trunk. Associated TrPs of the lower trapezius often occur in the latissimus dorsi and ipsilateral upper trapezius.

6. Note: The trapezius is considered to be the muscle most commonly found to have TrPs. Specifically, the upper trapezius has the most commonly found TrP in the body; further, the referral symptoms of this common TrP have occasionally spread to the other side of the body.

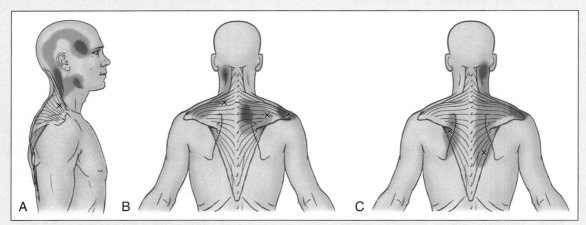

Figure 10-10 Common trapezius TrPs and their corresponding referral zones. **A** is a lateral view showing the location of a TrP in the most vertical fibers of the upper trapezius. **B** shows another upper trapezius TrP on the left side; the right side illustrates middle trapezius TrP locations. **C** shows two lower trapezius TrPs and their referral zones.

TRAPEZIUS—PRONE—cont'd

STRETCHING THE TRAPEZIUS

A   B   C

Figure 10-11 Stretches of the three functional parts of the right trapezius. **A** shows a stretch of the right upper trapezius. The client's head and neck are flexed, left laterally flexed, and (ipsilaterally) rotated to the right. To keep the shoulder girdle down, the right hand holds on to the bench. **B** shows a stretch of the right middle trapezius. A weight is held in the right hand; its traction force protracts and stretches the middle trapezius. Medially rotating the right arm will enhance the stretch. **C** shows a stretch of the right lower trapezius. A pole is grasped at approximately head height and the client leans back, causing protraction and elevation of the scapula.

10

RHOMBOIDS—PRONE

❑ **ATTACHMENTS:**

o Spinous processes of C7 through T5 *to the* medial border of the scapula from the root of the spine to the inferior angle

❑ **ACTIONS:**

o Retracts, elevates, and downwardly rotates the scapula at the scapulocostal joint

Starting position (Figure 10-13):

o Client prone with the hand resting in the small of the back
o Therapist standing to the side of the client
o Palpating hand placed between the spinal column and the scapula at the midscapular level

Palpation steps:

1. Ask the client to lift the hand away from the small of the back (Figure 10-14).
2. Look for the lower border of the rhomboids to become visible (Figure 10-15); make sure you are not covering the lower border with your palpating hand).
3. Palpate the rhomboids from the inferior aspect to the superior aspect. When palpating, strum perpendicular to the direction of the fibers.
4. Once the rhomboids have been located, have the client relax them and palpate to assess their baseline tone.

Figure 10-12 Posterior view of the right rhomboids major and minor. The levator scapulae has been ghosted in.

Rhomboid minor

Rhomboid major

Figure 10-13 Starting position for prone palpation of the right rhomboids. Note: The client's right hand is in the small of the back, as seen in Figure 10-15.

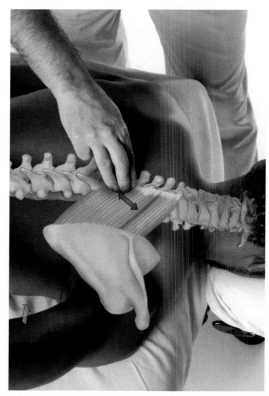

Figure 10-14 Palpating perpendicular to the fiber direction of the right rhomboids.

10

RHOMBOIDS—PRONE—cont'd

Palpation Notes:

1. Having the client place the hand in the small of the back requires extension of the arm at the shoulder joint. This requires the coupled action of downward rotation of the scapula at the scapulocostal joint, which will cause the trapezius to relax (because of reciprocal inhibition) so that we can palpate through it. It will also engage the rhomboids so that their contraction will be clearly felt.
2. The superior border of the rhomboids is more challenging to visualize and palpate than the inferior border. However, it can usually be palpated. Feel for a gap between the rhomboids and the levator scapulae.
3. It is usually not possible to clearly distinguish the border between the rhomboid major and rhomboid minor.

Alternate Palpation Position—Seated

Figure 10-15 The rhomboids can also be easily palpated in the seated position. Note that the inferior border of the rhomboids is often visible.

Palpation Key:
Client's hand in the small of the back.

TRIGGER POINTS

1. Trigger points (TrPs) in the rhomboids often result from or are perpetuated by acute or chronic overuse of the muscle (both as movers of scapular retraction and as stabilizers of the scapula when the arm is moved at the shoulder joint), a chronic stretch caused by a rounded-shoulder posture due to tight pectoralis muscles anteriorly, and TrPs in the trapezius.
2. TrPs in the rhomboids tend to produce pain that is felt superficially at rest and with use of the muscles; they can also cause joint dysfunction of the vertebrae to which they are attached.
3. The referral patterns of rhomboids TrPs must be distinguished from the referral patterns of TrPs in the levator scapulae, scalenes, middle trapezius, infraspinatus, latissimus dorsi, serratus posterior superior, thoracic transversospinalis, and serratus anterior.
4. TrPs in the rhomboids are often incorrectly assessed as fibromyalgia.
5. Associated TrPs often occur in the trapezius, levator scapulae, pectoralis major and minor, serratus anterior, and infraspinatus.

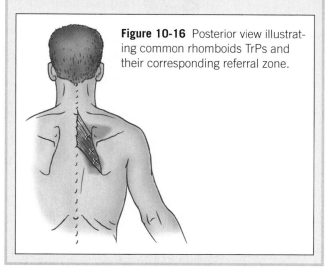

Figure 10-16 Posterior view illustrating common rhomboids TrPs and their corresponding referral zone.

STRETCHING THE RHOMBOIDS

Figure 10-17 A stretch of the right rhomboids. The client's arm is used to protract and depress the right scapula.

RHOMBOIDS—PRONE—cont'd

DETOUR

Serratus posterior superior (SPS) TrP notes:

1. Trigger points (TrPs) in the SPS often result from or are perpetuated by acute or chronic overuse of the muscle (e.g., in clients who have labored breathing due to chronic obstructive respiratory diseases, such as asthma, bronchitis, and emphysema) and TrPs in the scalenes.

2. TrPs in the SPS tend to produce a deep ache that is felt deep to the scapula (pain is often felt at rest, but increased with motions of the arm that cause the scapula to compress the SPS against the rib cage), difficulty sleeping on the affected side due to pressure on the TrP, a feeling of numbness in the little finger of the hand, or C7 to T3 spinal joint dysfunction.

3. The referral patterns of SPS TrPs must be distinguished from the referral patterns of TrPs in the erector spinae and transversospinalis muscles of the trunk, scalenes, rhomboids, levator scapulae, posterior deltoid, supraspinatus, infraspinatus, teres minor, latissimus dorsi, teres major, subscapularis, triceps brachii, all three wrist extensors, and extensor digitorum.

4. TrPs in the SPS are often incorrectly assessed as cervical disc syndrome, thoracic outlet syndrome, or elbow joint dysfunction.

5. Associated TrPs often occur in the scalenes, rhomboids, and erector spinae and transversospinalis muscles of the trunk.

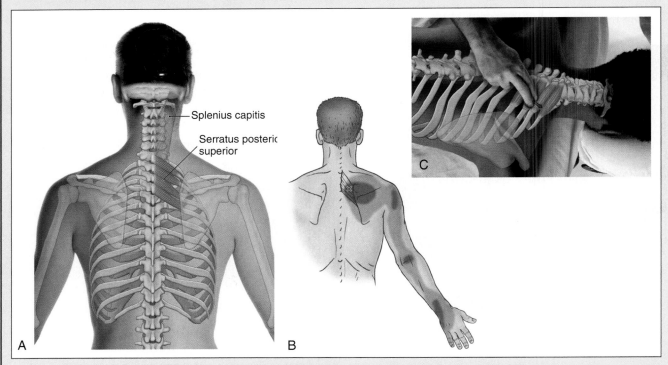

Splenius capitis

Serratus posterior superior

A

B

C

Figure 10-18 Serratus posterior superior (SPS). **A** is a posterior view of the right SPS; the splenius capitis has been ghosted in. The SPS attaches from the spinous processes of C7-T3 to ribs two through five. **B** is a posterior view illustrating a common SPS TrP and its corresponding referral zone. **C** illustrates palpation of the SPS. The arm is hanging off the table to protract the scapula at the scapulocostal joint, exposing the entire SPS.

Figure 10-19 Palpation of the right erector spinae group in the thoracic region. The client is asked to extend the head, neck, and trunk to engage the erector spinae musculature. For more information on palpation of the erector spinae, please see page 359 (Tour #7, Chapter 16).

LEVATOR SCAPULAE—PRONE   10-2 10-3

❏ **ATTACHMENTS:**
o Transverse processes of C1 through C4 *to the* medial border of the scapula from the root of the spine to the superior angle

❏ **ACTIONS:**
o Elevates and downwardly rotates the scapula at the scapulocostal joint;
o Extends, laterally flexes, and ipsilaterally rotates the neck at the spinal joints

Starting position (Figure 10-21):
o Client prone with hand resting in the small of the back
o Therapist standing or seated to the side of the client
o Palpating hand placed just superior and medial to the superior angle of the scapula

Palpation steps:
1. With the client's hand in the small of the back, the client is asked to perform a gentle, very short range of motion of elevation of the scapula at the scapulocostal joint. Feel for the levator scapulae's contraction deep to the trapezius (Figure 10-22, A).
2. Continue palpating the levator scapulae toward its superior attachment by strumming perpendicular to its fibers.
3. Once you are palpating the levator scapulae in the posterior triangle (superior to the trapezius), the client's hand no longer needs to be in the small of the back. It is also possible to ask the client to elevate the scapula more forcefully now; resistance can also be added (Figure 10-22, B).
4. Palpate the levator scapulae as far superiorly as possible (near its superior attachment, it goes deep to the sternocleidomastoid).
5. Once the levator scapulae has been located, have the client relax it and palpate to assess its baseline tone.

Figure 10-20 Posterior view of the right levator scapulae. The trapezius has been ghosted in.

Levator scapulae
Trapezius

Figure 10-21 Starting position for prone palpation of the right levator scapulae.

Palpation Key: Client's hand in the small of the back.

10

LEVATOR SCAPULAE—PRONE—cont'd

Figure 10-22 Palpation of the right levator scapulae. **A** shows palpation near the superior angle of the scapula (where the levator scapulae is deep to the trapezius). **B** shows palpation where the levator scapulae is superficial in the posterior triangle of the neck.

Palpation Notes:

1. Having the client place the hand in the small of the back requires extension and adduction of the arm at the shoulder joint. This requires the coupled action of downward rotation of the scapula at the scapulocostal joint, which will cause the upper trapezius to relax (because of reciprocal inhibition) so that the inferior attachment of the levator scapulae can be clearly felt when it contracts. It will also engage the levator scapulae, so its contraction will be more clearly felt.

2. Do not have the client perform a forceful elevation of the scapula or the reflex of reciprocal inhibition will be overcome and the upper trapezius will contract, blocking palpation of the levator scapulae at its inferior attachment.

3. Once the levator scapulae is being palpated in the posterior triangle of the neck, the client can remove the hand from the small of the back because it is no longer necessary to inhibit (relax) the upper trapezius. Furthermore, once we are palpating the levator scapulae in the posterior triangle, a forceful contraction of the levator scapulae can be engaged to better palpate and locate it.

4. In middle-aged or older adults, the levator scapulae is often visible in the posterior triangle of the neck (Figure 10-23).

5. It can be difficult to palpate the most superior aspect of the levator scapulae deep to the sternocleidomastoid (SCM). To do so, slacken the SCM by slightly flexing and ipsilaterally laterally flexing the neck and try to palpate deep to the SCM, reaching for the transverse processes of C1 through C4 (see Figure 11-39 on page 205).

6. Note that the transverse process of C1 is directly inferior to the ear (between the mastoid process and the ramus of the mandible)!

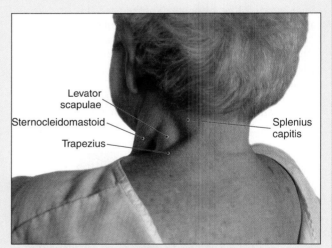

Figure 10-23 Posterolateral view showing the levator scapulae and splenius capitis in the posterior triangle of the neck.

LEVATOR SCAPULAE—PRONE—cont'd

Alternate Palpation Position—Seated

Figure 10-24 The levator scapulae can also be easily palpated with the client seated.

TRIGGER POINTS

1. Trigger points (TrPs) in the levator scapulae often result from or are perpetuated by acute or chronic overuse of the muscle (e.g., carrying a bag or purse on the shoulder, crimping a phone between the shoulder and ear, excessive exercise such as playing tennis, holding the shoulders uptight), chronic shortening or stretching of the muscle due to poor work or leisure postures (e.g., having a poorly placed computer monitor, reading with the head inclined forward), motor vehicle accidents, having a cold draft on the neck, or being overly stressed psychologically.
2. TrPs in the levator scapulae tend to produce a classic stiff neck (often called *torticollis* or *wry neck*) with restricted contralateral rotation of the neck.
3. The referral patterns of levator scapulae TrPs must be distinguished from the referral patterns of TrPs in the scalenes, rhomboids, supraspinatus, and infraspinatus.
4. TrPs in the levator scapulae are often incorrectly assessed as joint dysfunction of the cervical spine.
5. Associated TrPs often occur in the upper trapezius, splenius cervicis, scalenes, and erector spinae of the cervical spine.

Figure 10-25 Posterior view illustrating common levator scapulae TrPs and their corresponding referral zone.

STRETCHING THE LEVATOR SCAPULAE

Figure 10-26 A stretch of the right levator scapulae. The client's neck is flexed, left laterally flexed, and rotated (contralaterally) to the left. To keep the shoulder girdle down, the right hand holds on to the bench.

POSTERIOR DELTOID—PRONE

❏ ATTACHMENTS:
o Spine of the scapula *to the* deltoid tuberosity of the humerus

❏ ACTIONS:
o Extends, abducts, laterally rotates, and horizontally extends the arm at the shoulder joint

Starting position (Figure 10-28):
o Client prone with arm abducted 90 degrees to the side and resting on the table, and the forearm hanging off the table
o Therapist standing or seated to the side of the client
o Palpating hand placed just inferior to the lateral end of the spine of the scapula
o Support hand placed on the distal end of the client's arm

Palpation steps:
1. Ask the client to horizontally extend the arm at the shoulder joint (by lifting it straight up toward the ceiling) and feel for the contraction of the posterior fibers of the deltoid. Resistance can be added (Figure 10-29).
2. Palpate from the spine of the scapula to the deltoid tuberosity.
3. Once the posterior deltoid has been located, have the client relax it and palpate to assess its baseline tone.

Figure 10-27 Posterior view of the right deltoid. The trapezius has been ghosted in.

Figure 10-28 Starting position for prone palpation of the right posterior deltoid.

Figure 10-29 Palpation of the right posterior deltoid as the client horizontally extends the arm against resistance.

Palpation Notes:
1. Even though the posterior fibers of the deltoid laterally rotate the arm at the shoulder joint, when palpating the posterior deltoid, do not ask the client to do this action because the infraspinatus and teres minor muscles will also be engaged, making it more difficult to discern the inferior border of the posterior deltoid from these muscles.
2. The posterior deltoid attaches on the spine of the scapula nearly to the root of the spine of the scapula at the medial border.

Palpation Key:
Resist horizontal
extension of
the arm.

POSTERIOR DELTOID—PRONE—cont'd

TRIGGER POINTS

1. Trigger points (TrPs) in the posterior deltoid often result from or are perpetuated by acute or chronic overuse (e.g., holding the arm up in abduction or extension for prolonged periods, such as when working at a computer keyboard), direct trauma (e.g., impact during sports), and TrPs in the infraspinatus.
2. TrPs in the posterior deltoid tend to produce weakness when performing abduction or extension of the arm at the shoulder joint.
3. The referral patterns of posterior deltoid TrPs must be distinguished from the referral patterns of TrPs in the levator scapulae, scalenes, supraspinatus, infraspinatus, teres minor, subscapularis, teres major, triceps brachii, and serratus posterior superior.
4. TrPs in the posterior deltoid are often incorrectly assessed as a rotator cuff tear, subdeltoid/subacromial bursitis, or glenohumeral or acromioclavicular joint arthritis.
5. Associated TrPs often occur in the supraspinatus, teres major, infraspinatus, teres minor, triceps brachii, and latissimus dorsi.

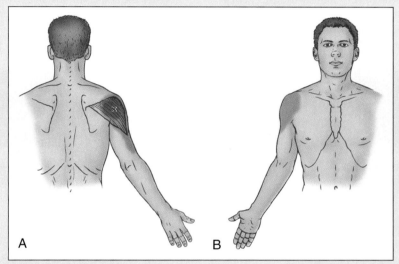

A   B

Figure 10-31 A is a posterior view illustrating a common posterior deltoid TrP and its corresponding referral zone. **B** is an anterior view showing the remainder of the referral zone.

Alternate Palpation Position—Seated

Figure 10-30 The posterior deltoid can also be easily palpated with the client seated or standing. To engage the posterior fibers of the deltoid, have the client horizontally extend the arm at the shoulder joint against resistance.

STRETCHING THE POSTERIOR DELTOID

Figure 10-32 A stretch of the right posterior deltoid. The client's right arm is horizontally flexed, keeping the trunk facing forward.

INFRASPINATUS AND TERES MINOR—PRONE

❑ ATTACHMENTS:

o Infraspinatus: infraspinous fossa of the scapula *to the* greater tubercle of the humerus
o Teres minor: superior $^2/_3$ of the dorsal surface of the lateral border of the scapula *to the* greater tubercle of the humerus

❑ ACTIONS:

o Infraspinatus: laterally rotates the arm at the shoulder joint
o Teres minor: laterally rotates and adducts the arm at the shoulder joint

Starting position (Figure 10-34):

o Client prone with arm resting on the table and the forearm hanging off the table
o Therapist seated to the side of the client, with the client's forearm between the knees
o Palpating hand placed just inferior to the spine of the scapula in the infraspinous fossa

Palpation steps:

1. Ask the client to laterally rotate the arm at the shoulder joint against the resistance of your knee, and feel for the contraction of the infraspinatus in the infraspinous fossa (Figure 10-35, A).
2. Continue palpating the infraspinatus distally toward the greater tubercle attachment on the humerus by strumming perpendicular to its fibers.
3. Locate the superior aspect of the lateral border of the scapula, and feel for the contraction of the teres minor as the client laterally rotates the arm at the shoulder joint against your knee (Figure 10-35, B).
4. Continue palpating its distal tendon toward the greater tubercle by strumming perpendicular to it.
5. Once the infraspinatus and teres minor have been located, have the client relax them and palpate to assess their baseline tone.

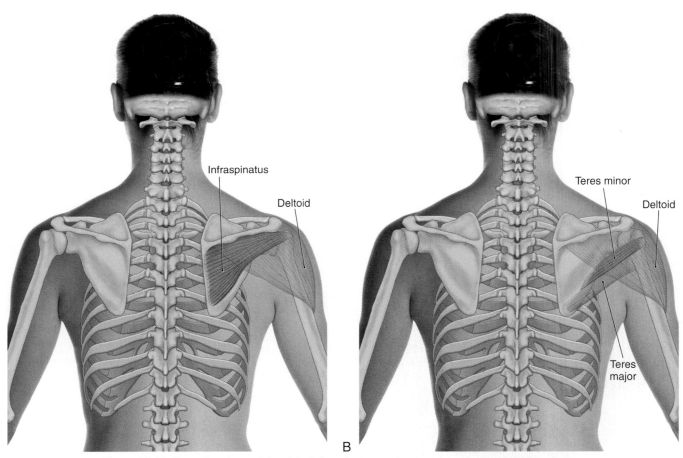

A   B

Figure 10-33 Posterior views of the right infraspinatus and teres minor. **A** shows the infraspinatus; the deltoid has been ghosted in. **B** shows the teres minor; the deltoid and teres major have been ghosted in.

INFRASPINATUS AND TERES MINOR—PRONE—cont'd

Figure 10-34 Starting position for prone palpation of the right infraspinatus.

Figure 10-35 Palpation of the right infraspinatus and teres minor as the client laterally rotates the arm against resistance. **A** shows palpation of the infraspinatus. **B** shows teres minor palpation.

Palpation Notes:

1. It can be difficult to palpate the distal tendons of the infraspinatus and teres minor all the way to the greater tubercle of the humerus, because they run deep to the posterior deltoid, which also contracts with lateral rotation of the arm at the shoulder joint. To better palpate the distal tendons, either ask the client to do a very gentle lateral rotation contraction of the arm so that the posterior deltoid is not engaged, or place the client's arm in flexion (This requires the client to be seated instead of lying prone.) to reciprocally inhibit the posterior deltoid as the gentle lateral rotation of the arm contraction is performed.

2. Discerning the infraspinatus from the teres minor (i.e., locating the border between the two muscles) is sometimes challenging.

3. It is easy to discern the inferior border of the teres minor from the superior border of the teres major. To do so, simply have the client alternate between lateral rotation of the arm and medial rotation of the arm at the shoulder joint (in each case against the resistance of your knee). The teres minor will be felt to contract with lateral rotation and the teres major will be felt to contract with medial rotation.

Alternate Palpation Position—Seated

Figure 10-36 The infraspinatus and teres minor can also be easily palpated with the client seated. To engage these muscles, have the client perform lateral rotation of the arm at the shoulder joint against resistance. Note: Given that it is usually uncomfortable to resist rotation of the arm by resisting motion of the arm itself, the client can be asked to flex the elbow joint to 90 degrees and then the resistance can be given to the forearm. It is important that the client's resistance against the therapist's hand is not coming from horizontal extension of the arm at the shoulder joint, but rather lateral rotation of the arm.

10

TRIGGER POINTS

1. Trigger points (TrPs) in the infraspinatus and teres minor often result from or are perpetuated by acute or chronic overuse of the muscle (e.g., reaching behind the body with lateral rotation of the arm at the shoulder joint) and trauma (e.g., shoulder joint dislocation).

2. TrPs in the infraspinatus and teres minor both tend to restrict medial rotation of the arm at the shoulder joint (e.g., reaching behind to the lower back) and cause discomfort when sleeping on the affected side. TrPs in the infraspinatus tend to also produce strong deep pain in the anterior shoulder or discomfort sleeping on the back due to pressure on the TrPs (when sleeping on the unaffected side, it may be necessary to support the affected arm on a pillow). TrPs in the teres minor tend to also produce deep pain that is well localized, altered sensation in the ring and little fingers, or cause quadrilateral space syndrome (entrapment of the axillary nerve between the teres minor and teres major).

3. Infraspinatus: The referral patterns of infraspinatus TrPs must be distinguished from the referral patterns of TrPs in the teres minor, supraspinatus, latissimus dorsi, teres major, subscapularis, rhomboids, deltoid, coracobrachialis, biceps brachii, triceps brachii, scalenes, pectoralis major and minor, subclavius, serratus posterior superior, and thoracic transversospinalis.

Teres minor: The referral patterns of teres minor TrPs must be distinguished from the referral patterns of TrPs in the infraspinatus, supraspinatus, teres major, subscapularis, deltoid, triceps brachii, serratus posterior superior, levator scapulae, and scalenes.

4. TrPs in the infraspinatus and teres minor are often incorrectly assessed as rotator cuff lesions or cervical disc syndrome. TrPs in the infraspinatus are also often incorrectly assessed as osteoarthritis of the shoulder joint, entrapment of the suprascapular nerve, or bicipital tendinitis. TrPs in the teres minor are also often incorrectly assessed as shoulder bursitis or cervical disc syndrome.

5. Associated TrPs of the infraspinatus and teres minor often occur in each other, as well as the teres major, supraspinatus, anterior deltoid, subscapularis, and pectoralis major.

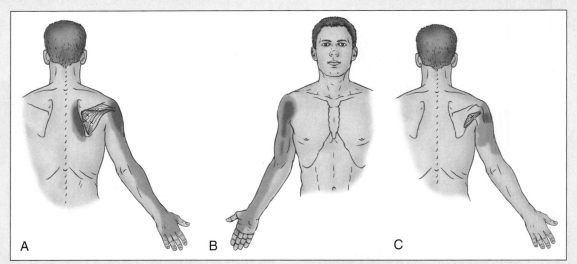

Figure 10-37 A is a posterior view illustrating common infraspinatus TrPs and their corresponding referral zone. **B** is an anterior view showing the remainder of the referral zone. **C** is a posterior view illustrating a common teres minor TrP and its corresponding referral zone.

INFRASPINATUS AND TERES MINOR—PRONE—cont'd

STRETCHING THE INFRASPINATUS AND TERES MINOR

Palpation Key:
Place client's forearm between your knees; use your knee to provide resistance.

10

Figure 10-38 A stretch of the right infraspinatus and teres minor. The client's right arm is medially rotated and pulled upward and away from the back using a towel.

TERES MAJOR—PRONE

❏ **ATTACHMENTS:**
o Inferior angle and inferior ¹/₃ of the dorsal surface of the lateral border of the scapula *to the* medial lip of the bicipital groove of the humerus

❏ **ACTIONS:**
o Medially rotates, adducts, and extends the arm at the shoulder joint
o Upwardly rotates the scapula at the glenohumeral and scapulocostal joints

Starting position (Figure 10-40):
o Client prone with arm resting on the table and the forearm hanging off the table
o Therapist seated to the side of the client, with the client's forearm between the knees
o Palpating hand placed just lateral to the lower aspect of the lateral border of the scapula

Palpation steps:
1. Ask the client to medially rotate the arm at the shoulder joint against the resistance of your knee, and feel for the contraction of the teres major at the inferior aspect of the lateral border of the scapula (Figure 10-41).
2. Continue palpating the teres major distally toward the humerus by strumming perpendicular to its fibers.
3. Once the teres major muscle has been located, have the client relax it and palpate to assess its baseline tone.

Figure 10-39 Posterior view of the right teres major. The deltoid and teres minor have been ghosted in.

Figure 10-40 Starting position for prone palpation of the right teres major.

Figure 10-41 Palpation of the right teres major as the client medially rotates the arm against resistance.

Palpation Notes:
1. It is easy to discern the superior border of the teres major from the inferior border of the teres minor. To do so, simply have the client alternate between medial rotation of the arm and lateral rotation of the arm at the shoulder joint (in each case against the resistance of your knee). The teres major will contract with medial rotation, and the teres minor will contract with lateral rotation.

2. It is sometimes challenging to discern the border between the bellies of the teres major and latissimus dorsi. They are located next to each other and they engage with the same actions of the arm at the shoulder joint. On the humerus, the latissimus dorsi attaches more anteriorly on the humerus than the teres major, but the teres major does attach slightly further distal.

TERES MAJOR—PRONE—cont'd

Alternate Palpation Position—Seated

The teres major can also be easily palpated with the client seated. This palpation should be carried out in a similar manner to the seated palpation of the teres minor and infraspinatus (see Figure 10-36), except that medial rotation of the arm at the shoulder joint is resisted. If the resistance is given to the forearm (with the elbow joint flexed to 90 degrees), be sure that the client is providing the resistance with medial rotation of the arm at the shoulder joint and not horizontal flexion of the arm at the shoulder joint.

TRIGGER POINTS

1. Trigger points (TrPs) in the teres major often result from or are perpetuated by acute or chronic overuse of the muscle (e.g., forceful extension of the arm, such as when rowing).
2. TrPs in the teres major tend to produce deep pain in the posterior shoulder when contracting or stretching the muscle, restricted arm abduction at the shoulder joint, or winging (lateral tilt) of the scapula.
3. The referral patterns of teres major TrPs must be distinguished from the referral patterns of TrPs in the deltoid, triceps brachii, serratus posterior superior, supraspinatus, infraspinatus, teres minor, and subscapularis.
4. TrPs in the teres major are often incorrectly assessed as joint dysfunction of the glenohumeral or acromioclavicular joints, deltoid strain, or rotator cuff disease.
5. Associated TrPs often occur in the latissimus dorsi, triceps brachii, posterior deltoid, teres minor, subscapularis, rhomboids, middle trapezius, or serratus anterior.

Figure 10-42 Posterior view illustrating common teres major TrPs and their corresponding referral zone.

Palpation Key:
Place client's forearm between your knees; use your knee to provide resistance.

Figure 10-43 A stretch of the right teres major. The client passively moves his arm into lateral rotation, flexion, and adduction in front of the body. Note: This also stretches the latissimus dorsi.

DETOUR

Latissimus dorsi: With the client prone, it is easy to palpate the latissimus dorsi along with the teres major. To do so, have the client perform either resisted extension or medial rotation of the arm at the shoulder joint (medial rotation shown in Figure 10-44). Even though the teres major and latissimus dorsi both attach together onto the medial lip of the bicipital groove of the humerus, the distal tendon of the latissimus dorsi is more easily palpated at the humerus because it is the more anterior (superficial) of the two tendons. For more information on palpation of the latissimus dorsi, please see page 353 (Tour #7, Chapter 16).

Figure 10-44 Palpation of the right latissimus dorsi as the client medially rotates the arm against resistance. The teres major is ghosted in.

SUPRASPINATUS—PRONE

❑ ATTACHMENTS:

o Supraspinous fossa of the scapula *to the* greater tubercle of the humerus

❑ ACTIONS:

o Abducts and flexes the arm at the shoulder joint

Starting position (Figure 10-46):

o Client prone with the arm resting on the table at the side of the client
o Therapist seated to the side of the client
o Palpating hand placed just superior to the spine of the scapula in the supraspinous fossa
o Support hand placed on distal arm (just proximal to the elbow joint); only needed if resistance is given

Palpation steps:

1. Ask the client to perform a very short range of motion of abduction of the arm at the shoulder joint (approximately 10 to 20 degrees) and feel for the contraction of the belly of the supraspinatus in the supraspinous fossa of the scapula (Figure 10-47, A).
2. To further bring out the contraction of the supraspinatus, the therapist can provide gentle resistance with the support hand to the client's arm abduction.
3. The distal tendon can be palpated deep to the deltoid. This can be done by locating the acromion process of the scapula and dropping just distally and laterally off it onto the distal tendon of the supraspinatus (see Palpation Note #2). Strum perpendicular to the distal tendon with

the supraspinatus either relaxed or contracting gently (Figure 10-47, B).

4. Once the supraspinatus muscle has been located, have the client relax it and palpate to assess its baseline tone.

Figure 10-45 Posterior view of the right supraspinatus. The trapezius has been ghosted in.

Figure 10-46 Starting position for prone palpation of the right supraspinatus.

Figure 10-47 Palpation of the right supraspinatus. **A** shows palpation of the belly superior to the spine of the scapula. **B** shows palpation of the distal tendon just distal to the acromion process of the scapula.

10

SUPRASPINATUS—PRONE—cont'd

Palpation Notes:

1. One difficulty with palpating the belly of the supraspinatus is that the upper trapezius, which lies superficial to it, contracts to stabilize the scapula whenever the arm is abducted. To minimize contraction of the upper trapezius, the client can be asked to actively move the arm halfway between abduction and flexion. This is difficult with the client prone unless the entire arm is hanging off the table, but it can be easily done if the supraspinatus is palpated with the client seated (see Figure 10-48).
2. There are two ways to find the distal tendon of the supraspinatus. One method is to follow the line of the spine of the scapula to the head of the humerus (just distal to the acromion process) and then palpate just anterior to that line. The other method is to find the bicipital groove (see page 76) and then palpate just posterior to that point on the greater tubercle.
3. Medially rotating the arm at the shoulder joint may help increase access to the greater tubercle attachment of the supraspinatus.

Alternate Palpation Position—Seated

Figure 10-48 The supraspinatus can also be easily palpated with the client seated. To engage the supraspinatus, have the client either perform a very short range of motion (approximately 10 to 20 degrees) of abduction of the arm at the shoulder joint with the hand in the small of the back (to reciprocally inhibit the upper trapezius), or perform a short range of motion (approximately 10 to 20 degrees) of the arm halfway between abduction and flexion at the shoulder joint as seen here.

10

YOU ARE HERE

SUPRASPINATUS—PRONE—cont'd

TRIGGER POINTS

1. Trigger points (TrPs) in the supraspinatus often result from or are perpetuated by acute or chronic overuse of the muscle (e.g., postures requiring the arm to be held in abduction for extended periods, especially at or above shoulder height), holding heavy objects in the hand when the arm is hanging down by the side of the body or walking a dog that constantly pulls at the leash (both of which require the supraspinatus to contract to hold the head of the humerus in the glenoid fossa), and trauma (e.g., shoulder dislocation).

2. TrPs in the supraspinatus tend to produce joint crepitus, difficulty performing and strong pain during shoulder abduction, dull pain at rest, stiff shoulder, difficulty sleeping because of pain, and extreme tenderness at the humeral attachment.

3. The referral patterns of supraspinatus TrPs must be distinguished from the referral patterns of TrPs in the infraspina-

tus, teres minor, teres major, deltoid, coracobrachialis, biceps brachii, triceps brachii, brachioradialis, extensor carpi radialis longus, extensor digitorum, supinator, pectoralis major, pectoralis minor, subclavius, scalenes, and serratus posterior superior.

4. TrPs in the supraspinatus are often incorrectly assessed as rotator cuff tendinitis or tears, shoulder bursitis, cervical disc syndrome, frozen shoulder, or lateral epicondylitis/epicondylosis.

5. Associated TrPs often occur in the infraspinatus, teres minor, subscapularis, upper trapezius, deltoid, and latissimus dorsi.

6. Note: The supraspinatus and infraspinatus share the referral zone at the outside of the shoulder joint. However, referral pain from the infraspinatus is usually experienced as a deeper ache than is the referral pain of the supraspinatus.

Figure 10-49 A is a posterior view illustrating common supraspinatus TrPs and their corresponding referral zone. **B** is an anterior view showing the remainder of the referral zone.

STRETCHING THE SUPRASPINATUS

Figure 10-50 A stretch of the right supraspinatus. The client's right arm is extended and adducted behind the body. See also Figure 13-10, C, for another stretch of the supraspinatus.

Palpation Key:
Client gently abducts the arm only a few degrees.

ANTERIOR DELTOID—SUPINE

❑ **ATTACHMENTS:**

o Lateral ¹/₃ of the clavicle *to the* deltoid tuberosity of the humerus

❑ **ACTIONS:**

o Flexes, abducts, medially rotates, and horizontally flexes the arm at the shoulder joint

Starting position (Figure 10-52):

o Client supine with arm resting on table against the body
o Therapist seated at the head of the table
o Palpating hand placed just inferior to the lateral end of the clavicle
o Support hand placed on the distal end of the arm (just proximal to the elbow joint)

Palpation steps:

1. Ask the client to lift the arm at the shoulder joint halfway between flexion and abduction and feel for the contraction of the anterior deltoid (Figure 10-53).
2. To further bring out the contraction of the anterior deltoid, the therapist can provide gentle resistance with the support hand.
3. Strum the fibers of the anterior deltoid perpendicularly from the lateral clavicle to the deltoid tuberosity.
4. Once the anterior deltoid has been located, have the client relax it and palpate to assess its baseline tone.

Pectoralis major
clavicular head (cut)

Brachialis (cut)

Figure 10-51 Anterior view of the right deltoid. The brachialis and pectoralis major have been cut and ghosted in.

10

Figure 10-52 Starting position for supine palpation of the right anterior deltoid.

Figure 10-53 Palpation of the right anterior deltoid as the client moves the arm obliquely into flexion and abduction.

ANTERIOR DELTOID—SUPINE—cont'd

Palpation Notes:

1. In the supine position, the anterior deltoid can also be engaged and palpated by asking the client to horizontally flex the arm at the shoulder joint. In this position, gravity often provides adequate resistance, but further resistance may be added with the therapist's hand.
2. The clavicular head of the pectoralis major also usually contracts with horizontal flexion of the arm at the shoulder joint.
3. When the anterior deltoid and the clavicular head of the pectoralis major are contracted, there is usually a small gap located between them that is visible.

Alternate Palpation Position—Seated or Standing

Figure 10-54 The anterior deltoid can also be easily palpated with the client seated or standing. To engage the anterior fibers of the deltoid, have the client perform horizontal flexion of the arm at the shoulder joint against resistance.

STRETCHING THE DELTOID

Figure 10-56 A stretch of the right anterior deltoid. With the arm horizontal, the client leans into a doorway, causing horizontal extension of the right arm. Note: This also stretches the pectoralis major.

TRIGGER POINTS

1. Trigger points (TrPs) in the anterior deltoid often result from or are perpetuated by acute overuse, chronic overuse (e.g., holding the arm up in abduction or flexion for prolonged periods, such as when working at a computer keyboard), direct trauma (e.g., impact during sports), and TrPs in the supraspinatus.
2. TrPs in the anterior deltoid may produce weakness when performing abduction or flexion of the arm at the shoulder joint.
3. The referral patterns of anterior deltoid TrPs must be distinguished from the referral patterns of TrPs in the scalenes, pectoralis major, pectoralis minor, coracobrachialis, supraspinatus, infraspinatus, and biceps brachii.
4. TrPs in the anterior deltoid are often incorrectly assessed as a rotator cuff tear, bicipital tendinitis, subdeltoid/subacromial bursitis, glenohumeral or acromioclavicular joint arthritis, or C5 nerve compression.
5. Associated TrPs often occur in the clavicular head of the pectoralis major, supraspinatus, biceps brachii, latissimus dorsi, and teres major.

Figure 10-55 Anterior view illustrating a common anterior deltoid TrP and its corresponding referral zone.

Palpation Key:
Arm moves halfway between flexion and abduction.

SUBSCAPULARIS—SUPINE 10-4

❑ **ATTACHMENTS:**

o Subscapular fossa of the scapula *to the* lesser tubercle of the humerus

❑ **ACTIONS:**

o Medially rotates the arm at the shoulder joint

Starting position (Figure 10-58):

o Client supine with the arm resting on the trunk and the other side hand gently holding the elbow of the side being palpated
o Therapist seated to the side of the client
o Palpating finger pads placed against the anterior surface of the scapula
o Support hand reaching under the client's body to grip the medial border of the scapula

Palpation steps:

1. Passively retract the client's scapula with your support hand.
2. Ask the client to take in a deep breath and as the client exhales, slowly but firmly press your finger pads in against the anterior surface of the client's scapula (Figure 10-59, A) (see Palpation Note #1).
3. To verify that you are on the subscapularis, ask the client to medially rotate the arm at the shoulder joint (this will cause the arm to lift slightly) (Figure 10-59, B).
4. Palpate as much of the subscapularis as possible by pressing in deeper toward the medial border of the scapula.
5. Once the subscapularis has been located, have the client relax it and palpate to assess its baseline tone.

Figure 10-57 Anterior view of the right subscapularis. The coracobrachialis and cut deltoid and pectoralis major have been ghosted in.

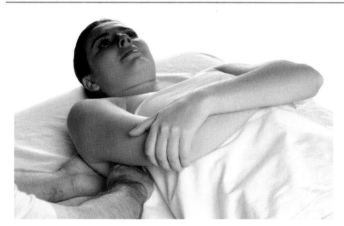

Figure 10-58 Starting position for supine palpation of the right subscapularis.

SUBSCAPULARIS—SUPINE—cont'd

Figure 10-59 Palpation of the right subscapularis. **A** shows palpation of the belly. Note: The client's arm is up so that the reader can visualize the belly of the muscle; the arm may be down and resting on the chest as seen in **B**, which shows the client medially rotating the arm to engage the subscapularis.

Palpation Notes:

1. Working deep to access the subscapularis need not be painful for the client if you have the client breathe and you sink into the tissue *slowly* with a firm confident touch.
2. To locate the subscapularis tendon's distal attachment on the lesser tubercle of the humerus, have the client rest the arm on your shoulder and follow the muscle from the subscapular fossa toward the humerus in baby steps, confirming that you are still on it by asking the client to medially rotate the arm at the shoulder joint. When you have reached the site of distal attachment, have the client fully relax the subscapularis and the rest of the musculature of the arm so that it is easier to feel the lesser tubercle attachment and discern it from the distal tendon of the subscapularis (Figure 10-60).
3. The subscapularis and serratus anterior are both located between the scapula and the rib cage. To palpate the subscapularis, orient your finger pads against the anterior surface of the scapula; to palpate the serratus anterior, orient your finger pads against the rib cage wall.
4. The humeral attachment of the subscapularis can also be palpated through the anterior deltoid. This can be done by locating the lesser tubercle of the humerus (see page 76)

and then strumming vertically along it, feeling for the tendon of the subscapularis. Alternately, locate the two heads of the biceps brachii and then palpate between them for the subscapularis tendon.

Figure 10-60 Palpation of the humeral tendon of the right subscapularis as the client medially rotates the arm against resistance (see Palpation Note #2).

SUBSCAPULARIS—SUPINE—cont'd

Alternate Palpation Position: Side Lying

Figure 10-61 The subscapularis can also be palpated with the client side lying.

TRIGGER POINTS

1. Trigger points (TrPs) in the subscapularis often result from or are perpetuated by acute or chronic overuse of the muscle (e.g., swimming), trauma (e.g., shoulder joint dislocation), prolonged immobilization (e.g., when the arm is held medially rotated in a sling or cast), and chronic shortening of the muscle (e.g., when the client has chronic rounded shoulders posture with the arms medially rotated).

2. TrPs in the subscapularis tend to produce restricted and painful lateral rotation of the arm at the shoulder joint (because lateral rotation of the arm is required for full abduction of the arm, arm abduction is also often restricted), pain when the client is at rest, or extreme tenderness at the humeral attachment.

3. The referral patterns of subscapularis TrPs must be distinguished from the referral patterns of TrPs in the scalenes, teres minor, teres major, posterior deltoid, triceps brachii, extensor carpi radialis brevis, extensor carpi ulnaris, extensor carpi radialis longus, extensor indicis, and serratus posterior superior.

4. TrPs in the subscapularis are often incorrectly assessed as frozen shoulder, rotator cuff lesions, cervical disc syndrome, or thoracic outlet syndrome.

5. Associated TrPs often occur in the pectoralis major, latissimus dorsi, teres major, and anterior deltoid.

Figure 10-62 Posterior view illustrating a common subscapularis TrP and its corresponding referral zone.

10

SUBSCAPULARIS—SUPINE—cont'd

STRETCHING THE SUBSCAPULARIS

Palpation Key:
Client rests in peace; pull scapula out with support hand.

Figure 10-63 A stretch of the right subscapularis. The client laterally rotates the right arm and reaches for the ceiling.

SERRATUS ANTERIOR—SUPINE

10-5

❏ ATTACHMENTS:

o Anterolateral surfaces of ribs one through nine *to the* anterior surface of the entire medial border of the scapula

❏ ACTIONS:

o Protracts and upwardly rotates the scapula at the scapulocostal joint
o Upper fibers can also elevate and lower fibers can also depress the scapula

Starting position (Figure 10-65):

o Client supine with the arm straight up in the air pointed toward the ceiling
o Therapist seated to the side of the client
o Palpating hand placed with finger pads oriented against the lateral rib cage wall, directly inferior to the axilla (armpit)
o Support hand placed on top of the client's fist; only needed if resistance is given

Palpation steps:

1. Ask the client to reach the hand toward the ceiling (this requires protraction of the scapula at the scapulocostal joint) and feel for the contraction of the serratus anterior (Figure 10-66).
2. If desired, resistance to the client's action can be given with your support hand.
3. Continue palpating as much of the serratus anterior as possible (see Figure 10-67).
4. Once the serratus anterior has been located, have the client relax it and palpate to assess its baseline tone.

Figure 10-64 Lateral view of the right serratus anterior.

10

Figure 10-65 Starting position for supine palpation of the right serratus anterior.

Figure 10-66 Palpation of the right serratus anterior against the lateral rib cage wall.

SERRATUS ANTERIOR—SUPINE—cont'd

Palpation Notes:

1. To palpate the upper fibers at their rib cage attachment, slowly but firmly sink in against the rib cage deep to the pectoralis major (Figure 10-67); it can be extremely challenging to access the fibers on the upper two ribs. To palpate the upper fibers closer to the scapular attachment, slowly but firmly sink in against the rib cage between the scapula and rib cage.

2. To better engage the upper fibers of the serratus anterior, have the client angle the arm upward (approximately 135 degrees of flexion) so that the scapula protracts and elevates at the scapulocostal joint (Figure 10-68, A). Similarly, to better engage the lower fibers, have the client angle the arm downward (approximately 45 degrees of flexion) so that the scapula protracts and depresses at the scapulocostal joint (Figure 10-68, B).

3. The serratus anterior and subscapularis are both located between the scapula and rib cage. To palpate the serratus anterior, orient your finger pads against the rib cage wall; to palpate the subscapularis, orient your finger pads against the anterior surface of the scapula.

Figure 10-67 Palpation of the right serratus anterior deep to the pectoralis major.

Figure 10-68 To better engage the upper fibers of the serratus anterior, orient the client's arm more superiorly as it is protracted, as seen in **A**. To better engage the lower fibers of the serratus anterior, orient the client's arm more inferiorly during protraction, as seen in **B**.

Alternate Palpation Position—Side Lying

The serratus anterior can also be easily palpated with the client side lying. As with the supine palpation, the client's upper extremity should be moved to allow access to the serratus anterior.

SERRATUS ANTERIOR—SUPINE—cont'd

TRIGGER POINTS

1. Trigger points (TrPs) in the serratus anterior often result from or are perpetuated by acute or chronic overuse of the muscle (e.g., push ups or any motion that requires the scapula to protract, such as throwing a punch in martial arts, swinging a tennis racquet, throwing a ball, or forceful pushing motions) or labored breathing (because of its accessory role in breathing).
2. TrPs in the serratus anterior tend to restrict scapular retraction at the scapulocostal joint; make it difficult to sleep if lying on the affected side due to compression on the TrP(s), or on the other side if the scapula falls (protracts) forward, resulting in shortening of the muscle; make it difficult to take a deep breath; or cause a "stitch in the side" when "pumping the arms" while running fast.
3. The referral patterns of serratus anterior TrPs must be distinguished from the referral patterns of TrPs in the intercostal muscles, middle trapezius, rhomboids, erector spinae/transversospinalis muscles of the thoracic spine, latissimus dorsi, infraspinatus, and diaphragm.
4. TrPs in the serratus anterior are often incorrectly assessed as angina pectoris or heart attack referral pain (if the muscle on the left side is affected), rib joint dysfunction or fracture, entrapment of the intercostal nerves, costochondritis, cervical disc syndrome, thoracic outlet syndrome, herpes zoster, and TrPs of the intercostal muscles.
5. Associated TrPs often occur in the erector spinae/transversospinalis muscles of the thoracic spine, rhomboids, middle trapezius, serratus posterior superior, latissimus dorsi, scalenes, and sternocleidomastoid.
6. Notes: Central and attachment TrPs can occur in any of the nine digitations of the serratus anterior. TrPs of the serratus anterior may also refer down the ulnar side of the entire upper extremity.

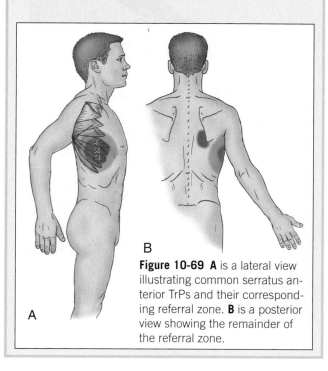

Figure 10-69 A is a lateral view illustrating common serratus anterior TrPs and their corresponding referral zone. **B** is a posterior view showing the remainder of the referral zone.

STRETCHING THE SERRATUS ANTERIOR

Figure 10-70 A stretch of the right serratus anterior. The client extends the arm to hold onto the back of the bench and rotates the body to the opposite side (causing retraction of the scapula).

Palpation Key: Reach for the ceiling.

PECTORALIS MAJOR—SUPINE

❏ ATTACHMENTS:

o Medial half of the clavicle, sternum, and the costal cartilages of ribs one through seven *to the* lateral lip of the
   bicipital groove of the humerus

❏ ACTIONS:

o Entire muscle: adducts, medially rotates, and horizontally
   flexes the arm at the shoulder joint; protracts the scapula
   at the scapulocostal joint
o Clavicular head: flexes the arm at the shoulder joint
o Sternocostal head: extends the arm at the shoulder joint
   (from a position of flexion to anatomic position);
   depresses the scapula at the scapulocostal joint

Starting position (Figure 10-72):

o Client supine with the arm resting at the side
o Therapist seated to the side of the client
o Palpating hand placed over the lower aspect of the anterior axillary fold of tissue
o Support hand placed on the distal arm, just proximal to
   the elbow joint

Palpation steps:

1. Begin by palpating the sternocostal head. Ask the client to
   adduct the arm at the shoulder joint against resistance.
   Resistance can be added either with your support hand or
   simply by having the client adduct against his body wall
   (Figure 10-73, A).
2. Feel for the contraction of the sternocostal head and
   palpate toward its proximal (medial) attachment.
3. To palpate the clavicular head, place the palpating hand
   just inferior to the medial clavicle, and ask the client to
   obliquely move the arm at the shoulder joint between

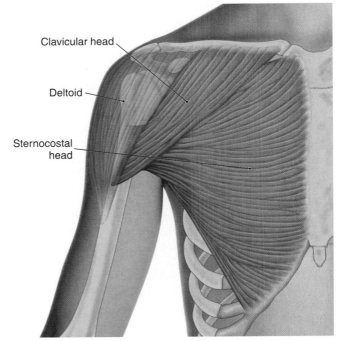

Figure 10-71 Anterior view of the right pectoralis major. The deltoid has been ghosted in.

flexion and adduction against resistance. Resistance can be
added with your support hand (Figure 10-73, B).
4. Feel for the contraction of the clavicular head and palpate
   toward the distal attachment by strumming perpendicular
   to the fibers.
5. Once the pectoralis major has been located, have the
   client relax it and palpate to assess its baseline tone.

Figure 10-72 Starting position for supine palpation of the right
pectoralis major (sternocostal head).

Figure 10-73 Palpation of the right pectoralis major. **A** shows palpation of the sternocostal head as the client performs adduction
against resistance. **B** shows palpation of the clavicular head as the
client performs an oblique plane motion of flexion and adduction
against resistance.

PECTORALIS MAJOR—SUPINE—cont'd

Palpation Notes:

1. Ask the client to abduct the arm at the shoulder joint, and grab the anterior axillary fold of tissue; then have the client relax the arm back against the body. You have the client's pectoralis major in your hand (Figure 10-74, A).
2. There is usually a discernable and visible groove between the clavicular head of the pectoralis major and the anterior deltoid.
3. To engage the entire pectoralis major, ask the client to horizontally flex the arm at the shoulder joint against resistance. (Note: This will also engage the anterior deltoid.) This is most easily done with the client seated (Figure 10-74, B).
4. When the client horizontally flexes the arm against resistance, there is usually a discernable and visible groove between the clavicular and sternocostal heads of the pectoralis major.

Figure 10-74 If the arm is abducted away from the body, the anterior axillary fold of tissue containing the pectoralis major can be easily grasped between palpating fingers, as seen in **A**. The entire pectoralis major can be easily palpated with the client seated by resisting the client's horizontal flexion of the arm at the shoulder joint, as seen in **B**.

TRIGGER POINTS

1. Trigger points (TrPs) in the pectoralis major often result from or are perpetuated by acute or chronic overuse of the muscle (e.g., repetitive lifting in front of the body, any repetitive adduction of the arm at the shoulder joint), prolonged postures that shorten the muscle (e.g., a chronic rounded shoulder posture, use of a sling or cast, sleeping on the back with the arms folded across the chest, sleeping on the affected side with the shoulder girdle protracted), use of a cane or crutches, excessively tight bra strap that compresses the muscle, or myocardial infarction.
2. TrPs in the pectoralis major tend to produce a rounded shoulder posture (which may cause pain in the interscapular region and may cause costoclavicular syndrome), restricted abduction and horizontal extension of the arm at the shoulder joint or retraction of the scapula at the scapulocostal joint, difficulty sleeping (due to pain), or breast pain or swelling. Additionally, a TrP in the right side of the pectoralis major between the fifth and sixth ribs has been attributed to causing cardiac arrhythmia.
3. The referral patterns of pectoralis major TrPs must be distinguished from the referral patterns of TrPs in the pectoralis minor, subclavius, intercostals, scalenes, anterior deltoid, supraspinatus, infraspinatus, coracobrachialis, and biceps brachii.
4. TrPs in the pectoralis major are often incorrectly assessed as angina pectoris or myocardial infarction (for left-sided TrPs), rib joint dysfunction, costochondritis, hiatal hernia, bicipital tendinitis, shoulder joint bursitis, cervical disc syndrome, or medial epicondylitis/epicondylosis.
5. Associated TrPs often occur in the anterior deltoid, coracobrachialis, latissimus dorsi, subscapularis, serratus anterior, rhomboids, middle trapezius, sternocleidomastoid, infraspinatus, teres minor, and posterior deltoid.

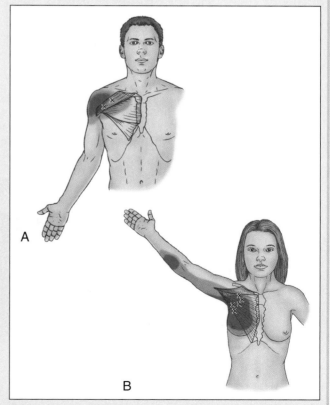

Figure 10-75 Anterior views illustrating common pectoralis major TrPs and their corresponding referral zones. **A** shows the clavicular head; **B** shows the sternocostal head.

PECTORALIS MAJOR—SUPINE—cont'd

STRETCHING THE PECTORALIS MAJOR

A   B

Figure 10-76 Stretches of the two heads of the right pectoralis major. **A** shows a stretch of the sternocostal head. The arm is abducted to approximately 90 degrees and the client leans into a doorway. **B** shows a stretch of the clavicular head. The arm is abducted to approximately 45 degrees and the client leans into a doorway. Note the difference in positions of the arm.

Palpation Key:
Palpate the anterior axillary fold of tissue.

PECTORALIS MINOR—SUPINE   10-6 10-7

❏ ATTACHMENTS:

o Ribs three through five *to the* medial surface of the coracoid process of the scapula

❏ ACTIONS:

o Protracts, depresses, and downwardly rotates the scapula at the scapulocostal joint
o Elevates ribs three through five at the sternocostal and costospinal joints

Starting position (Figure 10-78):

o Client supine with the hand under the body in the small of the back
o Therapist seated at the head of the table
o Palpating hand placed just inferior to the coracoid process of the scapula

Palpation steps:

1. Ask the client to press the hand and forearm down against the table, and feel for the contraction of the pectoralis minor through the pectoralis major (Figure 10-79).
2. Continue palpating toward the rib attachments by strumming perpendicular to the fibers.
3. Once the pectoralis minor has been located, have the client relax it and palpate to assess its baseline tone.

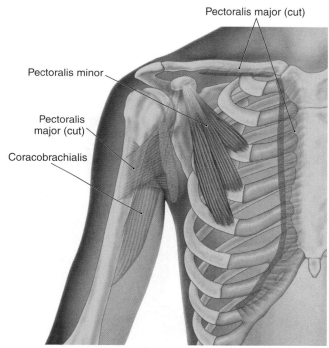

Figure 10-77 Anterior view of the right pectoralis minor. The coracobrachialis and cut pectoralis major have been ghosted in.

Figure 10-78 Starting position for supine palpation of the right pectoralis minor.

Figure 10-79 Palpation of the right pectoralis minor perpendicular to the fibers as the client presses the hand and forearm down against the table.

Palpation Notes:

1. The client is asked to press the hand and forearm against the table because this requires extension of the arm at the shoulder joint, which requires the coupled action of downward rotation of the scapula at the scapulocostal joint, an action of the pectoralis minor. This is easiest to perform with the client seated (see Figure 10-80).

2. It is usually possible to individually palpate and discern each of the three slips of the pectoralis minor.
3. An alternate method to palpate the lateralmost fibers of the pectoralis minor is to access it from the side by pressing in deep to the pectoralis major. This method does work but it can be uncomfortable for the client and is not necessary because the pectoralis minor can be easily palpated and worked through the pectoralis major.

10

PECTORALIS MINOR—SUPINE—cont'd

Alternate Palpation Position—Seated

Figure 10-80 Having the client seated is the easiest position for palpating the pectoralis minor, because the client can comfortably place the hand in the small of the back and easily move it posteriorly when asked to do so by the therapist.

STRETCHING THE PECTORALIS MINOR

Figure 10-82 A stretch of the right pectoralis minor. The arm is abducted to approximately 135 degrees and the client leans into a doorway.

TRIGGER POINTS

1. Trigger points (TrPs) in the pectoralis minor often result from or are perpetuated by acute or chronic overuse of the muscle, prolonged postures that shorten the muscle (e.g., a chronic rounded shoulder posture, use of a sling or cast, sleeping on the back with the arms folded across the chest, sleeping on the affected side with the shoulder girdle protracted), use of a cane or crutches, myocardial infarction, labored breathing, compression of the muscle (e.g., due to the straps of a heavy backpack), or from TrPs in the pectoralis major or scalenes.
2. TrPs in the pectoralis minor tend to produce pectoralis minor syndrome (causing neurologic or vascular symptoms in the upper extremity), a rounded shoulder posture (which may cause pain in the interscapular region and may cause costoclavicular syndrome), restricted retraction of the scapula at the scapulocostal joint, or winging of the scapula.
3. The referral patterns of pectoralis minor TrPs must be distinguished from the referral patterns of TrPs in the pectoralis major, deltoid, coracobrachialis, scalenes, supraspinatus, infraspinatus, biceps brachii, and triceps brachii.
4. TrPs in the pectoralis minor are often incorrectly assessed as cervical disc syndrome, anterior scalene syndrome, costoclavicular syndrome, carpal tunnel syndrome, bicipital tendinitis, medial epicondylitis/epicondylosis, or angina pectoris or myocardial infarction (for left-sided TrPs).
5. Associated TrPs often occur in the pectoralis major, anterior deltoid, scalenes, and sternocleidomastoid.

Figure 10-81 Anterior view illustrating common pectoralis minor TrPs and their corresponding referral zone.

Palpation Key:
Client's hand in the small of the back.

SUBCLAVIUS—SUPINE

❑ ATTACHMENTS:

o First rib at the junction with its costal cartilage *to the* middle ⅓ of the inferior surface of the clavicle

❑ ACTIONS:

o Depresses, protracts, and downwardly rotates the clavicle at the sternoclavicular joint
o Elevates the first rib at the sternocostal and costospinal joints

Starting position (Figure 10-84):

o Client supine with the arm medially rotated at the shoulder joint and resting on the table at the side of the body
o Therapist seated at the head of the table
o Palpating fingers curled around the clavicle so that the finger pads are on the inferior surface of the clavicle

Palpation steps:

1. The subclavius can be challenging to palpate.
2. With the musculature of the region relaxed, feel for the subclavius on the underside of the clavicle.
3. To palpate while engaged, ask the client to depress the clavicle at the sternoclavicular joint (i.e., to depress the shoulder girdle [scapula and clavicle]) and feel for the contraction of the subclavius (Figure 10-85).

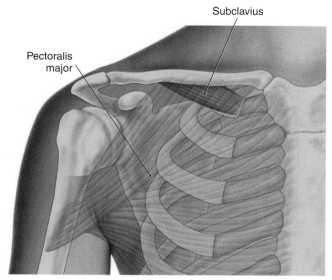

Figure 10-83 Anterior view of the right subclavius. The pectoralis major has been ghosted in.

4. Palpate from attachment to attachment.
5. Once the subclavius has been located, have the client relax it and palpate to assess its baseline tone.

Figure 10-84 Starting position for supine palpation of the right subclavius.

Figure 10-85 Palpation of the right subclavius as the client depresses the shoulder girdle.

Palpation Notes:

1. Asking the client to have the arm passively medially rotated at the shoulder joint helps to slacken the pectoralis major, which lies superficial to the subclavius. Also, having the arm in adduction further slackens the pectoralis major.
2. When palpating the subclavius, it can also be helpful to hold the client's arm in passive abduction. Abducting the arm at the shoulder joint requires the clavicle to upwardly rotate at the sternoclavicular joint, exposing more of the inferior surface of the clavicle to palpation. It is important that the client's arm is passively abducted so that the musculature of the region is relaxed.

Alternate Palpation Position
The subclavius can also be palpated with the client side lying or seated.

SUBCLAVIUS—SUPINE—cont'd

TRIGGER POINTS

1. Trigger points (TrPs) in the subclavius often result from or are perpetuated by acute or chronic overuse of the muscle, prolonged postures that shorten the muscle (e.g., a chronic rounded shoulder posture, use of a sling or cast, sleeping on the affected side with the shoulder girdle protracted), or use of a cane or crutches.
2. TrPs in the subclavius tend to produce costoclavicular syndrome (causing neurologic or vascular symptoms in the upper extremity).

3. The referral patterns of subclavius TrPs must be distinguished from the referral patterns of TrPs in the biceps brachii, brachialis, scalenes, supraspinatus, infraspinatus, brachioradialis, extensor carpi radialis longus, extensor digitorum, supinator, opponens pollicis, and adductor pollicis.
4. TrPs in the subclavius are often incorrectly assessed as cervical disc syndrome, anterior scalene syndrome, pectoralis minor syndrome, or lateral epicondylitis/epicondylosis.
5. Associated TrPs are likely to occur in the pectoralis major and pectoralis minor.

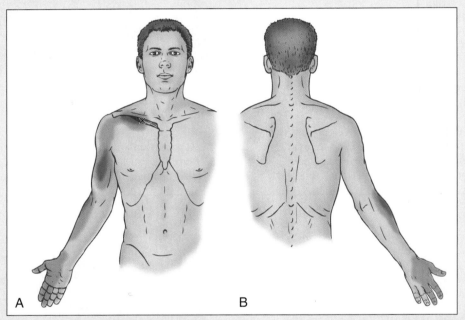

Figure 10-86 A is an anterior view illustrating a common subclavius TrP and its corresponding referral zone. **B** is a posterior view showing the remainder of the referral zone.

STRETCHING THE SUBCLAVIUS

Figure 10-87 A stretch of the right subclavius. The arm is abducted, laterally rotated, and extended back while the trunk remains facing forward.

Palpation Key:
Curl your fingertips around the clavicle.

Muscles of the Shoulder Girdle

Client Prone:

1. **Trapezius:** Begin with the client prone with the arm abducted to 90 degrees and resting on the table and the forearm hanging off the table; you are standing to the side of the client. Ask the client to abduct the arm at the shoulder joint with the forearm extended at the elbow joint, and to slightly retract the scapula at the scapulocostal joint. First look for and then feel for the lateral border of the lower trapezius. Once felt, palpate the entirety of the lower trapezius by strumming perpendicular to its fibers as the client alternately contracts and relaxes the muscle. Next, palpate the middle trapezius by strumming perpendicular to its fibers as the client alternately contracts and relaxes the muscle. Then ask the client to slightly extend the head and upper neck at the spinal joints and feel for the contraction of the upper trapezius. Once felt, palpate the entire upper trapezius by strumming perpendicular to its fibers as the client alternately contracts and relaxes the muscle.

2. **Rhomboids:** The client is prone and places the hand in the small of the back; you are standing to the side of the client. Ask the client to lift the hand up, away from the small of the back, and look for the rhomboids to contract and become visible (especially the lower border). Then palpate all of the rhomboids by strumming perpendicular to its fibers as the client alternately contracts and relaxes the muscle. Remember that the most superior aspect of the medial attachment is C7 at the base of the neck.

3. **Levator scapulae:** The client is prone with the hand in the small of the back; you are standing or seated to the side of the client. Ask the client to perform a gentle, very short range of motion of elevation of the scapula and feel for the contraction of the levator scapulae deep to the trapezius at the superior angle of the scapula. Once felt, strum perpendicular to the fibers, palpating the muscle superiorly as the client gently contracts and relaxes the muscle. Once you are palpating the levator scapulae in the posterior triangle, the hand does not need to be in the small of the back and the client can elevate the scapula more forcefully. Continue strumming perpendicularly with the client contracting and relaxing the muscle until you reach the transverse processes attachment. Remember that the transverse process of C1 is directly below the client's ear.

4. **Posterior deltoid:** The client is prone with the arm abducted to 90 degrees and resting on the table and the forearm hanging off the table; you are standing or seated to the side of the client. Ask the client to horizontally extend the arm at the shoulder joint and feel for the contraction of the posterior deltoid. Resistance can be added. Once felt, palpate from the spine of the scapula to the deltoid tuberosity, strumming perpendicularly as the client alternately contracts and relaxes the muscle.

5. **Infraspinatus and teres minor:** To palpate the infraspinatus, have the client prone with the arm abducted to 90 degrees and resting on the table, and the forearm hanging off the table; you are seated to the side of the client with the client's forearm between your knees. Ask the client to laterally rotate the arm at the shoulder joint and feel for the contraction of the infraspinatus immediately inferior to the spine of the scapula. Once felt, palpate the entire infraspinatus in the infraspinous fossa as the client alternately contracts and relaxes the muscle. Continue palpating it toward the greater tubercle attachment by strumming perpendicularly as the client contracts and relaxes it. To palpate the teres minor, ask the client to laterally rotate the arm at the shoulder joint and palpate for the contraction of the teres minor at the superior aspect of the lateral border of the scapula. Once felt, palpate it toward the greater tubercle attachment by strumming perpendicularly as the client alternately contracts and relaxes it. Note: It can be challenging to locate the border between the infraspinatus and teres minor; however, it is easy to locate the border between the teres minor and the teres major by simply asking the client to alternately perform lateral rotation and medial rotation of the arm (the teres minor contracts with laterally rotation; the teres major contracts with medial rotation).

6. **Teres major:** The client is prone; you are seated to the side of the client with the client's forearm between your knees. Palpate as for the teres minor, except that the palpating fingers are placed at the inferior aspect of the lateral border of the scapula and the client is asked to medially rotate the arm at the shoulder joint. Once the contraction of the teres major is felt, continue palpating it toward the humeral attachment by strumming perpendicularly as the client alternately contracts and relaxes the muscle. To reach the attachment on the medial lip of the bicipital groove, it is necessary to palpate within the axillary region. Note: It can be challenging to discern the teres major from the latissimus dorsi.

7. **Supraspinatus:** The client is prone with the arm resting at the side of the body; you are seated to the side of the client. Ask the client to perform a very short range of motion of abduction of the arm (approximately 10 to 15 degrees) at the shoulder joint and feel for the contraction of the supraspinatus immediately superior to the spine of the scapula (gentle resistance can be given). Once felt, palpate the entire belly in the supraspinous fossa. To palpate the distal tendon, drop just off the acromion process of the scapula onto the distal tendon (draw an imaginary line along the spine of the scapula onto the humerus and place your palpating fingers just anterior to that point on the humerus). Strum perpendicular to the distal tendon and feel for it deep to the deltoid; this may be done with the supraspinatus either relaxed or gently contracted.

Client Supine:

8. **Anterior deltoid:** The client is supine; you are seated at the head of the table. Ask the client to lift the arm at the shoulder joint halfway between flexion and abduction and feel for the contraction of the anterior deltoid; resistance can be added if needed. Once felt, palpate the

anterior deltoid from the lateral clavicle to the deltoid tuberosity by strumming perpendicular to the fibers as the client alternately contracts and relaxes the muscle.

9. **Subscapularis:** Have the client supine with the arm resting on the trunk and the other side hand gently holding the elbow of the upper extremity on the side being palpated; you are seated to the side of the client. Using your support hand under the client's body, passively protract the client scapula, ask the client to take in a deep breath and slowly but firmly palpate into the subscapularis as the client slowly exhales. Be sure to press your finger pads against the anterior surface of the client's scapula. To verify that you are palpating the client's subscapularis, ask the client to medially rotate the arm at the shoulder joint and feel for the muscle's contraction. Palpate as much of the subscapularis as possible by pressing deeper toward the medial border of the scapula. Note: To follow the subscapularis all the way to the lesser tubercle of the humerus, hold the client's arm passively in the air (in a position of flexion) and follow the subscapularis toward the humerus as the client alternately contracts and relaxes the muscle. To feel the lesser tubercle attachment, be sure that the muscle is relaxed.

10. **Serratus anterior:** Have the client supine with the arm straight up in the air, pointed toward the ceiling; you are seated to the side of the client. Ask the client to reach toward the ceiling as you palpate against the lateral rib cage wall. If desired, resistance can be given with your support hand. Continue palpating as much of the serratus anterior as possible (including palpating deep to the pectoralis major).

11. **Pectoralis major:** Have the client supine with the arm resting at their side; you are seated to the side of the client. For the sternocostal head, palpate the lower aspect of the axillary fold of tissue as you resist adduction of the client's arm at the shoulder joint. Palpate the entire sternocostal head by strumming perpendicular to the fibers. For the clavicular head, palpate just inferior to the medial aspect of the clavicle as the client moves the arm at the shoulder joint obliquely between flexion and adduction. Resistance can be added if desired. Palpate the entire clavicular head by strumming perpendicular to the fibers.

12. **Pectoralis minor:** Have the client supine with the hand under the body in the small of the back; you are seated at the head of the table. Palpate for the contraction of the pectoralis minor just inferior to the coracoid process of the scapula as the client presses the hand and forearm down against the table. Once felt, palpate all three slips of the pectoralis minor to the rib attachments by strumming perpendicular to the fibers as the client alternately contracts and relaxes the muscle.

13. **Subclavius:** Have the client supine with the arm medially rotated and resting at the side of the body; you are seated at the head of the table. Curl your palpating fingers around the clavicle so that your finger pads are on the inferior surface of the clavicle. With the muscle relaxed, feel for the subclavius on the inferior surface of the clavicle. To feel the subclavius while contracting, palpate the muscle while asking the client to depress the shoulder girdle.

Chapter 11

Tour #2—Palpation of the Neck Muscles

Overview

This chapter is a palpation tour of the muscles of the neck. The tour begins with anterior neck muscles and then moves to the posterior muscles of the neck. Palpation of anterior neck muscles is shown in the supine position. Palpation of most of the posterior neck muscles is shown with the client seated; a few are shown with the client supine. Alternate palpation positions are also described. The major muscles or muscle groups of the region are each given a separate layout; there are also a number of detours to other muscles of the region. Trigger point (TrP) information and stretching is given for each of the major muscles covered in this chapter. The chapter closes with an advanced *Whirlwind Tour* that explains the sequential palpation of all of the muscles of the chapter.

Chapter Outline

Chapter Objectives

After completing this chapter, the student should be able to perform the following for each of the muscles covered in this chapter:

1. State the attachments.
2. State the actions.
3. Describe the starting position for palpation.
4. Describe and explain the purpose of each of the palpation steps.
5. Palpate each muscle.
6. State the "Palpation Key."
7. Describe alternate palpation positions.
8. State the locations of the most common TrP(s).
9. Describe the TrP referral zones.
10. State the most common factors that create and/or perpetuate TrPs.
11. State the symptoms most commonly caused by TrPs.
12. Describe and perform a stretch.

Video demonstrations of the muscle palpations in this chapter are presented in Chapter 11 on DVD 1.

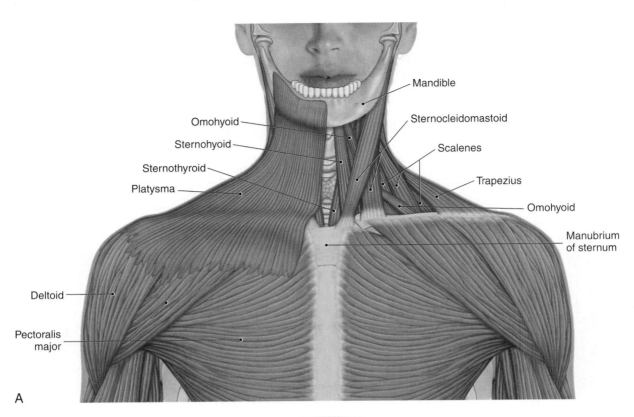

Mandible

Omohyoid

Sternohyoid

Sternothyroid

Platysma

Sternocleidomastoid

Scalenes

Trapezius

Omohyoid

Manubrium of sternum

Deltoid

Pectoralis major

A

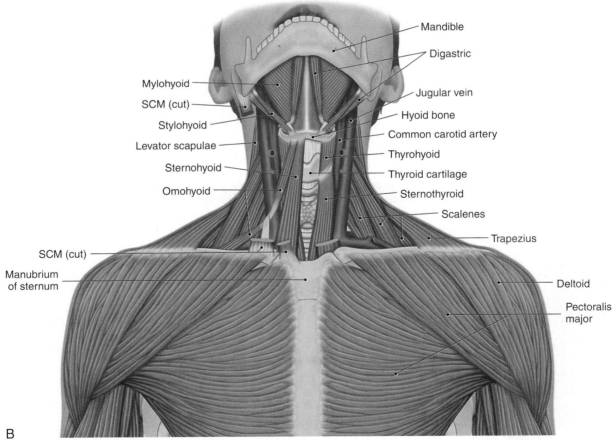

Mandible

Digastric

Mylohyoid

SCM (cut)

Stylohyoid

Levator scapulae

Sternohyoid

Omohyoid

Jugular vein

Hyoid bone

Common carotid artery

Thyrohyoid

Thyroid cartilage

Sternothyroid

Scalenes

Trapezius

SCM (cut)

Manubrium of sternum

Deltoid

Pectoralis major

B

Figure 11-1 Anterior views of the neck and upper chest region. **A** shows superficial views; the platysma has been removed on the left side. **B** shows intermediate views; the sternocleidomastoid has been cut on the right side; the sternocleidomastoid and omohyoid have been removed and the sternohyoid has been cut on the left side.

11

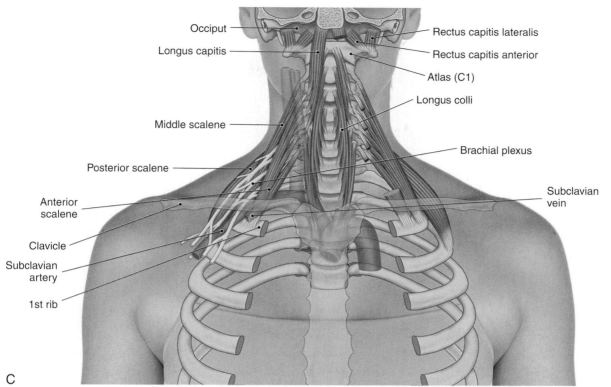

Occiput

Longus capitis

Middle scalene

Posterior scalene

Anterior scalene

Clavicle

Subclavian artery

1st rib

Rectus capitis lateralis

Rectus capitis anterior

Atlas (C1)

Longus colli

Brachial plexus

Subclavian vein

C

Figure 11-1, cont'd C shows deep views; the anterior scalene and longus capitis, as well as the brachial plexus of nerves and subclavian artery and vein, have been cut and/or removed on the left side.

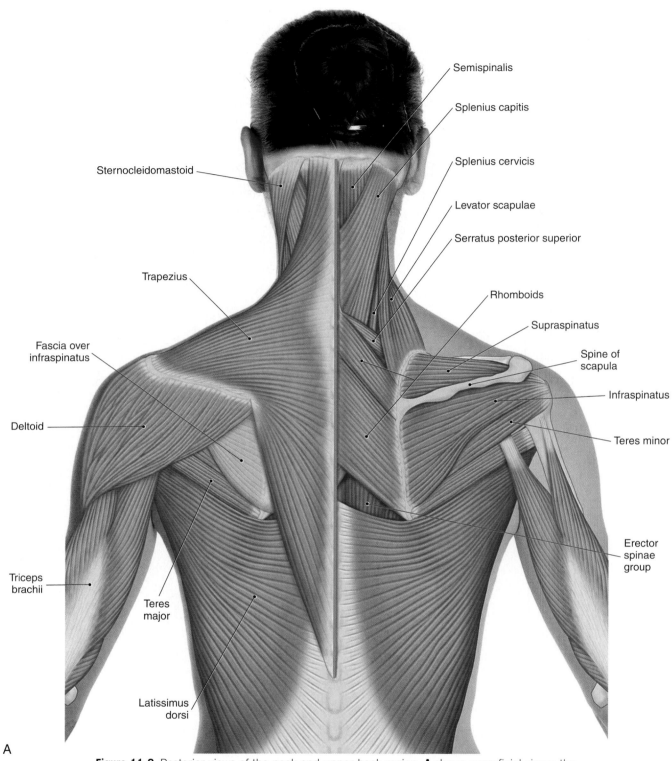

A

Figure 11-2 Posterior views of the neck and upper back region. **A** shows superficial views; the trapezius, sternocleidomastoid, and deltoid have been removed on the right side.

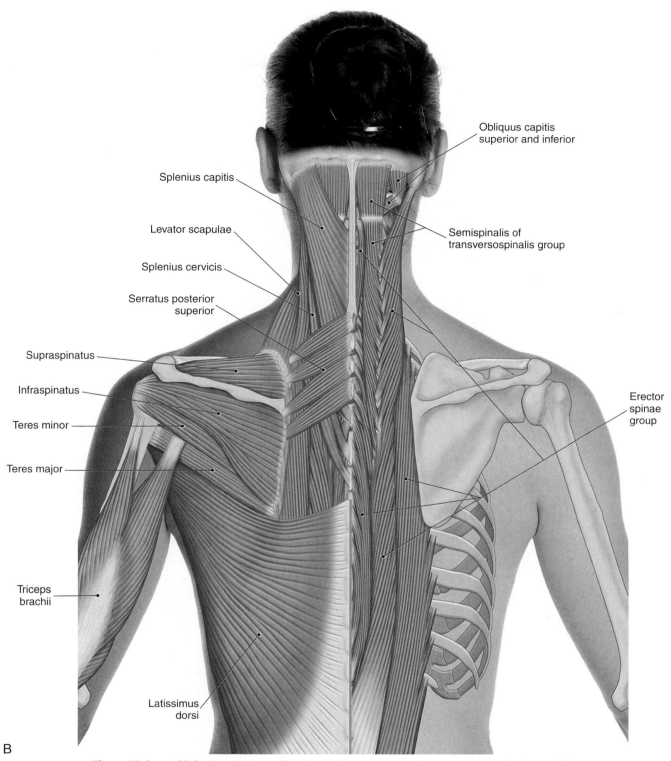

Obliquus capitis
superior and inferior

Splenius capitis

Levator scapulae

Splenius cervicis

Serratus posterior
superior

Semispinalis of
transversospinalis group

Supraspinatus

Infraspinatus

Teres minor

Teres major

Erector
spinae
group

Triceps
brachii

Latissimus
dorsi

B

Figure 11-2, cont'd B shows intermediate views; the serratus posterior superior, splenius capitis and cervicis, levator scapulae, supraspinatus, infraspinatus, teres minor and major, and triceps brachii have been removed on the right side.

YOU ARE HERE

11

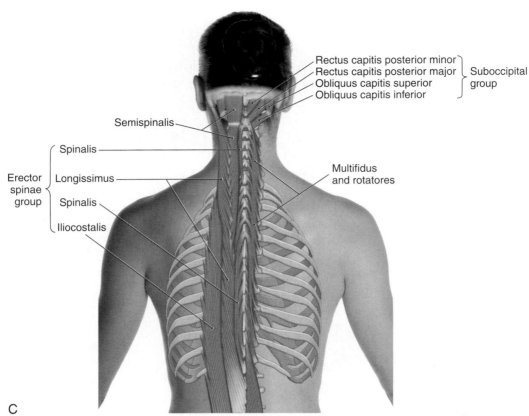

C

Figure 11-2, cont'd C shows deep views; the iliocostalis, longissimus, and spinalis of the erector spinae group and the semispinalis of the transversospinalis group have been removed on the right side.

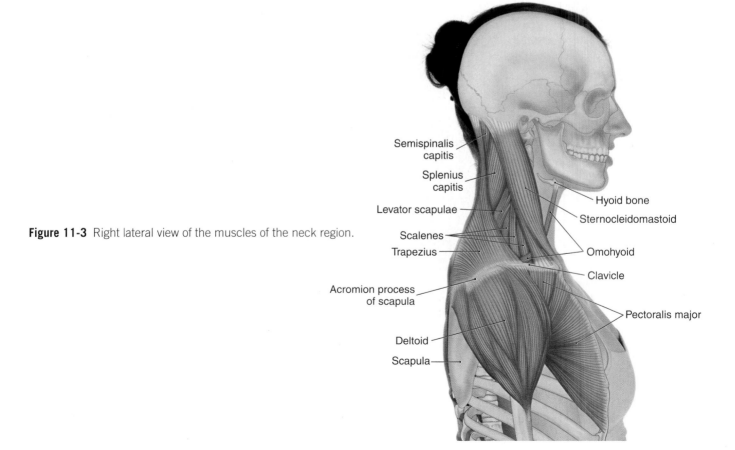

Figure 11-3 Right lateral view of the muscles of the neck region.

STERNOCLEIDOMASTOID (SCM)—SUPINE
11-1

❑ ATTACHMENTS:
o Manubrium of the sternum and the medial ⅓ of the clavicle *to the* mastoid process of the temporal bone and the lateral ½ of the superior nuchal line of the occiput

❑ ACTIONS:
o Flexes the lower neck and extends the head and upper neck at the spinal joints
o Laterally flexes and contralaterally rotates the head and neck at the spinal joints
o Elevates the sternum and clavicle

Starting position (Figure 11-5):
o Client supine with the head and neck contralaterally rotated
o Therapist seated at the head of the table
o Palpating hand placed just superior to the sternoclavicular joint

Palpation steps:
1. Ask the client to lift the head and neck from the table, and look for the SCM to become visible (Figure 11-6).
2. Although resistance could be added by the support hand, it is often unnecessary because lifting the head and neck against gravity usually provides sufficient resistance.
3. Palpate toward the superior attachment by strumming perpendicular to the fibers.
4. Once the SCM has been located, have the client relax it and palpate to assess its baseline tone.

Figure 11-4 Lateral view of the right SCM.

11

Figure 11-5 Starting position for supine palpation of the right SCM.

Figure 11-6 Supine palpation of the right SCM as the client raises the head and neck from the table. **A**, Palpation of the clavicular head. **B**, Palpation of the sternal head.

STERNOCLEIDOMASTOID (SCM)—SUPINE—cont'd

Palpation Notes:

1. The sternal head of the SCM is usually much more visible than the clavicular head. If the clavicular head is not visible, palpate for it just lateral to the inferior aspect of the sternal head. Note: Although it is common to have a small gap between the sternal and clavicular heads, some people have a large gap and other people have no gap at all.

2. **Palpation of the SCM must be done somewhat carefully, because the carotid sinus of the common carotid artery lies deep to the SCM (see Figure 11-1, B, on page 182), and pressure against the carotid sinus can create a reflex that lowers blood pressure. For this reason, pincer palpation is often recommended for palpating the SCM, rather than flat palpation.**

3. The SCM creates the anterior border of the posterior triangle of the neck, and forms an excellent landmark for locating the scalenes and the longus colli and longus capitis muscles.

Alternate Palpation Position—Seated

Figure 11-7 The SCM can be easily palpated with the client seated. Ask the client to rotate the head and neck to the opposite side (contralaterally rotate) and slightly laterally flex to the same side; then resist any further lateral flexion to the same side. The sternal head will often become visible with contralateral rotation. Resistance to same side lateral flexion will usually bring out the clavicular head (indicated). If the clavicular head is not visible, try increasing the resistance to lateral flexion.

Palpation Key:
Turn to the opposite side and lift the head.

TRIGGER POINTS

1. Trigger points (TrPs) in the sternocleidomastoid (SCM) often result from or are perpetuated by acute or chronic overuse of the muscle (e.g., chronic postures of sitting with the head turned to one side or looking upward to paint a ceiling, a chronic cough using the muscle for its respiratory function), chronic postures that result in shortening of the muscle (e.g., having a protracted head posture, looking downward to read a book in the lap by flexing the lower cervical spine, sleeping with a pillow that is too thick), irritation from wearing a tie or a shirt with a tight collar, or trauma (e.g., whiplash, fall).

2. TrPs in the SCM tend to produce headaches, altered posture of ipsilateral lateral flexion of the head and neck, restricted range of motion of the neck and head, a sore throat, autonomic nervous system symptoms (sternal head: eye symptoms, such as ptosis of the upper eyelid, loss of visual acuity, and excessive tear formation; clavicular head: localized vasoconstriction and increased sweating), proprioceptive symptoms (sternal head: dizziness, vertigo, nausea, and ataxia; clavicular head: hearing loss), and even entrapment of cranial nerve XI (spinal accessory nerve).

3. The referral patterns of SCM TrPs must be distinguished from the referral patterns of TrPs in the trapezius, semispinalis capitis, suboccipitals, temporalis, masseter, digastric (due to pain referral and possible throat symptoms), lateral and medial pterygoids, occipitofrontalis, platysma, longus colli and capitis (due to possible throat symptoms), and some muscles of facial expression.

4. TrPs in the SCM are often incorrectly assessed as swollen lymph nodes, sinus or migraine headaches, osteoarthritis of the sternoclavicular joint, trigeminal neuralgia, tic douloureux, or neurogenic spasmodic torticollis.

5. Associated TrPs often occur in the scalenes, platysma, levator scapulae, trapezius, splenius capitis and cervicis, semispinalis capitis, temporalis, masseter, digastric, and contralateral SCM.

6. The referral pain of SCM TrPs can cross over to the other side of the body.

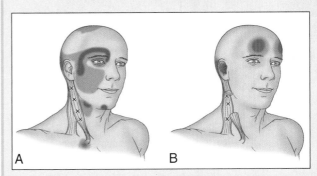

Figure 11-8 Anterolateral views illustrating common sternocleidomastoid (SCM) TrPs and their corresponding referral zones. **A**, Sternal head. **B**, Clavicular head.

STERNOCLEIDOMASTOID (SCM)—SUPINE—cont'd

STRETCHING THE SCM

Figure 11-9 A stretch of the right SCM. The client left laterally flexes and right rotates the head and neck, and extends the lower neck but tucks the chin (flexes the head).

DETOUR

Platysma: The platysma is a very thin superficial sheet of muscle that attaches from the subcutaneous fascia of the superior chest to the mandible and subcutaneous fascia of the lower face (Figure 11-10, A). When it contracts, it creates wrinkles in the skin of the neck. It can be engaged by asking the client to forcefully depress and draw the lower lip laterally while keeping the mandible in a position of slight depression (Figure 11-10, C).

Trigger Points:

1. Trigger points (TrPs) in the platysma often result from or are perpetuated by acute or chronic overuse of the muscle (e.g., habitual expression of disgust or horror) and TrPs in the SCM and scalene muscles.

2. TrPs in the platysma tend to produce prickly pain over the mandible.
3. The referral patterns of platysma TrPs must be distinguished from the referral patterns of TrPs in the SCM, masseter, temporalis, and medial pterygoid.
4. TrPs in the platysma are often incorrectly assessed as temporomandibular joint (TMJ) dysfunction.
5. Associated TrPs often occur in other muscles of facial expression.
6. Note: TrPs in the platysma are usually located over the SCM.

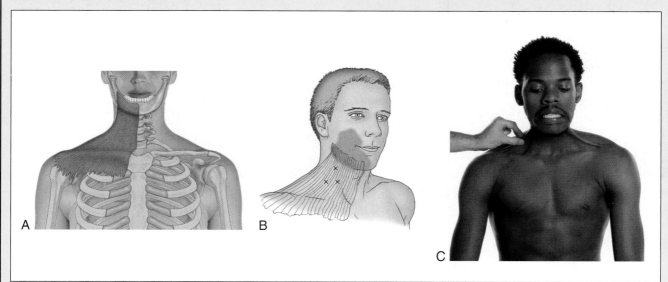

Figure 11-10 Views of the platysma. **A**, Anterior view of the right platysma. **B**, Anterolateral view illustrating common platysma TrPs and their corresponding referral zone. **C**, Anterior view of the platysma contracted and being palpated.

YOU ARE HERE

❏ ATTACHMENTS:

o Anterior scalene: first rib *to the* transverse processes of C3-C6
o Middle scalene: first rib *to the* transverse processes of C2-C7
o Posterior scalene: second rib *to the* transverse processes of C5-C7

❏ ACTIONS:

o Anterior scalene: flexes, laterally flexes, and contralaterally rotates the neck at the spinal joints; elevates the first rib at the sternocostal and costovertebral joints
o Middle scalene: flexes and laterally flexes the neck at the spinal joints; elevates the first rib at the sternocostal and costovertebral joints
o Posterior scalene: laterally flexes the neck at the spinal joints; elevates the second rib at the sternocostal and costovertebral joints

Starting position (Figure 11-12):

o Client supine
o Therapist seated at the head of the table
o Palpating hand placed in the posterior triangle of the neck, just superior to the clavicle and just lateral to the inferior aspect of the lateral border of the clavicular head of the sternocleidomastoid (SCM)

Palpation steps:

1. Begin by locating the lateral border of the clavicular head of the SCM muscle (see Figure 11-6, A, page 187); then drop immediately off it laterally onto the scalenes in the posterior triangle of the neck.

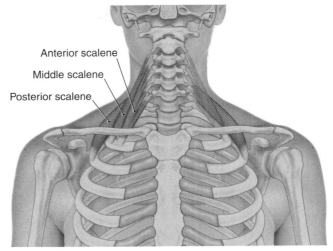

Figure 11-11 Anterior view of the scalenes. All three scalenes are seen on the right; the posterior scalene and ghosted-in middle scalene are seen on the left.

2. With your finger pads pressing into the scalene muscle group, ask the client to take in short, quick breaths through the nose and feel for the contraction of the scalene musculature (Figure 11-13).
3. Palpate as much of the scalenes in the posterior triangle of the neck between the SCM, upper trapezius, levator scapulae, and clavicle as possible. To best palpate the scalenes, remember to strum perpendicular to the fiber direction of the muscles.
4. Once the scalenes have been located, have the client relax them and palpate to assess their baseline tone.

Figure 11-12 Starting position for supine palpation of the right scalenes, lateral to the lateral border of the clavicular head of the SCM.

Figure 11-13 Palpation of the right scalenes as the client takes in short, quick breaths through the nose.

11

SCALENE GROUP—SUPINE—cont'd

Palpation Notes:

1. Taking in short, quick breaths requires the scalenes to contract to elevate the first and second ribs to expand the ribcage for inhalation.
2. It can be challenging to discern the anterior, middle, and posterior scalenes from each other. Knowing their location and the direction of their fibers helps. Much of the anterior scalene is deep to the SCM and its fibers are directed toward C3-C6. The middle scalene is located just lateral to the anterior scalene and has the greatest presence in the posterior triangle of the neck; its fibers are directed toward C2-C7. The posterior scalene is the most difficult to palpate of the three because it is mostly deep to other musculature. Feel for it just anterior to the upper trapezius and levator scapulae; its fibers are directed nearly horizontally toward C5-C7.
3. The scalene attachments on the transverse processes of the cervical spine can be palpated deep to the SCM if the SCM is first relaxed and slackened. To achieve this, passively move the client's head and neck into flexion and lateral flexion to the same side. Then slowly sink in deep to the SCM, pressing with your finger pads toward the transverse processes of the spine, and feel for the scalene attachments.
4. To better access the inferior attachments of the scalenes on the first and second ribs posterior to the clavicle, it can be helpful to slacken the scalenes by passively bringing the client's neck into lateral flexion to the side that is being palpated. This usually affords more space for the palpating fingers to reach down behind the clavicle toward the first and second ribs.
5. **Palpation of the scalenes must be done carefully because the brachial plexus of nerves and the subclavian artery are located between the anterior and middle scalenes (see Figure 11-1, C, on page 183).**

Alternate Palpation Position—Seated

Palpation Key:
Drop laterally off the SCM and have the client take in short, quick breaths through the nose.

11

Figure 11-14 The scalenes can be easily palpated with the client seated. Locate the lateral border of the clavicular head of the sternocleidomastoid (SCM) as explained on page 187; then drop off it onto the scalenes and follow the supine scalene palpation directions.

SCALENE GROUP—SUPINE—cont'd

TRIGGER POINTS

1. Trigger points (TrPs) in the scalenes often result from or are perpetuated by acute or chronic overuse of the muscles (e.g., coughing, labored breathing, especially due to chronic obstructive respiratory disease) or motor vehicle accidents.
2. TrPs in the scalenes tend to produce thoracic outlet syndrome (especially anterior scalene syndrome but also may contribute to costoclavicular syndrome, causing neurologic or vascular symptoms in the upper extremity), restricted lateral flexion and/or ipsilateral rotation of the neck, entrapment of nerve roots that contribute to the long thoracic nerve (that innervates the serratus anterior muscle), joint dysfunction of the first or second ribs, or painful sleeping.
3. The referral patterns of scalene TrPs must be distinguished from the referral patterns of TrPs in the levator scapulae, rhomboids, serratus posterior superior, subclavius, supraspinatus, infraspinatus, teres minor, subscapularis, latissimus dorsi, teres major, deltoid, coracobrachialis, biceps brachii, brachialis, triceps brachii, extensor carpi radialis brevis, extensor indicis, and supinator.
4. TrPs in the scalenes are often incorrectly assessed as cervical disc syndrome, cervical spine joint dysfunction, angina (from left-sided TrPs), costoclavicular syndrome, pectoralis minor syndrome, or carpal tunnel syndrome.
5. Associated TrPs often occur in the sternocleidomastoid, upper trapezius, splenius capitis, pectoralis major, pectoralis minor, deltoid, triceps brachii, posterior forearm extensor muscles, and brachialis.

Figure 11-15 A, Anterior view illustrating common scalene TrPs and their corresponding referral zone. **B**, Posterior view showing the remainder of the referral zone.

SCALENE GROUP—SUPINE—cont'd

STRETCHING THE SCALENE GROUP

Figure 11-16 A stretch of the right scalene group. The client extends, left laterally flexes, and right (ipsilaterally) rotates the neck. An additional stretch can be obtained by using the left hand to passively move the head and neck further in this direction.

DETOUR

Omohyoid inferior belly: The inferior belly of the omohyoid is fairly easily palpable in the posterior triangle of the neck. Palpate just lateral to the sternocleidomastoid (SCM) and superior to the clavicle, feeling for the horizontal fibers of the omohyoid as the client depresses the mandible at the temporomandibular joints (TMJs) against resistance. See page 197 for more on the palpation of the omohyoid and the rest of the hyoid group of muscles.

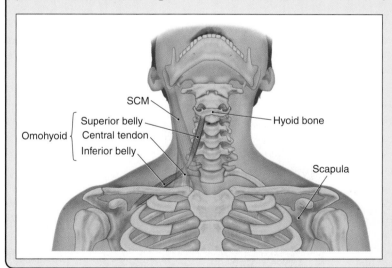

SCM
Superior belly
Omohyoid { Central tendon
Inferior belly
Hyoid bone
Scapula

Figure 11-17 Anterior view of the right omohyoid. The SCM has been ghosted in.

11

LONGUS COLLI AND LONGUS CAPITIS—SUPINE

❏ ATTACHMENTS:

o Longus colli: between T3 and C1, from transverse processes and anterior surfaces of vertebral bodies inferiorly
to the transverse processes and anterior surfaces of vertebral bodies superiorly

o Longus capitis: transverse processes of C3-C5 *to the*
occiput

❏ ACTIONS:

o Longus colli: flexes, laterally flexes, and contralaterally
rotates the neck at the spinal joints

o Longus capitis: flexes and laterally flexes the head and
neck at the spinal joints

Starting position (Figure 11-19):

o Client supine

o Therapist seated at the head of the table

o Place palpating hand just medial to the sternocleidomastoid (SCM) muscle

o Place support hand on the client's forehead (if resistance
will be added)

Palpation steps:

1. Begin by locating the medial border of the sternal head of
the SCM muscle (see page 187); then drop immediately
off it medially onto the longus muscles in the anterior
neck.

2. Gently and slowly but firmly sink in toward the anterior
surface of the vertebral bodies of the cervical spine. Note:
If you feel a pulse under your fingers, you are on the
common carotid artery; either gently move it out of the
way, or move your fingers slightly to one side of it or the
other, continuing to aim for the longus muscles.

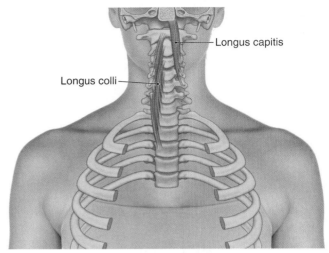

Figure 11-18 Anterior view of the longus colli and capitis. The longus colli is seen on the right; the longus capitis is seen on the left.

3. To confirm that you are on the longus musculature, ask
the client to flex the head and neck at the spinal joints by
lifting the head up from the table and feel for their contraction (Figure 11-20). Note: Lifting the head and neck up
into flexion against gravity usually creates a fairly strong
contraction of the longus muscles. However, if necessary,
resistance can be given with your support hand (as seen in
Figure 11-21).

4. Once located, strum perpendicular to the fibers and
palpate as far superiorly as possible and as far inferiorly as
possible.

5. Once the longus muscles have been located, have the
client relax them and palpate to assess their baseline tone.

Figure 11-19 Starting position for supine palpation of the right
longus colli and capitis.

Figure 11-20 Palpation of the right longus colli and capitis as
the client engages the muscles by lifting his head and neck into
flexion.

LONGUS COLLI AND LONGUS CAPITIS—SUPINE—cont'd

Palpation Notes:

1. The anterior neck has a number of fragile structures; therefore palpation into this region must be done carefully. When palpating, sink into the tissue slowly and gently, but with pressure that is firm enough to reach the longus musculature.
2. One precaution when palpating the longus musculature is the carotid sinus of the common carotid artery, located just lateral to the spine. Pressure against the carotid sinus can create a neurologic reflex that lowers blood pressure.
3. Another structure that requires careful palpation is the trachea. Be careful to not exert excessive pressure against the trachea or you may cause the client to involuntarily cough.
4. Even though there are many fragile and sensitive structures in the anterior neck, palpation/treatment of the longus muscles should not be avoided, because it can be very beneficial for the client.
5. If you find it difficult to discern the longus musculature from the SCM, ask the person to rotate the head and neck to the same side as where you are palpating; this will inhibit and relax the SCM.
6. The longus musculature of the spine is often injured in whiplash accidents.

TRIGGER POINTS

1. Trigger points (TrPs) in the longus muscles often result from or are perpetuated by acute or chronic overuse of the muscle, and trauma such as whiplash.
2. TrPs in the longus muscles tend to produce a sore throat, difficulty swallowing, and tight posterior neck muscles (working harder to oppose the tension of tight longus muscles).
3. The referral patterns of longus muscle TrPs must be distinguished from the referral patterns of TrPs in the anterior belly of the digastric and the SCM (due to the possible throat symptoms).
4. TrPs in the longus muscles are often incorrectly assessed as a sore throat.
5. Associated TrPs often occur in the posterior cervical muscles (e.g., upper trapezius, semispinalis capitis).
6. Note: Referral pain patterns for the longus colli and capitis have not been well mapped out.

STRETCHING THE LONGUS COLLI

Alternate Palpation Position—Seated

Figure 11-21 The longus muscles can be easily palpated with the client seated. Follow the supine directions; the only difference in this position is that it is necessary to resist flexion of the client's head and neck with your support hand to make the longus musculature contract (because flexion of the head and neck is not against gravity when seated).

Figure 11-22 A stretch of the right longus colli and capitis muscles. The client's head and neck are extended and laterally flexed to the opposite side.

Palpation Key:
Drop medially off the SCM and sink in toward the spine.

DETOUR

Rectus capitis anterior and lateralis: The rectus capitis anterior attaches from the occiput to the transverse process (TP) of the atlas (C1) and is extremely deep and usually not palpable; its action is flexion of the head at the atlanto-occipital joint. The rectus capitis lateralis also attaches from the occiput to the TP of the atlas and is also located quite deep, but can be sometimes be palpated; its action is lateral flexion of the head at the atlanto-occipital joint. To palpate the rectus capitis lateralis in the anterolateral neck, have the client supine or seated and palpate immediately superior to the TP of the atlas (Note:

The location of the TP of the atlas is often mistaken; it is located immediately posterior to the ramus of the mandible and inferior to the ear), between the atlas and the occiput. Press gently into the small depression that can often be felt here and feel for the rectus capitis lateralis (see Figure 11-24); it can be very difficult to discern this muscle from adjacent soft tissue. Notes: 1) Due to the presence of the facial nerve and styloid process located nearby, be careful to not press too forcefully. 2) Trigger point (TrP) pain referral zones for the rectus capitis anterior and lateralis have not been mapped out.

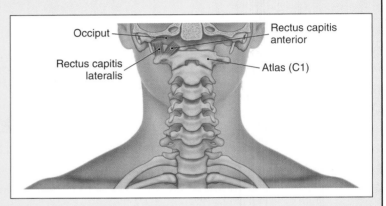

Figure 11-23 Anterior view of the right rectus capitis anterior and rectus capitis lateralis.

11

Figure 11-24 Palpation of the right rectus capitis lateralis superior to the transverse process of the atlas.

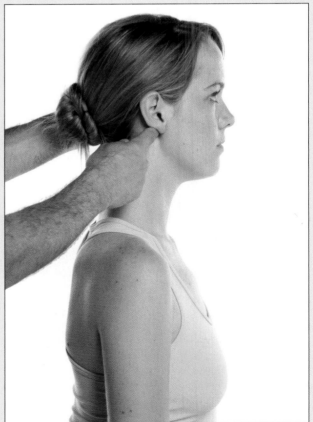

HYOID GROUP—SUPINE

❏ ATTACHMENTS:

o Infrahyoids:
  o Sternohyoid: sternum *to the* hyoid
  o Sternothyroid: sternum *to the* thyroid cartilage
  o Thyrohyoid: thyroid cartilage *to the* hyoid
  o Omohyoid: superior border of the scapula *to the* hyoid (with a central tendon attached to the clavicle)
o Suprahyoids:
  o Digastric: mastoid notch of the temporal bone *to the* mandible (with a central tendon attached to the hyoid)
  o Stylohyoid: styloid process of the temporal bone *to the* hyoid
  o Mylohyoid: hyoid *to the* inner surface of the mandible
  o Geniohyoid: hyoid *to the* inner surface of the mandible

❏ ACTIONS:

o Hyoid muscle group depresses the mandible at the temporomandibular joints (TMJs)
o Flexes the head and neck at the spinal joints
o Infrahyoids depress the hyoid bone; suprahyoids elevate the hyoid bone

Starting position (Figure 11-26):

o Client supine
o Therapist seated at the head of the table
o Palpating hand placed immediately inferior to the hyoid, just off center
o Support hand placed under the client's chin

Palpation steps:

1. Begin palpating the infrahyoid muscle group* by asking the client to depress the mandible at the TMJs while providing resistance with your support hand, and feel for the

---

*Palpation of the inferior belly of the omohyoid is shown as a detour when palpating the scalene muscle group on page 193.

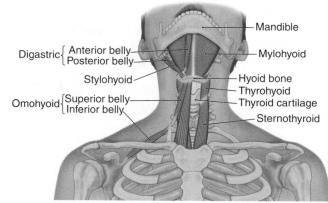

Figure 11-25 Anterior view of the hyoid muscle group. The sternohyoid, omohyoid, stylohyoid, and digastric have been removed on the left.

contraction of the infrahyoid muscles by strumming perpendicular to their fibers (Figure 11-27, A).

2. Continue palpating them inferiorly toward the sternum (strumming perpendicular to their fibers).
3. To palpate the suprahyoid muscle group, place your palpating hand just inferior to the mandible; add resistance to prevent the client from depressing the mandible at the TMJs, and feel for the contraction of the suprahyoid muscles (Figure 11-27, B).
4. Continue palpating them toward the hyoid bone while resisting mandibular depression by strumming perpendicular to their fibers.
5. To palpate the stylohyoid and the superior belly of the digastric of the suprahyoid group, continue palpating laterally from the hyoid toward the mastoid process of the temporal bone, while resisting mandibular depression and strumming perpendicular to the fibers (Figure 11-27, C).
6. Once the hyoid muscles have been located, have the client relax them and palpate to assess their baseline tone.

Figure 11-26 Starting position for supine palpation of the right hyoid muscles.

HYOID GROUP—SUPINE—cont'd

11

Figure 11-27 Palpation of the right hyoid muscles as the client depresses the mandible against resistance. **A**, Palpation of the right infrahyoids. **B**, Palpation of the right suprahyoids. **C**, Palpation of the right stylohyoid and superior belly of digastric (of the suprahyoid group).

HYOID GROUP—SUPINE—cont'd

Palpation Notes:

1. When depression of the mandible is resisted, all hyoid muscles contract. The digastric, mylohyoid, and genio-hyoid contract as movers to depress the mandible at the TMJs. The other hyoid muscles contract to stabilize the hyoid, providing a firm base from which the digastric, mylohyoid, and geniohyoid can pull upon the mandible.
2. If the hyoids contract as a group and the mandible is fixed to the temporal bone (by contraction of elevators of the mandible, such as the temporalis and/or masseter), the hyoids will exert their pull upon the head and cause flexion of the head and neck at the spinal joints.
3. Most of the hyoid muscles are small thin muscles and can be challenging to discern from each other.

Alternate Palpation Position

The hyoid muscles can be easily palpated with the client seated.

TRIGGER POINTS

Of all the hyoid muscles, the referral patterns for the digastric have been best mapped out. Each belly of the digastric has its own typical referral pattern.

1. Trigger points (TrPs) in the digastric often result from or are perpetuated by acute or chronic overuse of the muscle (e.g., having an open-mouthed posture, which is especially common for individuals who habitually breath through their mouth, perhaps because of nasal congestion; excessive tone to oppose tight elevators of the mandible, such as the temporalis, masseter, and medial pterygoid), protracted head posture (which causes a chronic pulling on all the hyoid muscles), or trauma such as whiplash.
2. TrPs in the inferior belly of the digastric tend to produce pain in the four lower incisor teeth (two on the same side as the TrP and two on the other side), tongue pain, throat discomfort, or difficulty swallowing. TrPs in the superior belly of the digastric tend to produce TrPs in the occipitofrontalis.
3. The referral patterns of digastric TrPs must be distinguished from the referral patterns of TrPs in the other hyoid muscles, sternocleidomastoid (SCM), upper trapezius,

medial pterygoid, longus colli and capitis (because of possible throat symptoms), and the suboccipitals.
4. TrPs in the digastric are often incorrectly assessed as dental conditions of the affected teeth (e.g., cavities) or tight SCM musculature.
5. Associated TrPs often occur in the ipsilateral occipitofrontalis or SCM. They also often occur ipsilaterally or contralaterally in other hyoid muscles and the masseter, temporalis, or medial pterygoid.
6. Notes: 1) The stylohyoid lies next to the posterior belly of the digastric, is difficult to discern from the digastric, and is assumed to have a similar referral pattern to the posterior digastric. Furthermore, the stylohyoid has been known to cause entrapment of the external carotid artery. 2) TrPs in the omohyoid are thought to create tension in the muscle that can press on the brachial plexus of nerves (causing thoracic outlet syndrome) and can contribute via its fascial attachments to dysfunction of the costospinal joints of the first rib. 3) Similar to the inferior belly of the digastric, the mylohyoid has also been reported to refer pain to the tongue.

Figure 11-28 Common digastric TrPs and their corresponding referral zones. **A**, Lateral view. **B**, Anterior view.

11

HYOID GROUP—SUPINE—cont'd

STRETCHING THE HYOID

Palpation Key:
Resist depression of the mandible.

Figure 11-29 A stretch of the right hyoids. The client's neck is extended and left laterally flexed.

11

UPPER TRAPEZIUS—SEATED

❏ ATTACHMENTS:

o External occipital protuberance and medial ⅓ of the superior nuchal line of the occiput, entire nuchal ligament, and the spinous process of C7 *to the* lateral clavicle and the acromion process of the scapula

❏ ACTIONS:

o Elevates, retracts, and upwardly rotates the scapula at the scapulocostal joint
o Extends, laterally flexes, and contralaterally rotates the head and neck at the spinal joints

Starting position (Figure 11-31):

o Client seated with the head and neck rotated to the opposite side (contralaterally) of the body
o Therapist standing to the side of the client
o Place palpating hand on the upper trapezius at the top of the shoulder region
o Place support hand on the back of the client's head

Palpation steps:

1. Resist extension of the client's head and neck at the spinal joints, and look and feel for the contraction of the upper trapezius (Figure 11-32).
2. Continue palpating the upper trapezius superiorly to the occiput and inferiorly to the scapula and clavicle (strumming perpendicular to its fibers).
3. Once the upper trapezius has been located, have the client relax it and palpate to assess its baseline tone.

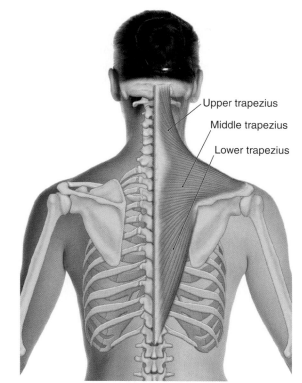

Figure 11-30 Posterior view of the right trapezius. The sternocleidomastoid, splenius capitis, and levator scapulae have been ghosted in.

11

Figure 11-31 Starting position for seated palpation of the right upper trapezius.

Figure 11-32 Palpation of the right upper trapezius as the client extends the head and neck against resistance.

UPPER TRAPEZIUS—SEATED—cont'd

Palpation Note:

1. All muscles in the posterior neck will contract with resisted extension of the head and neck at the spinal joints. By having the client contralaterally rotate the head and neck (to the opposite side), the splenius capitis and cervicis will be reciprocally inhibited (relaxed) and the upper trapezius will be more forcefully engaged and therefore easier to palpate.

Alternate Palpation Position—Prone

Figure 11-33 The upper trapezius can be palpated with the client prone (see page 142). Asking the client to lift her head up from the face cradle will engage the upper trapezius.

TRIGGER POINTS

1. Trigger points (TrPs) in the upper trapezius often result from or are perpetuated by acute or chronic overuse of the muscle (e.g., chronic postures of elevation of the shoulder girdle, anteriorly held head, or any chronic posture due to poor ergonomics, especially at the computer or with crimping the phone between the ear and shoulder; also when working to resist depression of the shoulder girdle when the upper extremity is hanging, and especially when the upper extremity is carrying a weight), trauma (e.g., whiplash), compression forces (e.g., carrying a heavy purse or backpack on the shoulder, having a tight bra strap), irritation from wearing a tie or a shirt with a tight collar, having a cold draft on the neck, or chronic stress/tension (holding the shoulder girdles uptight).

2. TrPs in the upper trapezius tend to produce a classic stiff neck with restricted contralateral lateral flexion and ipsilateral rotation of the neck at the spinal joints, a posture of elevated shoulder girdles, pain at the end of ipsilateral rotation of the neck, and tension headaches.

3. The referral patterns of upper trapezius TrPs must be distinguished from the referral patterns of TrPs in the sternocleidomastoid, masseter, temporalis, occipitalis, splenius cervicis, levator scapulae, semispinalis capitis, cervical multifidus, and lower trapezius.

4. TrPs in the trapezius are often incorrectly assessed as cervical disc syndrome, TMJ syndrome, or greater occipital neuralgia.

5. Associated TrPs of the upper trapezius often occur in the scalenes, splenius capitis and cervicis, levator scapulae, rhomboids, semispinalis capitis, temporalis, masseter, and contralateral upper trapezius.

6. Note: The upper trapezius has the most commonly found TrP in the body. Furthermore, the referral symptoms of this common TrP occasionally spread to the other side of the body.

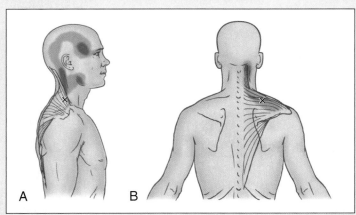

Figure 11-34 Common upper trapezius TrPs and their corresponding referral zones. **A**, Lateral view. **B**, Posterior view.

UPPER TRAPEZIUS—SEATED—cont'd

STRETCHING THE UPPER TRAPEZIUS

Palpation Key:
Contralaterally rotate and push back into extension.

Figure 11-35 A stretch of the right upper trapezius. The client's head and neck are flexed, left laterally flexed (to the opposite side), and (ipsilaterally) rotated to the right. To keep the shoulder girdle down, the right hand holds onto the bench.

11

LEVATOR SCAPULAE—SEATED

❑ **ATTACHMENTS:**

o Transverse processes of C1-C4 *to the* medial border of the scapula from the root of the spine to the superior angle

❑ **ACTIONS:**

o Elevates and downwardly rotates the scapula at the scapulocostal joint
o Extends, laterally flexes, and ipsilaterally rotates the neck at the spinal joints

Starting position (Figure 11-37):

o Client seated with the hand in the small of the back
o Therapist standing behind or to the side of the client
o Place palpating hand immediately superior and medial to the superior angle of the scapula
o Place support hand on top of the client's shoulder

Palpation steps:

1. With the client's hand in the small of the back, the client is asked to perform a gentle, very short range of motion of elevation of the scapula at the scapulocostal joint. Feel for the levator scapulae's contraction deep to the trapezius (Figure 11-38, A).
2. Continue palpating the levator scapulae toward its superior attachment by strumming perpendicular to its fibers.
3. Once you are palpating the levator scapulae in the posterior triangle of the neck (superior to the trapezius), the client's hand no longer needs to be in the small of the back. It is also possible to ask the client to elevate the scapula more forcefully now; resistance can also be added with your support hand (Figure 11-38, B).

Levator scapulae

Trapezius

Figure 11-36 Posterior view of the right levator scapulae. The trapezius has been ghosted in.

4. Palpate the levator scapulae as far superiorly as possible (near its superior attachment, it will go deep to the sternocleidomastoid).
5. Once the levator scapulae has been located, have the client relax it and palpate to assess its baseline tone.

Figure 11-37 Starting position for seated palpation of the right levator scapulae.

LEVATOR SCAPULAE—SEATED—cont'd

Figure 11-38 Palpation of the right levator scapulae. **A**, Palpation of the levator scapulae deep to the trapezius as the client performs gentle, short ranges of motion of elevation of the scapula with the hand in the small of the back; no resistance is given. **B**, Palpation in the posterior triangle of the neck; resistance can now be added to elevation of the scapula to better engage the levator scapulae.

11

Palpation Notes:

1. Having the client place the hand in the small of the back requires extension and adduction of the arm at the shoulder joint. This requires the coupled action of downward rotation of the scapula at the scapulocostal joint, which will cause the trapezius to relax (because of reciprocal inhibition) so that the inferior attachment of the levator scapulae can be clearly felt when the levator scapulae contracts. It will also engage the levator scapulae, so its contraction will be more clearly felt.

2. Do not have the client perform a forceful action of elevation of the scapula, or the reflex of reciprocal inhibition will be overcome and the upper trapezius will contract, blocking palpation of the levator scapulae at its inferior attachment.

3. Once the levator scapulae is being palpated in the posterior triangle of the neck, it is no longer necessary to have the client place the hand in the small of the back because it is no longer necessary to relax the trapezius. Furthermore, once we are palpating the levator scapulae in the posterior triangle, a forceful contraction of the levator scapulae can be engaged to better palpate and locate it.

4. In middle-aged and older people, the levator scapulae is often visible in the posterior triangle of the neck, even when they are not consciously contracting it (see Figure 10-23 on page 150).

5. It can be challenging to palpate the most superior aspect of the levator scapulae deep to the sternocleidomastoid (SCM). To do so, slacken the SCM by slightly flexing and ipsilaterally laterally flexing (same-side lateral flexion of) the neck and try to palpate deep to the SCM (Figure 11-39).

6. Note that the transverse process (TP) of C1 is directly inferior to the ear (between the mastoid process and the ramus of the mandible)! See Figure 11-39.

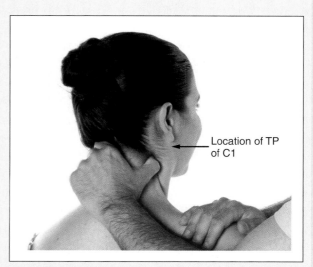

Location of TP of C1

Figure 11-39 The superior attachment of the levator scapulae is accessed by reaching under the SCM and pressing anteriorly and superiorly toward the TP of the atlas (C1). This is best accomplished by first passively slackening the SCM by moving the client's head and neck into flexion and ipsilateral (same side) lateral flexion (not shown). Note the location of the TP of C1.

LEVATOR SCAPULAE—SEATED—cont'd

Alternate Palpation Position

The levator scapulae can be palpated with the client prone (see Figures 10-21 and 10-22).

TRIGGER POINTS

1. Trigger points (TrPs) in the levator scapulae often result from or are perpetuated by acute or chronic overuse of the muscle (e.g., carrying a bag or purse on the shoulder, crimping a phone between the ear and shoulder, excessive exercise such as playing tennis, holding the shoulders uptight), chronic shortening or stretching of the muscle due to poor work or leisure postures (e.g., having a poorly placed computer monitor, reading with the head inclined forward), motor vehicle accidents, having a cold draft on the neck, or being overly stressed psychologically.
2. TrPs in the levator scapulae tend to produce a classic stiff neck (often called *torticollis* or *wry neck*) with restricted contralateral rotation of the neck.
3. The referral patterns of levator scapulae TrPs must be distinguished from the referral patterns of TrPs in the scalenes, rhomboids, supraspinatus, and infraspinatus.
4. TrPs in the levator scapulae are often incorrectly assessed as joint dysfunction of the cervical spine.
5. Associated TrPs often occur in the upper trapezius, splenius cervicis, scalenes, and erector spinae of the cervical spine.

Figure 11-40 Posterior view illustrating common levator scapulae TrPs and their corresponding referral zone.

Figure 11-41 A stretch of the right levator scapulae. The client's neck is flexed, left laterally flexed, and (ipsilaterally) rotated to the left. To keep the shoulder girdle down, the right hand holds onto the bench.

Palpation Key:
Client's hand in the small of the back.

SPLENIUS CAPITIS—SEATED

❑ ATTACHMENTS:

o Nuchal ligament from the level of C3-C6 and the spinous processes of C7-T4 *to the* mastoid process of the temporal bone and the lateral $^1/_3$ of the superior nuchal line of the occiput

❑ ACTIONS:

o Extends, laterally flexes, and ipsilaterally rotates the head and neck at the spinal joints

Starting position (Figure 11-43):

o Client seated with the head and neck ipsilaterally rotated
o Therapist standing behind the client
o Palpating hand placed at the upper aspect of the posterior triangle of the neck just inferior to the occiput and just posterior to the sternocleidomastoid (SCM); the splenius capitis is superficial here (see palpation of the SCM on page 187)
o Support hand placed on the back of the client's head

Palpation steps:

1. With palpating hand in position and the client's head and neck ipsilaterally rotated, resist the client from extending the head and neck at the spinal joints and feel for the contraction of the splenius capitis (Figure 11-44).
2. Strum perpendicular to the fibers of the splenius capitis in the posterior triangle until you reach the border of the upper trapezius.
3. While asking the client to alternately extend the head and neck against gentle resistance and then relax, feel for the

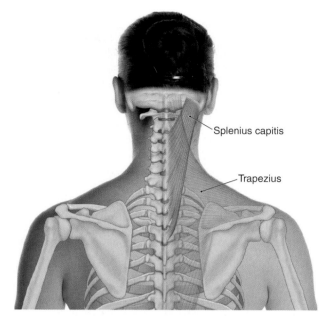

Figure 11-42 Posterior view of the right splenius capitis. The trapezius has been ghosted in.

contraction and relaxation of the splenius capitis deep to the upper trapezius. Continue palpating the splenius capitis deep to the trapezius as far inferiorly as possible.
4. Once the splenius capitis has been located, have the client relax it and palpate to assess its baseline tone.

Figure 11-43 Starting position for seated palpation of the right splenius capitis.

Figure 11-44 Palpation of the right splenius capitis in the posterior triangle of the neck as the client extends the head and neck against resistance.

SPLENIUS CAPITIS—SEATED—cont'd

Palpation Notes:

1. By having the client's head and neck ipsilaterally rotated, the splenius capitis is better engaged to contract. Ipsilateral rotation also reciprocally inhibits and therefore relaxes the sternocleidomastoid and upper trapezius. Relaxing the upper trapezius makes it easier to feel the contraction of the splenius capitis deep to it. However, only gentle resistance should be given to the client's head and neck extension, or the reciprocal inhibition of the upper trapezius will be overridden and it will contract, blocking the ability to palpate the splenius capitis deep to it.

2. The inferior attachment of the splenius capitis on the spinous processes of the upper thoracic spine can be directly accessed by palpating anterior to the border of the upper trapezius and pressing downward toward the spinous processes. Sink slowly into the tissue with your finger pads oriented anteriorly, using firm pressure to palpate deep toward the spinous processes (see Figure 11-45).

3. The client's hand can be place in the small of the back to inhibit and relax the upper trapezius. Placing the hand in this manner requires extension and adduction of the arm at the shoulder joint, which requires downward rotation of the scapula at the scapulocostal joint. Because the upper trapezius is an upward rotator of the scapula, it is inhibited and relaxed.

11

Alternate Palpation Position—Prone or Supine

Figure 11-45 The splenius capitis can also be palpated with the client prone or supine. The prone position especially allows easy access to the inferior attachment on the spinous processes, deep to the trapezius (as explained in Palpation Note #2).

Palpation Key:
Begin at the top of the posterior triangle.

TRIGGER POINTS

1. Trigger points (TrPs) in the splenius capitis often result from or are perpetuated by acute or chronic overuse of the muscle (e.g., prolonged forward head posture, or prolonged posture with the head and neck rotated to one side, for example when working on a computer in which the monitor is not located directly in front of the person; or when playing violin), a sudden excessive stretch (e.g., whiplash injury), or a cold draft on the neck.

2. TrPs in the splenius capitis tend to produce restricted flexion and contralateral rotation of the head and neck at the spinal joints, restricted active rotation to the same side (due to pain upon contraction), cervical joint dysfunction, or headaches.

3. The referral patterns of splenius capitis TrPs must be distinguished from the referral patterns of TrPs in the occipitofrontalis and sternocleidomastoid.

4. TrPs in the splenius capitis are often incorrectly assessed as cervical joint dysfunction, migraine headaches, or spasmodic torticollis.

5. Associated TrPs often occur in the splenius cervicis, upper trapezius, levator scapulae, and semispinalis capitis.

Figure 11-46 Lateral view illustrating a common splenius capitis TrP and its corresponding referral zone.

SPLENIUS CAPITIS—SEATED—cont'd

STRETCHING THE SPLENIUS CAPITIS

Figure 11-47 A stretch of the right splenius capitis and cervicis. The client flexes, left laterally flexes, and left (contralaterally) rotates the head and neck. Note: This stretch is identical to the levator scapulae stretch (Figure 11-41) except that there is no need to hold the scapula down with this stretch.

DETOUR

Splenius cervicis: The splenius cervicis attaches from the spinous processes of T3-T6 to the transverse processes of C1-C3 (Figure 11-48, A) and is deep to other musculature for its entire course; therefore it can be difficult to palpate and discern. The best place to first locate and palpate the splenius cervicis is between the levator scapulae and splenius capitis muscles (see Figure 11-2, A, right side). The actions of the splenius cervicis are the same as the splenius capitis, except that the splenius cervicis only moves the neck, not the head. Ask the client to ipsilaterally rotate the neck (against resistance if necessary) and feel for its contraction. Once located, try to follow toward both attachments.

Palpation Key: Palpate between the splenius capitis and levator scapulae.

Trigger Points:
1. Trigger points (TrPs) in the splenius cervicis often result from or are perpetuated by the same factors that create/perpetuate TrPs in the splenius capitis.
2. TrPs in the splenius cervicis tend to produce headaches, eye pain, or even blurriness of vision in the ipsilateral eye.
3. The referral patterns of splenius cervicis TrPs must be distinguished from the referral patterns of TrPs in the trapezius, sternocleidomastoid, suboccipitals, occipitofrontalis, temporalis, masseter, levator scapulae, and erector spinae and transversospinalis of the upper trunk.
4. TrPs in the splenius cervicis are often incorrectly assessed as cervical joint dysfunction, migraine headaches, or spasmodic torticollis.
5. Associated TrPs often occur in the splenius capitis, upper trapezius, levator scapulae, and semispinalis capitis.

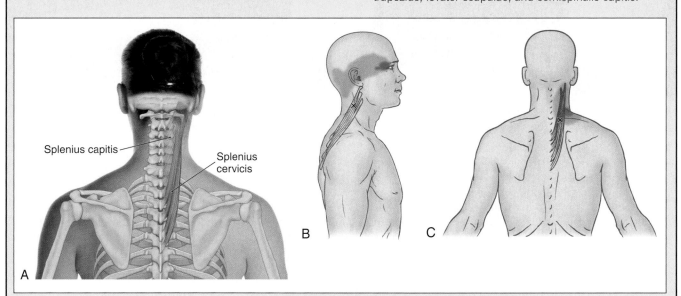

Splenius capitis

Splenius cervicis

A

B

C

Figure 11-48 The splenius cervicis. **A,** Posterior view of Tour right splenius cervicis; the splenius capitis has been ghosted in. Common splenius cervicis TrPs and their corresponding referral zones are shown in lateral view **(B)** and posterior view **(C).**

11

SEMISPINALIS CAPITIS—SUPINE

❏ ATTACHMENTS:

o Transverse processes of C7-T6 and articular processes of C4-6 *to the* medial $^1/_2$ of the occipital bone between the superior and inferior nuchal lines

❏ ACTIONS:

o Extends and laterally flexes the head and neck at the spinal joints

Starting position (Figure 11-50):

o Client supine with the hand in the small of the back and/ or the head and neck rotated to the same side (ipsilaterally rotated)
o Therapist seated at the head of the table
o Palpating hand placed just below the occiput and just lateral to the midline of the spine (i.e., over the laminar groove)

Palpation steps:

1. Ask the client to extend the head and neck at the spinal joints by gently pressing the head into the table, and feel for the contraction of the semispinalis capitis deep to the upper trapezius (Figure 11-51).
2. Once felt, continue palpating superiorly to the occiput and then inferiorly as far as possible by strumming perpendicular to its fibers.
3. Once the semispinalis capitis has been located, have the client relax it and palpate to assess its baseline tone.

Figure 11-49 Posterior view of the right semispinalis capitis. The semispinalis thoracis and cervicis are seen on the left. The semispinalis capitis is seen on the right; the erector spinae group has been ghosted in on the right.

Figure 11-50 Starting position for supine palpation of the right semispinalis capitis.

Figure 11-51 Palpation of the right semispinalis capitis as the client extends the head and neck down against the table.

Palpation Notes:

1. The hand is placed in the small of the back to extend and adduct the arm at the shoulder joint, which requires downward rotation of the scapula at the scapulocostal joint; this reciprocally inhibits and relaxes the upper trapezius, making it easier to palpate the semispinalis deep to it. Ipsilaterally rotating the head and neck also reciprocally inhibits the upper trapezius. Be sure that the client does not contract the head and neck into extension too forcefully, or the neurologic reflex of reciprocal inhibition will be overridden and the upper trapezius will contract, blocking the ability to palpate the semispinalis capitis deep to it.
2. Even though the upper trapezius is the best known muscle of the posterior neck, the semispinalis capitis muscle in the neck is appreciably larger and thicker; in fact, it is the largest muscle of the neck.

SEMISPINALIS CAPITIS—SUPINE—cont'd

Alternate Palpation Position—Prone

Figure 11-52 The semispinalis capitis can also be palpated with the client prone. In this position, it is also important to reciprocally inhibit the upper trapezius to relax it; this is accomplished by having the client ipsilaterally rotate the head and neck at the spinal joints. Then the head can be lifted up slightly into extension against gravity to engage the semispinalis capitis. Note: The upper trapezius can also be inhibited by having the client place the hand in the small of the back, as seen in Figure 11-50.

TRIGGER POINTS

1. Trigger points (TrPs) in the semispinalis capitis often result from or are perpetuated by acute or chronic overuse of the muscle (e.g., prolonged protracted head posture, or prolonged posture where the head and neck are flexed with their center of weight imbalanced anterior to the trunk), prolonged postures that result in shortening of the muscle (e.g., propping up on elbows to support the head when watching television or when lying prone and doing homework on a bed), trauma such as a whiplash or a fall, radiculopathy of the cervical spinal nerves, osteoarthritic changes of the cervical spine, irritation from wearing a tie or a shirt with a tight collar, a cold draft on the neck, or secondary to TrPs in the upper trapezius or splenius capitis.

2. TrPs in the semispinalis capitis tend to produce headaches, restricted head and neck flexion or contralateral lateral flexion, entrapment of the greater occipital nerve (which may result in altered sensation in the posterior scalp, such as tingling or pain), or joint dysfunction or osteoarthritis of the cervical spine.

3. The referral patterns of semispinalis capitis TrPs must be distinguished from the referral patterns of TrPs in the trapezius, sternocleidomastoid, temporalis, occipitofrontalis, and the suboccipitals.

4. TrPs in the semispinalis capitis are often incorrectly assessed as osteoarthritis of the cervical spine or sinus or migraine headaches.

5. Associated TrPs often occur in the upper trapezius, semispinalis cervicis, splenius capitis or cervicis, and erector spinae and transversospinalis muscles of the trunk.

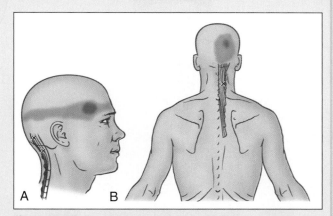

Figure 11-53 Common semispinalis capitis TrPs and their corresponding referral zones. **A**, Lateral view. **B**, Posterior view.

STRETCHING THE SEMISPINALIS CAPITIS

Figure 11-54 A stretch of the right semispinalis capitis. The client flexes and left laterally flexes the head and neck. Note: Flexion is the most important component of this stretch.

Palpation Key:
Reciprocally inhibit the upper trapezius and palpate deep to it.

11

SEMISPINALIS CAPITIS—SUPINE—cont'd

DETOUR

Longissimus capitis, semispinalis cervicis, and cervical multifidus and rotatores: The longissimus capitis of the erector spinae group attaches from the transverse or articular processes of C5-T5 to the mastoid process of the temporal bone; it is deep for its entire course and therefore challenging to palpate and discern. Its actions are extension and ipsilateral rotation of the neck and head at the spinal joints. To locate it, with the client supine, palpate lateral to the splenius capitis, and deep to the levator scapulae and upper trapezius. Gentle extension of the head against the table with the head and neck ipsilaterally rotated will cause it to contract (and reciprocally inhibit the upper trapezius).

The semispinalis cervicis attaches from the transverse processes of T1-T5 to the spinous processes of C2-C5; it is also deep (primarily to the semispinalis capitis) and challenging to palpate and discern.

The cervical multifidus and rotatores are located very deep within the laminar groove of the cervical spine and are also very challenging to palpate and discern.

The semispinalis, multifidus, and rotatores are members of the transversospinalis group and extend and contralaterally rotate the neck at the spinal joints.

Trigger Points:
1. Trigger points (TrPs) in the longissimus capitis usually refer pain posterior to the ear. Pain referral may also occur in the neck or around the eye. These TrPs are also often involved in joint dysfunction of the costospinal joints of the first rib (Figure 11-55, B).
2. TrPs in the semispinalis cervicis likely refer pain to the occipital region in a pattern similar to the semispinalis capitis (see Figure 11-53, B).
3. TrPs in the multifidus of the cervical spine usually refer pain superiorly to the suboccipital region and inferiorly to the medial border of the scapula (Figure 11-55, C).
4. TrPs in the rotatores of the cervical spine usually refer pain to the midline of the spine at the segmental level of the TrP (similar to rotatores TrPs in the thoracic and lumbar regions) (Figure 11-55, D).

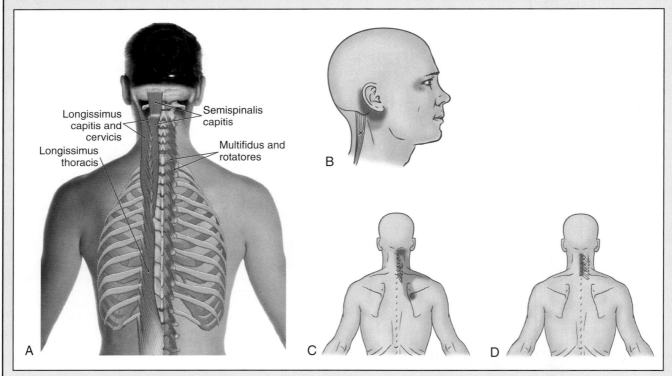

Figure 11-55 A, Posterior view of the longissimus, semispinalis, multifidus, and rotatores. The longissimus and semispinalis are seen on the left; the multifidus (ghosted in) and rotatores are seen on the right. **B, C,** and **D,** Common TrPs and their corresponding referral zones. **B,** Lateral view of a common TrP in the longissimus capitis and its referral zone. **C,** Posterior view of a common TrP in the cervical multifidus and its referral zone. **D,** Posterior view of common TrPs in the cervical rotatores and their referral zone.

SUBOCCIPITAL GROUP—SUPINE

11-3   11-4

The suboccipital group is composed of the following:

o Rectus capitis posterior major (RCPMaj)
o Rectus capitis posterior minor (RCPMin)
o Obliquus capitis inferior (OCI)
o Obliquus capitis superior (OCS)

❏ ATTACHMENTS:

o RCPMaj: spinous process of C2 *to the* lateral ½ of the inferior nuchal line of the occiput
o RCPMin: posterior tubercle of C1 *to the* medial ½ of the inferior nuchal line of the occiput
o OCI: spinous process of C2 *to the* transverse process of C1
o OCS: transverse process of C1 *to the* lateral occiput between the superior and inferior nuchal lines

❏ ACTIONS:

o As a group, the suboccipital muscles extend and anteriorly translate the head at the atlanto-occipital joint.
o The obliquus capitis inferior ipsilaterally rotates the atlas at the atlantoaxial joint.

Starting position (Figure 11-57):

o Client supine
o Therapist seated at the head of the table
o Palpating hand placed just superior and slightly lateral to the spinous process of C2 (the axis)

Palpation steps:

1. The easiest suboccipital muscle to palpate is the rectus capitis posterior major (RCPMaj). Begin by finding the spinous process of C2, an easy landmark to locate in the upper neck. Then palpate just superolateral to it and feel for the RCPMaj by strumming perpendicular to its fibers.
2. If located, continue strumming perpendicularly, following it superolaterally toward its occipital attachment (Figure 11-58, A).
3. Repeat the same steps for the rectus capitis posterior minor (RCPMin) by starting just superolateral to the posterior tubercle of C1. Strum perpendicular to locate the muscle; then follow toward the occipital attachment (Figure 11-58, B). It may be helpful to have the RCPMin contract by asking the client to anteriorly translate the head at the atlanto-occipital joint (see Palpation Note #3).
4. To palpate the obliquus capitis inferior (OCI), palpate between the spinous process of C2 and the transverse process of C1, strumming perpendicular to the fibers. It may be helpful to have the OCI contract by gently resisting the client's ipsilateral rotation of the head.
5. The obliquus capitis superior is extremely challenging to palpate and discern from adjacent musculature. To attempt its palpation, feel for it just lateral to the superior attachment of the RCPMaj; if felt, try to continue palpating it inferiorly by strumming perpendicular to it.
6. Once the suboccipital muscles have been located, have the client relax them and palpate to assess their baseline tone.

11

Rectus capitis posterior minor

Rectus capitis posterior major

Obliquus capitis superior

Obliquus capitis inferior

A

OCS

RCPMin

B

Figure 11-56 Views of the right suboccipital group. **A,** Posterior view. **B,** Lateral view. Note the anterior to posterior horizontal direction of the rectus capitis posterior minor (RCPMin) and the obliquus capitis superior (OCS). This fiber direction is ideal for anterior translation of the head at the atlanto-occipital joint.

SUBOCCIPITAL GROUP—SUPINE—cont'd

Figure 11-57 Starting position for supine palpation of the right suboccipital muscles.

Figure 11-58 Palpation of the suboccipital muscles. **A**, Palpation of the right RCPMaj between the spinous process of the axis (C2) and the occiput. **B**, Palpation of the right RCPMin between the posterior tubercle of the atlas (C1) and the occiput.

SUBOCCIPITAL GROUP—SUPINE—cont'd

Palpation Notes:

1. Generally it is best to palpate the suboccipital muscles when they are relaxed. They are deep and can be challenging to palpate and discern. However, if the superficial muscles are loose and the suboccipitals are tight, they can be fairly easily palpated.

2. The easiest suboccipital muscle to palpate is the rectus capitis posterior major. The obliquus capitis superior is usually the most difficult to palpate.

3. **A certain amount of caution must be exercised when palpating and pressing into the region known as the *suboccipital triangle* (bounded by the RCPMaj and the two obliquus capitis muscles), because of the presence of the vertebral artery and suboccipital nerve. The greater occipital nerve is also located nearby.**

4. Anterior translation of the head involves the head gliding directly anterior at the atlanto-occipital joint. Asking the client to create this action will cause the rectus capitis posterior minor to contract and become more easily palpable.

Palpation Key:

Begin at the spinous process of C2 for the rectus capitis posterior major.

TRIGGER POINTS

1. Trigger points (TrPs) in the suboccipitals often result from or are perpetuated by acute or chronic overuse of the muscle (e.g., sustained extension of the head at the atlanto-occipital joint, perhaps while painting a ceiling or bird-watching, or sustained posture with the head rotated to one side [for the OCI]), chronic forward (anterior translation) head posture, trauma such as whiplash, having a cold draft on the neck, or joint dysfunction of the atlanto-occipital or atlantoaxial joints.

2. TrPs in the suboccipitals tend to produce headache pain that is diffuse and difficult to localize, restrict flexion or contralateral lateral flexion of the head at the atlanto-occipital joint, restrict contralateral rotation of the axis at the atlantoaxial joint (OCI), or cause joint dysfunction of the atlanto-occipital or atlantoaxial joints.

3. The referral patterns of suboccipital TrPs must be distinguished from the referral patterns of TrPs in the sternocleidomastoid, temporalis, splenius cervicis, and semispinalis capitis.

4. TrPs in the suboccipitals are often incorrectly assessed as migraines or greater occipital neuralgia.

5. Associated TrPs often occur in the other posterior cervical muscles or the occipitalis.

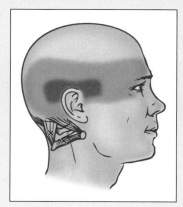

Figure 11-59 Lateral view illustrating common suboccipital TrPs and their corresponding referral zone.

11

SUBOCCIPITAL GROUP—SUPINE—cont'd

STRETCHING THE SUBOCCIPITALS

Figure 11-60 Stretches of the suboccipital muscles. **A**, Stretch of the bilateral rectus capitis posterior major and minor muscles as well as the bilateral obliquus capitis superior muscles. The client both flexes the head (by tucking the chin toward the chest) and posteriorly translates the head at the atlanto-occipital joint. To focus this stretch to the right suboccipitals, add left lateral flexion (not shown). **B**, Stretch of the right obliquus capitis inferior. The client rotates as far as possible to the (contralateral) left side.

11

Muscles of the Neck

Client Supine:

1. **Sternocleidomastoid (SCM):** The client is supine with the head and neck contralaterally rotated; you are seated at the head of the table. Before palpating, first visualize the contraction of the SCM as the client lifts the head from the table. Then palpate the contraction of the SCM just superior to the sternoclavicular joint as the client again lifts the head from the table. Once felt, continue palpating the SCM to the mastoid process of the temporal bone and the superior nuchal line of the occipital bone by strumming perpendicular to the fibers as the client alternately contracts and relaxes the muscle. Note: Look and palpate carefully for the clavicular head; it is usually less obvious than the sternal head.

2. **Scalene group:** The client is supine; you are seated at the head of the table. Locate the lateral border of the clavicular head of the SCM (be sure that it is the lateral border of the clavicular head, not the sternal head that you have located). Place palpating fingers just lateral to the lateral border of the clavicular head of the SCM and just superior to the clavicle, and feel for the contraction of the scalenes as the client takes in short, quick breaths through the nose. Once felt, palpate as much of the scalenes as possible in the posterior triangle of the neck by strumming perpendicular to the fibers. The transverse processes attachment of the scalenes can usually be palpated by pressing in deep to the SCM if it is first slackened by passively flexing and ipsilaterally laterally flexing the client's head and neck. Note: It can be challenging to discern the anterior, middle, and posterior scalenes from each other. The best way to achieve this is to try to feel for the different direction of fibers that each one has. Remember: the anterior scalene goes to C3-C6; the middle scalene goes to C2-C7; and the posterior scalene goes to C5-C7. Also, keep in mind that the posterior scalene is located in the posterior triangle of the neck immediately anterior to the upper trapezius and levator scapulae.

3. **Longus colli/longus capitis:** The client is supine; you are seated at the head of the table. Locate the medial border of the sternal head of the SCM, and then drop off it and place palpating fingers immediately medial to that. Sink in toward the anterior surface of the vertebral bodies slowly and gently, but firmly. If you feel a pulse under your fingers, move your fingers to one side or the other and continue palpating for the vertebral bodies. Once you have reached the vertebral bodies, confirm that you are on the longus colli by asking the client to flex the head and neck by lifting the head up off the table. Palpate as much of the longus colli and capitis as possible superiorly and inferiorly by strumming perpendicular to the fibers. Note: The carotid tubercle on the transverse process of C6 (see page 100) is a good landmark for determining the segmental level of the palpating fingers.

4. **Hyoid group:** For the purpose of palpation, the hyoid group can be divided into the infrahyoid group and the suprahyoid group. The client is supine; you are seated at the head of the table. To palpate the infrahyoids, place your palpating fingers immediately inferior to the hyoid bone and just off center and feel for their contraction as the client is resisted from depressing the mandible at the temporomandibular joints (TMJs). Once felt, palpate these muscles toward their inferior attachments on the sternum by strumming perpendicular to the fibers as the client alternately contracts and relaxes them. The inferior belly of the omohyoid can be palpated in the posterior triangle of the neck by strumming perpendicular to it as the client is resisted from depressing the mandible at the TMJs. To palpate the suprahyoids, place your palpating fingers immediately inferior to the mandible and again feel for their contraction as the client is resisted from depressing the mandible at the TMJs. Once felt, palpate these muscles toward the hyoid bone by strumming perpendicular to the fibers as the client alternately contracts and relaxes them. Palpate the stylohyoid and superior belly of the digastric by strumming perpendicular to their fibers from the hyoid bone toward the mastoid process of the temporal bone as the client alternately contracts and relaxes them.

Client Seated:

5. **Upper trapezius:** The client is seated with the head and neck contralaterally rotated; you are standing to the side of the client. Feel for the contraction of the upper trapezius at the top of the shoulder as the client is resisted from extending the head and neck against the resistance of your support hand on the back of their head (Note: The contraction of the upper trapezius is often visible and palpable; be sure to look for it as well). Continue palpating the upper trapezius toward its medial attachment on the head and neck and its lateral attachment on the lateral clavicle and acromion process by strumming perpendicular to its fibers as the client alternately contracts and relaxes it. Note: The superior aspect of the upper trapezius is actually quite narrow and only attaches to the medial 1/3 of the superior nuchal line of the occipital bone.

6. **Levator scapulae:** Note: The palpation of the levator scapulae can be divided into three parts: when it is deep to the upper trapezius near its scapular attachment, when it is superficial in the posterior triangle of the neck, and when it is deep to the SCM near its spinal attachment. The client is seated with the hand in the small of the back; you are standing behind or to the side of the client. Locate the superior angle of the scapula and place your palpating hand immediately superior and medial to it. Feel for the contraction of the levator scapulae deep to the upper trapezius as the client performs a gentle, short range of motion of elevation of the scapula at the scapulocostal joint. Once felt, continue palpating it until it enters the posterior triangle of the neck (i.e., until it is no longer deep to the upper trapezius) by strumming perpendicular to its fibers as the client alternately gently

11

contracts and relaxes the muscle. Once the levator scapulae is located in the posterior triangle, it is superficial and easily palpable, and sometimes visible as well. It is no longer necessary for the client to have the hand in the small of the back, and the client can be asked to perform a more forceful contraction (against resistance if desired) of elevation of the scapula. Continue palpating it superiorly by strumming perpendicular to its fibers as the client alternately contracts and relaxes the muscle. As it approaches its spinal attachment (transverse processes of C1-C4), the levator scapulae will go deep to the SCM. To palpate it all the way to its spinal attachments deep to the SCM, the SCM must be slackened by passively moving the client's head and neck into flexion and ipsilateral lateral flexion. Note: When following the levator scapulae superiorly, be sure that you follow it toward the transverse process of C1, which is located more anteriorly than most people realize; the transverse process of C1 is located immediately inferior to the ear.

7. **Splenius capitis:** The client is seated with the head and neck ipsilaterally rotated; you are standing behind the client. Palpate in the uppermost aspect of the posterior triangle of the neck, just inferior to the occiput and posterior to the SCM. Now feel for the contraction of the splenius capitis as the client is resisted from extending the head and neck at the spinal joints. Once felt, strum perpendicular to its fibers and try to follow it inferiorly as the client alternately contracts and relaxes the muscle. Once you are no longer in the posterior triangle of the neck, the splenius capitis can be palpated two ways: (1) feel for it through the upper trapezius by asking the client to extend the head and neck against *gentle* resistance; once felt, try to follow it as far inferiorly as possible; or (2) feel for it directly: this requires you to palpate deep (anterior) to the border of the upper trapezius and press anteriorly toward the upper thoracic spinous processes by reaching with your palpating fingers between the upper trapezius and the splenius capitis. To accomplish this, it is best to stand more to the front of the client so that your finger pads are oriented anteriorly toward the splenius capitis. Furthermore, it is important

that the upper trapezius is relaxed and slackened; it can be slackened by passively moving the client's head and neck into extension, contralateral rotation, and/or ipsilateral lateral flexion.

Client Supine:

8. **Semispinalis capitis:** The client is supine with the hand in the small of the back, and/or the head and neck rotated to the same side (ipsilaterally rotated); you are seated at the head of the table. Ask the client to extend the head and neck at the spinal joints by gently pressing the head into the table and feel for the contraction of the semispinalis capitis deep to the upper trapezius, just below the occiput and just lateral to the spine. Once felt, continue palpating the semispinalis capitis inferiorly as far as possible as the client alternately contracts and relaxes the muscle.

9. **Suboccipital group (rectus capitis posterior major [RCPMaj], rectus capitis posterior minor [RCPMin], obliquus capitis inferior [OCI], obliquus capitis superior [OCS]):** The client is supine; you are seated at the head of the table. Begin by palpating the RCPMaj; palpate just superior and slightly lateral to the spinous process of C2 and strum perpendicular to it fibers. Once felt, continue palpating the RCPMaj to the occiput by strumming perpendicular to its fibers. Palpate the RCPMin in the same manner by strumming perpendicular to it, beginning just superolateral to the posterior tubercle of C1. Once felt, continue palpating the RCPMin to the occiput by strumming perpendicular to it. To palpate the OCI, palpate between the spinous process of C2 and the transverse process of C1, strumming perpendicular to the fibers. It may be helpful to have the OCI contract by gently resisting the client from ipsilaterally rotating the head. The OCS is extremely challenging to palpate and discern from adjacent musculature. To attempt its palpation, feel for it just lateral to the superior attachment of the RCPMaj; if felt, try to continue palpating it inferiorly by strumming perpendicular to it.

Chapter 12

Tour #3—Palpation of the Muscles of the Head

Overview

This chapter is a palpation tour of the muscles of the head. The tour begins with the scalp muscles, then addresses the muscles of mastication, and then concludes with palpation of the muscles of facial expression. Palpation for each of the muscles is shown in the supine position. Alternate palpation positions are also described. The major muscles or muscle groups of the region are each given a separate layout; there is also a detour to other muscles of the scalp. Trigger point (TrP) information and stretching is given for each of the muscles covered in this chapter. The chapter closes with an advanced *Whirlwind Tour* that explains the sequential palpation of all of the muscles of the chapter.

Chapter Outline

Chapter Objectives

After completing this chapter, the student should be able to perform the following for each of the muscles covered in this chapter:

1. State the attachments.
2. State the actions.
3. Describe the starting position for palpation.
4. Describe and explain the purpose of each of the palpation steps.
5. Palpate each muscle.
6. State the "Palpation Key."
7. Describe alternate palpation positions.

8. State the locations of the most common TrP(s).
9. Describe the TrP referral zones.
10. State the most common factors that create and/or perpetuate TrPs.
11. State the symptoms most commonly caused by TrPs.
12. Describe and perform a stretch.

Video demonstrations of the muscle palpations in this chapter are presented in Chapter 12 on DVD 1.

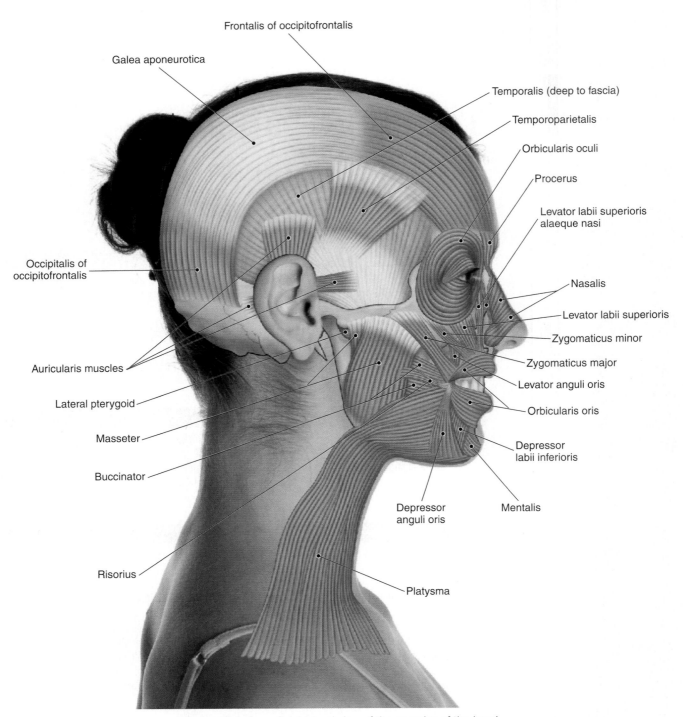

Figure 12-1 Superficial lateral view of the muscles of the head.

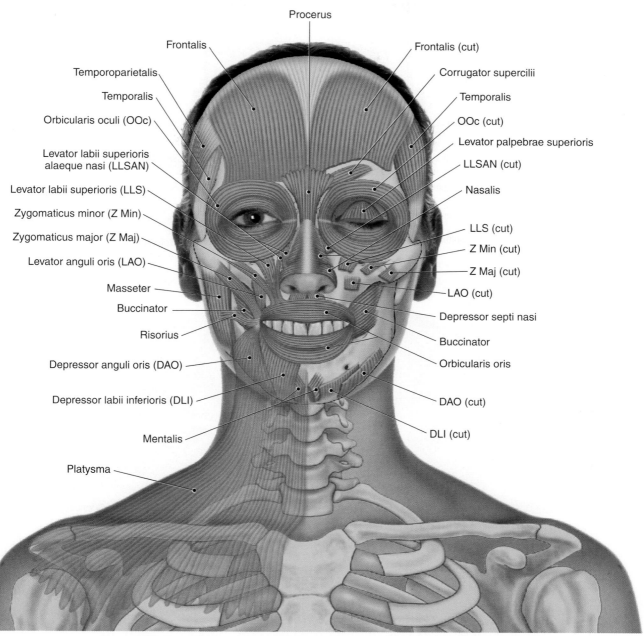

Figure 12-2 Superficial and intermediate anterior views of the muscles of the head.

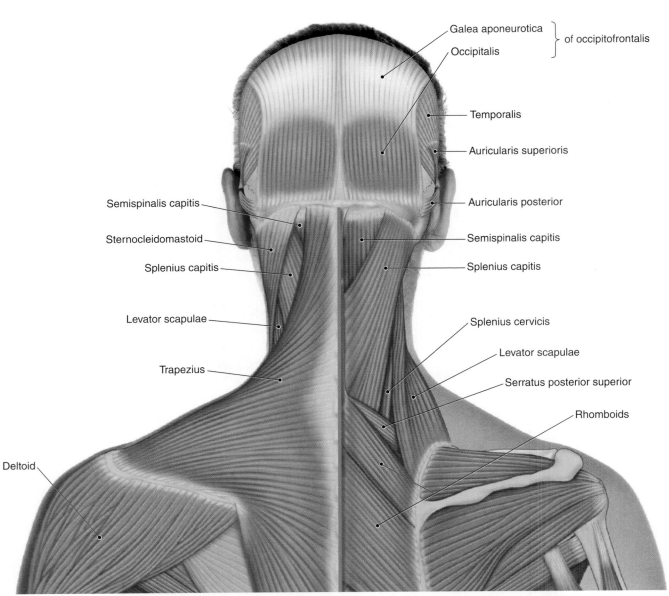

Figure 12-3 Superficial posterior view of the muscles of the head.

OCCIPITOFRONTALIS—SUPINE

❑ **ATTACHMENTS:**

o Highest nuchal line of the occiput and the mastoid region of the temporal bone *to the* galea aponeurotica *to the* fascia overlying the frontal bone

❑ **ACTIONS:**

o Draws the anterior scalp posteriorly (elevates the eyebrows); draws the posterior scalp anteriorly

Starting Position (Figure 12-5):

o Client supine
o Therapist seated at head of table
o Place palpating fingers on the forehead of the client

Palpation steps:

1. With your palpating fingers on the client's forehead, ask the client to elevate the eyebrows and feel for the contraction of the frontalis (see Figure 12-5). Once felt, palpate the entire frontalis belly.
2. Now palpate over the client's occipital bone and ask the client to elevate the eyebrows and feel for the contraction of the occipitalis (Figure 12-6). Once felt, palpate the entire occipitalis.
3. Once the occipitofrontalis has been located, have the client relax it and palpate to assess its baseline tone.

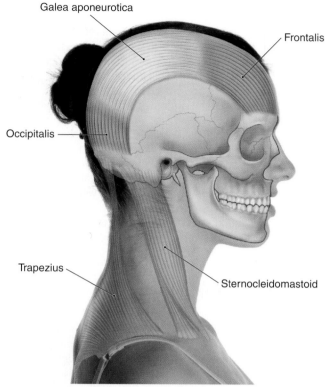

Figure 12-4 Lateral view of the right occipitofrontalis. The trapezius and sternocleidomastoid have been ghosted in.

12

Figure 12-5 Palpation of the right frontalis belly of the occipitofrontalis.

Figure 12-6 Palpation of the right and left occipitalis bellies of the occipitofrontalis muscles.

OCCIPITOFRONTALIS—SUPINE—cont'd

Palpation Notes:

1. The occipitofrontalis consists of two bellies: the frontalis overlies the frontal bone; the occipitalis overlies the occipital bone. These two bellies are connected to each other by a large aponeurosis called the *galea aponeurotica*.

2. The entire occipitofrontalis is superficial and easily palpable.

3. Because the occipitofrontalis is a thin fascial muscle, feeling its contraction is not always as obvious as feeling the contraction of a thicker larger muscle. For this reason, locating the entire occipitofrontalis by feeling its contraction is not as useful as it is with most other muscles.

4. The occipitofrontalis is often tight in clients who suffer from tension headaches.

Alternate Palpation Position

Both bellies of the occipitofrontalis (the frontalis and the occipitalis) are easily accessible with the client seated. The occipitalis belly can also be easily palpated with the client prone.

Palpation Key:
Palpate over the frontal and occipital bones.

TRIGGER POINTS

1. Trigger points (TrPs) in the occipitofrontalis often result from or are perpetuated by acute or chronic overuse of the muscle (from the chronic habit of wrinkling the forehead) or direct trauma. Furthermore, TrPs in the occipitalis belly often result from or are perpetuated by TrPs in the posterior cervical musculature; and TrPs in the frontalis belly often result from or are perpetuated by TrPs in the clavicular head of the sternocleidomastoid (SCM).

2. TrPs in the occipitalis belly tend to produce headache pain in the back of the head and behind the eye, discomfort having pressure against the back of the head (e.g., with pressure against a pillow at night or the back of a chair), and perhaps even an earache. TrPs in the frontalis belly tend to produce headache pain in the forehead and can also entrap the supraorbital nerve (resulting in headache pain in the forehead with symptoms more characteristic of nerve entrapment, such as more of a tingling and prickling pain).

3. The referral patterns of occipitalis TrPs must be distinguished from the referral patterns of TrPs in the splenius cervicis and temporalis; the referral patterns of frontalis TrPs must be distinguished from the referral patterns of TrPs in the SCM, temporalis, masseter, orbicularis oculi, and zygomaticus major.

4. TrPs in the occipitofrontalis are often incorrectly assessed as migraine headaches; furthermore, TrPs in the occipitalis belly are often incorrectly assessed as greater occipital neuralgia.

5. Associated TrPs of the occipitalis often occur in the upper trapezius, semispinalis capitis, and posterior belly of the digastric; associated TrPs of the frontalis often occur in the clavicular head of the SCM.

Figure 12-7 Common occipitofrontalis TrPs and their corresponding referral zones. **A**, Anterior view. **B**, Lateral view.

OCCIPITOFRONTALIS—SUPINE—cont'd

DETOUR

Temporoparietalis and Auricularis Muscles: The temporoparietalis and the three auricularis muscles (auricularis anterior, superior, and posterior) are other muscles of the scalp. The temporoparietalis attaches from the fascia superior to the ear to the galea aponeurotica; its action is to elevate the ear. The anterior and superior auricularis muscles attach from the galea aponeurotica to the ear; they move the ear anteriorly and superiorly, respectively. The auricularis posterior attaches from the mastoid bone to the ear; it moves the ear posteriorly. The temporoparietalis and all three auricularis muscles can also act to tighten the scalp. Because these scalp muscles are superficial, they are easy to palpate. However, if the client cannot voluntarily control the contraction of these muscles (engaging these muscles requires the ability to move the ear,

which most people are unable to do), then they must be palpated based upon location only. However, it can be difficult to be sure of their exact location and discern them from adjacent soft tissue.

To palpate the temporoparietalis, palpate 1 to 2 inches (2.5 to 5 cm) superior and slightly anterior to the ear; ask the client to elevate the ear and feel for the muscle's contraction (Figure 12-8, B).

To palpate the auricularis muscles, palpate either immediately anterior, superior, or posterior to the ear, and ask the client to move the ear in that direction, feeling for the contraction of that particular auricularis muscle. Again, very few people can consciously contract these muscles, so it is usually necessary to palpate them by location while they are relaxed.

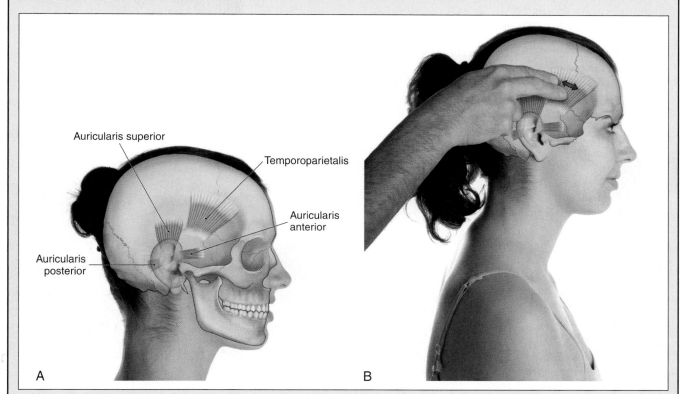

Auricularis superior
Temporoparietalis
Auricularis anterior
Auricularis posterior

A

B

Figure 12-8 Other muscles of the scalp. **A**, Lateral view of the right temporoparietalis and auricularis muscles. **B**, Palpation of the right temporoparietalis.

12

TEMPORALIS—SUPINE

❏ **ATTACHMENTS:**

o Temporal fossa *to the* coronoid process and the anterosuperior aspect of the ramus of the mandible

❏ **ACTIONS:**

o Elevates and retracts the mandible at the temporomandibular joints (TMJs)

Starting Position (Figure 12-10):

o Client supine
o Therapist seated at head of table
o Palpating fingers placed over the temporal fossa

Palpation steps:

1. With palpating fingers over the temporal fossa, ask the client to alternately contract and relax the temporalis; this is accomplished by alternately clenching the teeth and then relaxing the jaw. Feel for the contraction of the temporalis as the client clenches the teeth (Figure 12-11).
2. Once the contraction of the temporalis has been felt, palpate the entire muscle as the client continues to contract and relax it as indicated in Step 1.
3. Once the temporalis has been located, have the client relax it and palpate to assess its baseline tone.

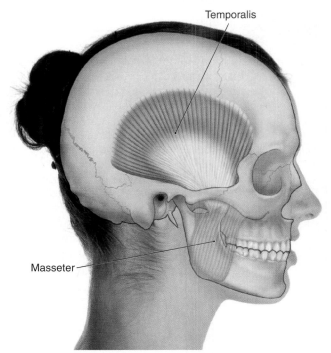

Figure 12-9 Lateral view of the right temporalis. The masseter has been ghosted in.

Figure 12-10 Starting position for supine palpation of the right temporalis.

Figure 12-11 Palpation of the right temporalis as the client clenches the teeth.

Palpation Key:
Clench the teeth.

12

TEMPORALIS—SUPINE

Palpation Notes:

1. Clenching the teeth requires elevation of the mandible at the temporomandibular joints, thereby engaging the temporalis.
2. The vast majority of the temporalis is superficial and easily palpable. Only a small portion at its inferior end (the portion of it that is deep to the zygomatic arch and the inferior attachment on the mandible) is not easily palpable.
3. The inferior attachment of the temporalis on the mandible can be accessed and palpated, especially if the client opens the mouth widely, causing the coronoid process of the mandible to drop down from behind the zygomatic arch. However, if the client is asked to contract the temporalis by elevating the mandible at the TMJs, the more superficial masseter will also contract, making palpation of the mandibular attachment of the temporalis difficult. For this reason, palpation of the mandibular attachment of the temporalis is best attempted with the musculature relaxed.
4. The mandibular attachment of the temporalis is also palpable from inside the mouth. With a gloved hand or a finger cot on your index finger, reach posteriorly into the vestibule of the client's mouth (between the cheeks and the teeth) and feel for the coronoid process of the mandible with the musculature relaxed. Once found, palpate on the anterior and medial surfaces of the coronoid process for the temporalis attachment (Figure 12-12). While palpating the mandibular attachment inside the mouth, it is awkward but possible to have the client contract the temporalis by asking the client to elevate the mandible.

TRIGGER POINTS

1. Trigger points (TrPs) in the temporalis often result from or are perpetuated by acute or chronic overuse of the muscle (e.g., chronic clenching or grinding of the teeth, excessive gum chewing or fingernail biting), prolonged stretching (e.g., keeping the mouth open during long dental procedures), occlusal asymmetry (poor bite), protracted head posture (creating pull on the hyoid muscles, which then pull on the mandible, requiring the temporalis to contract), temporomandibular joint (TMJ) dysfunction, direct trauma, having a cold draft on the head, emotional stress, or TrPs in the upper trapezius or sternocleidomastoid (SCM).
2. TrPs in the temporalis tend to produce headaches, pain and hypersensitivity of the upper teeth and the adjacent gums, occlusal asymmetry, or pain in the TMJ.
3. The referral patterns of temporalis TrPs must be distinguished from the referral patterns of TrPs in the upper trapezius, SCM, masseter, lateral and medial pterygoids, semispinalis capitis, orbicularis oculi, and buccinator.
4. TrPs in the temporalis are often incorrectly assessed as headaches, dental disease, or a TMJ disorder (e.g., osteoarthritis or other internal joint derangement).
5. Associated TrPs often occur in the contralateral temporalis, ipsilateral and contralateral masseters, lateral and medial pterygoids, upper trapezius, and SCM.

Figure 12-13 Lateral view illustrating common temporalis TrPs and their corresponding referral zones.

Figure 12-12 Palpation of the mandibular attachment of the right temporalis from inside the mouth.

Alternate Palpation Position—Seated
The temporalis is also easily palpated with the client seated.

STRETCHING THE TEMPORALIS

Figure 12-14 A stretch of the right temporalis and masseter. The client opens the jaw as widely as possible; assistance is given with the hand.

12

MASSETER—SUPINE

❏ ATTACHMENTS:

o Inferior margins of the zygomatic bone and the zygomatic arch of the temporal bone *to the* anterior surfaces of the angle, ramus, and coronoid process of the mandible

❏ ACTIONS:

o Elevates, protracts, and retracts the mandible at the temporomandibular joints (TMJs)

Starting position (Figure 12-16):

o Client supine
o Therapist seated at head of table
o Palpating fingers placed between the zygomatic arch and the angle of the mandible

Palpation steps:

1. Ask the client to alternately contract and relax the masseter; this is accomplished by alternately clenching the teeth and then relaxing the jaw. Feel for the contraction of the masseter as the client clenches the teeth (Figure 12-17).
2. Once the contraction of the masseter has been felt, palpate the entire muscle from the zygomatic arch to the angle of the mandible as the client continues to contract and relax it as indicated in Step 1.
3. Once the masseter has been located, have the client relax it and palpate to assess its baseline tone.

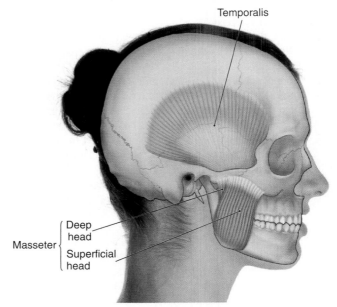

Figure 12-15 Lateral view of the right masseter. The temporalis has been ghosted in.

Figure 12-16 Starting position for supine palpation of the right masseter.

Figure 12-17 Palpation of the right masseter as the client clenches the teeth.

MASSETER—SUPINE—cont'd

Palpation Notes:

1. The entire masseter is superficial and easily palpated and discerned from adjacent musculature.
2. When the client clenches the teeth, the contraction of the masseter becomes extremely obvious and the masseter often visibly bulges.
3. The masseter is also easily palpated from within the mouth. Wearing a glove or finger cot on your index finger, pinch the masseter between your index finger and thumb, with the index finger in the vestibule of the client's mouth (between the cheeks and the teeth) and the thumb outside the mouth (Figure 12-18). To engage and contract the masseter, the client can be asked to clench the teeth.

Figure 12-18 Palpation of the right masseter by pinching it between the index finger and thumb.

Alternate Palpation Position
The masseter can be easily palpated with the client seated.

TRIGGER POINTS

1. Trigger points (TrPs) in the masseter often result from or are perpetuated by acute or chronic overuse of the muscle (e.g., chronic clenching or grinding of the teeth, excessive gum chewing or fingernail biting), prolonged stretching (e.g., keeping the mouth open during long dental procedures), occlusal asymmetry (poor bite), protracted head posture (creating pull on the hyoid muscles, which then pull on the mandible, requiring the masseter to contract), temporomandibular joint (TMJ) dysfunction, direct trauma, emotional stress, or TrPs in the upper trapezius or sternocleidomastoid (SCM).
2. TrPs in the masseter tend to produce restricted depression of the mandible at the TMJs, pain and hypersensitivity of the upper and lower molar teeth and the adjacent gums, pain in the TMJ, occlusal asymmetry, puffiness of the ipsilateral eye (due to possible entrapment of the maxillary vein), or tinnitus or deeply felt pain in the ipsilateral ear.
3. The referral patterns of masseter TrPs must be distinguished from the referral patterns of TrPs in the upper trapezius, SCM, semispinalis capitis, temporalis, lateral and medial pterygoids, platysma, buccinator, and orbicularis oculi.
4. TrPs in the masseter are often incorrectly assessed as a TMJ disorder (e.g., osteoarthritis or other internal joint derangement), dental disease, headaches, or sinusitis.
5. Associated TrPs often occur in the contralateral masseter, ipsilateral and contralateral temporalis, lateral and medial pterygoids, upper trapezius, and SCM.

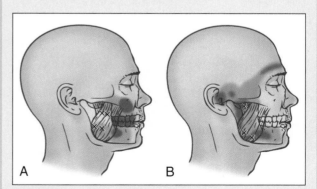

A   B

Figure 12-19 Lateral views illustrating common masseter TrPs and their corresponding referral zones.

12

MASSETER—SUPINE—cont'd

STRETCHING THE MASSETER

Palpation Key:
Clench the teeth and the masseter jumps out.

Figure 12-20 A stretch of the right masseter and temporalis. The client opens the jaw as widely as possible; assistance is given with the hand.

12

LATERAL PTERYGOID—SUPINE   12-1

❏ **ATTACHMENTS:**

o Sphenoid bone *to the* neck of the mandible and the capsule and articular disc of the temporomandibular joint (TMJ)

❏ **ACTIONS:**

o Protracts and contralaterally deviates the mandible at the TMJs

Starting position (Figure 12-22, A):

o Client supine
o Therapist seated at the head or the side of the table
o Wearing either a glove or a finger cot, place your palpating finger inside the vestibule of the client's mouth (between the cheeks and the teeth), run along the external surfaces of the upper teeth until you reach the back molars; then press posteriorly and superiorly into a little pocket in the tissue between the gum above the upper teeth and the condyle of the mandible (see Palpation Note #2). You will be on the internal surface of the lateral pterygoid (Figure 12-22, B).

Palpation steps:

1. With the palpating finger positioned inside the vestibule of the mouth, ask the client to either protract the mandible at the TMJs or to slowly and carefully contralaterally deviate the mandible (deviate it to the opposite side of the

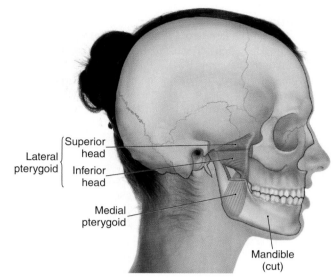

Figure 12-21 Lateral view of the right lateral pterygoid. The medial pterygoid has been ghosted in. Note: The mandible has been cut to better show the lateral pterygoid.

body), and feel for the contraction of the lateral pterygoid (Figure 12-23).

2. Once felt, palpate as much of the lateral pterygoid as possible, from the condyle of the mandible to the inside wall of the mouth (above the gum of the upper teeth).

12

Figure 12-22 Starting position for supine palpation of the right lateral pterygoid. **A**, Palpation with a client. **B**, Palpation with a skull.

Figure 12-23 Supine palpation of the right lateral pterygoid as the client protracts the mandible.

LATERAL PTERYGOID—SUPINE—cont'd

Palpation Notes:

1. In addition to the neck of the mandible, the lateral pterygoid also attaches into the capsule and disc of the temporomandibular joint (TMJ).

2. When placing your palpating finger inside the vestibule of the client's mouth to locate the lateral pterygoid, press posteriorly and superiorly from the back molars, and search for what feels like a little pocket between the upper teeth and the condyle of the mandible. (Food such as peanut butter often gets stuck here!)

3. If you ask the client to contralaterally deviate the mandible at the TMJs, the client must do so slowly and carefully; otherwise your palpating finger may be pinched between the client's mandible and upper teeth.

4. The lateral and medial pterygoids are often quite sensitive to palpation. One reason for this is that they are covered only by a thin layer of mucosa.

5. Some sources state that the lateral pterygoid can be palpated from outside the mouth between the condyle and coronoid process of the mandible. However, it is difficult to palpate and discern the lateral pterygoid here because it is deep to the masseter. If you do attempt this palpation, ask the client to contralaterally deviate the mandible and feel for the contraction of the lateral pterygoid.

TRIGGER POINTS

1. Trigger points (TrPs) in the lateral pterygoid often result from or are perpetuated by acute or chronic overuse of the muscle (e.g., chronic grinding of the teeth, excessive gum chewing or fingernail biting, using the jaw to help hold a violin when playing), occlusal asymmetry (poor bite), or protracted head posture (creating pull on the hyoid muscles, which then pull on the mandible, requiring the lateral pterygoid to contract).

2. TrPs in the lateral pterygoid tend to produce pain felt deeply in the temporomandibular joint (TMJ), joint crepitus in the TMJ, restricted ipsilateral deviation of the mandible at the TMJs, occlusal asymmetry, tingling in the cheek or weakness of the buccinator muscle (if the buccal nerve is entrapped by the lateral pterygoid), or tinnitus.

3. The referral patterns of lateral pterygoid TrPs must be distinguished from the referral patterns of TrPs in the temporalis, masseter, medial pterygoid, sternocleidomastoid (SCM), and zygomaticus major.

4. TrPs in the lateral pterygoid are often incorrectly assessed as TMJ disorder (e.g., osteoarthritis or other internal joint derangement), sinusitis, tic douloureux, or ear infections.

5. Associated TrPs often occur in the contralateral lateral and medial pterygoids, the ipsilateral temporalis and masseter, and the SCM.

6. Notes: 1) The lateral pterygoid is the muscle of mastication most likely to have TrPs. 2) Unlike the temporalis and masseter, the lateral and medial pterygoids do not usually refer pain to the teeth.

Figure 12-25 Lateral view illustrating common lateral pterygoid TrPs and their corresponding referral zones.

Alternate Palpation Position—Seated

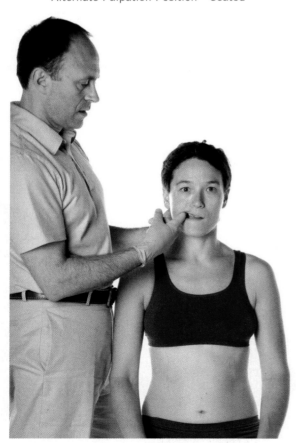

Figure 12-24 The lateral pterygoid is also easily accessed and palpated with the client seated.

12

LATERAL PTERYGOID—SUPINE—cont'd

STRETCHING THE LATERAL PTERYGOID

Palpation Key:
Find the pocket in the upper vestibule of the mouth where peanut butter gets stuck.

Figure 12-26 A stretch of the right lateral pterygoid. The client uses his hand to laterally deviate the jaw to the right (same) side.

12

MEDIAL PTERYGOID—SUPINE

❏ **ATTACHMENTS:**

o Sphenoid and maxillary bones *to the* internal surface of the mandible at the angle and inferior aspect of the ramus

❏ **ACTIONS:**

o Elevates, protracts, and contralaterally deviates the mandible at the temporomandibular joints (TMJs)

Starting position (Figure 12-28):

o Client supine
o Therapist seated at the head or the side of the table
o Palpating fingers curled around to the inside surface of the angle of the mandible

Palpation steps:

1. With palpating fingers hooked around to the internal surface of the angle of the mandible, ask the client to elevate the mandible at the TMJs by clenching the teeth, and feel for the contraction of the medial pterygoid (Figure 12-29).
2. Once felt, palpate the medial pterygoid as far superiorly as possible.
3. Once the medial pterygoid has been located, have the client relax it and palpate to assess its baseline tone.

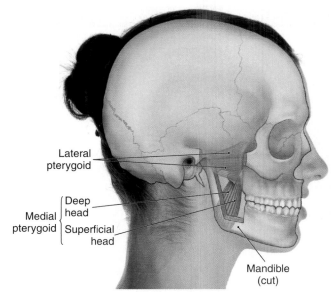

Figure 12-27 Lateral view of the right medial pterygoid. The lateral pterygoid has been ghosted in. Note: The mandible has been cut to better show the medial pterygoid.

12

Figure 12-28 Starting position for supine palpation of the right medial pterygoid.

Figure 12-29 Palpation of the right medial pterygoid as the client clenches the teeth.

MEDIAL PTERYGOID—SUPINE—cont'd

Palpation Notes:

1. The inferior attachment of the medial pterygoid can be easily palpated from outside the mouth. However, the vast majority of the muscle is palpable only from inside the mouth.

2. To palpate the medial pterygoid from inside the mouth, wearing a glove or finger cot, place your palpating finger along the internal surfaces of the lower teeth until you reach the back molars, then press posterolaterally until you reach the inside wall of the mouth. Now ask the client to protract the mandible and feel for the contraction of the medial pterygoid. Palpate as much of the medial pterygoid as possible by following it toward its attachments as the client alternately contracts and relaxes the muscle (Figure 12-30).

3. When palpating the medial pterygoid toward its attachments from within the mouth, it helps to visualize it as running identically to the masseter (except that the masseter is located on the external surface of the mandible and the medial pterygoid is located on the internal surface of the mandible).

4. The medial and lateral pterygoids are often quite sensitive to palpation. One reason for this is that they are covered only by a thin layer of mucosa.

Alternate Palpation Position—Seated

Figure 12-31 The medial pterygoid is also easily accessed and palpated with the client seated.

Figure 12-30 Palpation of the right medial pterygoid from inside the mouth (see Palpation Note #2).

12

MEDIAL PTERYGOID—SUPINE—cont'd

TRIGGER POINTS

1. Trigger points (TrPs) in the medial pterygoid often result from or are perpetuated by acute or chronic overuse of the muscle (e.g., chronic clenching or grinding of the teeth, excessive gum chewing or fingernail biting, using the jaw to help hold a violin when playing), prolonged stretching (e.g., keeping the mouth open during long dental procedures), occlusal asymmetry (poor bite), protracted head posture (creating pull on the hyoid muscles, which then pull on the mandible, requiring the medial pterygoid to contract), temporomandibular joint (TMJ) dysfunction, direct trauma, emotional stress, or TrPs in the other muscles of mastication.

2. TrPs in the medial pterygoid tend to produce a diffuse aching pain in the mouth (including the tongue) and the throat, TMJ pain, occlusal asymmetry (poor bite), pressure (often described as stuffiness) or pain felt deeply in the ear (when present, the pressure is caused by a eustacian tube blocked by a tight medial pterygoid that prevents the tensor veli palatini from opening the eustacian tube), pain or difficulty when swallowing, or restricted depression of the mandible at the TMJs.

3. The referral patterns of medial pterygoid TrPs must be distinguished from the referral patterns of TrPs in the lateral pterygoid, temporalis, masseter, sternocleidomastoid (SCM), longus colli and capitis, and inferior belly of the digastric.

4. TrPs in the medial pterygoid are often incorrectly assessed as a TMJ disorder (e.g., osteoarthritis or other internal joint derangement), headaches, an ear infection, a head cold, or a sore throat.

5. Associated TrPs often occur in the contralateral medial pterygoid, the ipsilateral and contralateral temporalis, masseter, lateral pterygoids, SCM, longus colli and capitis, and digastric.

6. Note: Unlike the temporalis and masseter, the medial and lateral pterygoids do not usually refer pain to the teeth.

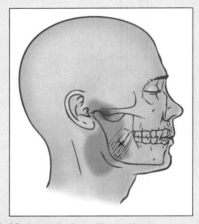

Figure 12-32 Lateral view illustrating a common medial pterygoid TrP and its corresponding referral zone.

STRETCHING THE MEDIAL PTERYGOID

Figure 12-33 A stretch of the right medial pterygoid. The client uses his hand to depress and slightly deviate the jaw laterally to the right (same) side.

Palpation Key:

Curl your palpating fingers around to the internal surface of the angle of the mandible.

MUSCLES OF FACIAL EXPRESSION—SEATED

Muscles of facial expression are thin superficial muscles located within the skin and fascia of the face. These muscles can be divided into three groups: those that move the eye (three muscles), the nose (three muscles), and the mouth (eleven muscles).

All facial muscle palpations are shown in this chapter with the client seated. These muscles can also be palpated with the client supine and the therapist seated at the head of the table. Furthermore, only the index finger is shown palpating the target muscle, so that less of the target muscle is obstructed for the reader. It is often preferable to palpate the muscles of facial expression using the finger pads of two fingers, the index and middle fingers. Palpating facial expression muscles requires gentle pressure and a sensitive touch.

Because muscles of facial expression are small, it may seem unimportant to stretch them. However, like any muscle, a facial expression muscle can become tight, especially if

the same facial expression is habitually created, requiring its repeated contraction. When a muscle of facial expression becomes tight, it pulls the overlying fascia and skin in toward its center, thereby creating wrinkles that are oriented perpendicularly to the direction of the muscle fibers. Examination of the typical pattern of facial wrinkles reveals that the wrinkles are perpendicular to the underlying muscles of facial expression. To stretch the muscles of facial expression, it is necessary to move the face by making a wide variety of strong expressions. Each expression will stretch the muscles that create the opposite expression. For this reason, it is especially important to make facial expressions that you do not normally make.

Note: Trigger points and their referral patterns have not been mapped out for all the muscles of facial expression. Facial expression muscles that have been investigated and mapped are the orbicularis oculi, zygomaticus major, levator labii superioris, and buccinator.

12

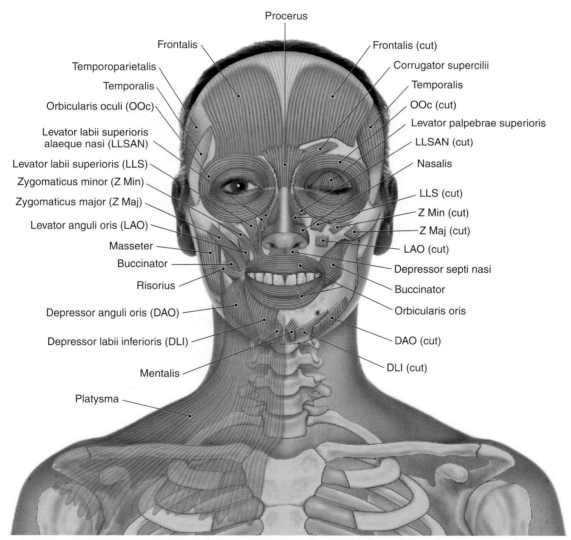

Figure 12-34 Superficial and intermediate anterior views of the muscles of the head.

MUSCLES OF FACIAL EXPRESSION—SEATED—cont'd

Facial Expression Muscles of the Eye:

Orbicularis Oculi:

❑ **ATTACHMENTS:**

o The orbicularis oculi encircles the eye (Figure 12-35, A).

❑ **ACTIONS:**

o Closes and squints the eye; depresses the upper eyelid, elevates the lower eyelid

Palpation steps:

1. Gently place palpating finger(s) on the tissue around the client's eye.
2. Ask the client to somewhat forcefully close the eye and feel for the contraction of the orbicularis oculi (Figure 12-35, C).
3. Once felt, palpate the entire muscle as the client alternately contracts and relaxes it. Note: Be sure to distinguish the orbicularis oculi from the nearby corrugator supercilii by having the client try to isolate the actions of closing and squinting the eye, and not also drawing the eyebrows down into a frown.

A

B

C

Figure 12-35 A, Anterior view of the right orbicularis oculi. **B**, Anterolateral view illustrating a common orbicularis oculi TrP and its corresponding referral zone. **C**, Palpation of the right orbicularis oculi as the client somewhat forcefully closes the eye as if to squint.

TRIGGER POINTS

1. Trigger points (TrPs) in the orbicularis oculi often result from or are perpetuated by acute or chronic overuse of the muscle (e.g., habitual squinting or frowning) or TrPs in the sternal head of the sternocleidomastoid (SCM).
2. TrPs in the orbicularis oculi tend to produce pain in the nose.
3. The referral patterns of orbicularis oculi TrPs must be distinguished from the referral patterns of TrPs in the other muscles of facial expression, SCM, temporalis, masseter, and frontalis.
4. TrPs in the orbicularis oculi are often incorrectly assessed as sinusitis or headache.
5. Associated TrPs often occur in the other muscles of facial expression, muscles of mastication (temporalis, masseter, and the lateral and medial pterygoids), SCM, and upper trapezius.

MUSCLES OF FACIAL EXPRESSION—SEATED—cont'd

Corrugator Supercilii:

❑ **ATTACHMENTS:**

o Inferior aspect of the frontal bone *to the* fascia and skin deep to the medial portion of the eyebrow (Figure 12-36, A)

❑ **ACTIONS:**

o Draws the eyebrow inferomedially

Palpation steps:

o Gently place palpating finger(s) on the medial portion of the client's eyebrow.
o Ask the client to frown, bringing the eyebrows down, and feel for the contraction of the corrugator supercilii (Figure 12-36, B).
o Once felt, palpate the entire muscle as the client alternately contracts and relaxes it. Note: Be sure to distinguish the corrugator supercilii from the nearby orbicularis oculi, which can also draw the eyebrow downward when it contracts.

A

B

Figure 12-36 A, Anterior view of the right corrugator supercilii. **B**, Palpation of the right corrugator supercilii as the client frowns.

12

Levator Palpebrae Superioris:

❏ **ATTACHMENTS:**

o Sphenoid bone *to the* fascia and skin of the upper eyelid (Figure 12-37, A)

❏ **ACTIONS:**

o Elevates the upper eyelid

Palpation steps:

o Gently place palpating finger(s) on the client's upper eyelid; ask the client to elevate the upper eyelid and feel for the contraction of the levator palpebrae superioris (Figure 12-37, B).

o Once felt, palpate as much of the muscle as possible as the client alternately contracts and relaxes it.

A

B

Figure 12-37 A, Lateral view of the right levator palpebrae superioris. **B**, Palpation of the right levator palpebrae superioris in the upper eyelid as the client elevates the upper eyelid.

MUSCLES OF FACIAL EXPRESSION—SEATED—cont'd

Facial Expression Muscles of the Nose:

Procerus:

❑ **ATTACHMENTS:**

o Fascia over the nasal bone *to the* fascia and skin between the eyes (Figure 12-38, A)

❑ **ACTIONS:**

o Draws down the medial eyebrow; wrinkles the skin of the nose upward

Palpation steps:

o Gently place palpating finger(s) on the bridge of the client's nose.

o Ask the client to make a look of disdain, bringing the eyebrows down and/or wrinkling the skin of the nose upward, and feel for the contraction of the procerus (Figure 12-38, B).

o Once felt, palpate the entire muscle as the client alternately contracts and relaxes it. Note: Be sure to distinguish the procerus from the nearby corrugator supercilii, which can also result in drawing the medial eyebrow downward when it contracts.

A

B

Figure 12-38 A, Anterior view of the right procerus. **B**, Palpation of the right procerus as the client makes a look of disdain.

MUSCLES OF FACIAL EXPRESSION—SEATED—cont'd

Nasalis:

❏ **ATTACHMENTS:**

o Maxilla *to the* cartilage of the nose (and the opposite-side nasalis muscle) (Figure 12-39, A)

❏ **ACTIONS:**

o Flares the nostril (alar part)
o Constricts the nostril (transverse part)

Palpation steps:

1. Gently place palpating finger(s) on the inferolateral aspect of the client's nose.
2. Ask the client to flare the nostril (as when taking in a deep breath) and feel for the contraction of the nasalis (Figure 12-39, B).
3. Once felt, palpate the entire muscle as the client alternately contracts and relaxes it. Note: Be sure to distinguish the nasalis from the nearby procerus by making sure that the client does not also elevate the skin of the nose when flaring the nostril. Also, distinguish from the nearby levator labii superioris alaeque nasi, which can also flare the nostril.

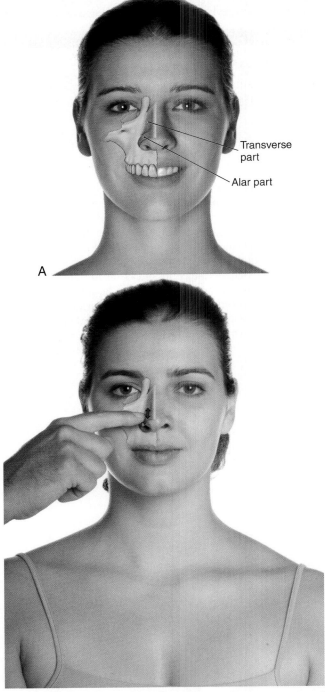

Transverse part

Alar part

A

B

Figure 12-39 A, Anterior view of the right nasalis. **B**, Palpation of the right nasalis as the client flares her nostril.

MUSCLES OF FACIAL EXPRESSION—SEATED—cont'd

Depressor Septi Nasi:

❏ **ATTACHMENTS:**

o Maxilla *to the* cartilage of the nose (Figure 12-40, A)

❏ **ACTIONS:**

o Constricts the nostril

Palpation steps:

1. Gently place palpating finger(s) directly inferior to the client's nose.
2. Ask the client to constrict the nostril (as if pulling the middle of the nose down toward the mouth) and feel for the contraction of the depressor septi nasi (Figure 12-40, B).
3. Once felt, palpate the entire muscle as the client alternately contracts and relaxes it. Note: Be sure to distinguish the depressor septi nasi from the nearby orbicularis oris by making sure that the client does not also close and/or protract (protrude) the lips when constricting the nostril.

A

B

Figure 12-40 A, Anterior view of the right depressor septi nasi. **B**, Palpation of the right depressor septi nasi as the client constricts her nostril.

12

MUSCLES OF FACIAL EXPRESSION—SEATED—cont'd

Facial Expression Muscles of the Mouth:

Levator Labii Superioris Alaeque Nasi:

❑ **ATTACHMENTS:**

o Maxilla *to the* fascia and muscle tissue of the upper lip and the fascia and cartilage of the nose (Figure 12-41, A)

❑ **ACTIONS:**

o Elevates and everts the upper lip; flares the nostril

Palpation steps:

1. Gently place palpating finger(s) just lateral to the client's nose.
2. Ask the client to either elevate the upper lip to show you the upper gum or flare the nostril, and feel for the contraction of the levator labii superioris alaeque nasi (Figure 12-41, B).
3. Once felt, palpate the entire muscle as the client alternately contracts and relaxes it. Note: It can be difficult to distinguish the levator labii superioris alaeque nasi from the nearby nasalis medially (which also flares the nostril), and the nearby levator labii superioris laterally (which also elevates the upper lip).
4. Additional note: The levator labii superioris alaeque nasi is considered to be a muscle of facial expression of the nose as well as of the mouth.

A

B

Figure 12-41 A, Anterior view of the right levator labii superioris alaeque nasi (LLSAN). The orbicularis oris (OOr) and levator labii superioris (LLS) have been ghosted in. **B,** Palpation of the right LLSAN as the client elevates the upper lip and flares the nostril.

12

MUSCLES OF FACIAL EXPRESSION—SEATED—cont'd

Levator Labii Superioris:

❏ **ATTACHMENTS:**

o Maxilla *to the* fascia and muscular tissue of the upper lip (Figure 12-42, A)

❏ **ACTIONS:**

o Elevates and everts the upper lip

Palpation steps:
1. Gently place palpating finger(s) approximately ½ inch (1 cm) lateral to the center of the upper lip, at its superior margin.
2. Ask the client to elevate the upper lip to show you the upper gum, and feel for the contraction of the levator labii superioris (Figure 12-42, C).
3. Once felt, palpate the entire muscle toward the eye as the client alternately contracts and relaxes it. Note: It can be difficult to distinguish the levator labii superioris from the nearby levator labii superioris alaeque nasi (medially) and zygomaticus minor (laterally), both of which contract with elevation of the upper lip.

LLSAN
LLS
OOr

A

B

C

Figure 12-42 A, Anterior view of the right levator labii superioris (LLS). The orbicularis oris (OOr) and levator labii superioris alaeque nasi (LLSAN) have been ghosted in. **B,** Anterolateral view illustrating a common LLS TrP and its corresponding referral zone. **C,** Palpation of the right LLS as the client elevates her upper lip.

12

TRIGGER POINTS

1. Trigger points (TrPs) in the levator labii superioris often result from or are perpetuated by acute or chronic overuse of the muscle (e.g., habitual smiling).
2. TrPs in the levator labii superioris may produce allergy symptoms (sneezing, itchy eyes) and apparent sinus pain.
3. The referral patterns of levator labii superioris TrPs must be distinguished from the referral patterns of TrPs in the other muscles of facial expression, sternocleidomastoid (SCM), temporalis, masseter, and frontalis.
4. TrPs in the levator labii superioris are often incorrectly assessed as sinusitis, a cold, or headache.
5. Associated TrPs often occur in the other muscles of facial expression, muscles of mastication (temporalis, masseter, and the lateral and medial pterygoids), SCM, and upper trapezius.

Zygomaticus Minor:

❏ ATTACHMENTS:

o Zygomatic bone *to the* fascia and muscular tissue of the upper lip (Figure 12-43, A)

❏ ACTIONS:

o Elevates and everts the upper lip

Palpation steps:

1. Gently place palpating finger(s) approximately ½ to ¾ inch (1 to 2 cm) lateral to the center of the upper lip, at its superior margin.
2. Ask the client to elevate the upper lip to show you the upper gum, and feel for the contraction of the zygomaticus minor (Figure 12-43, B).
3. Once felt, palpate the entire muscle toward the zygomatic bone as the client alternately contracts and relaxes it. Note: It can be difficult to distinguish the zygomaticus minor from the nearby levator labii superioris (medially), which contracts with elevation of the upper lip, and the nearby zygomaticus major (laterally), which contracts with elevation of the corner of the mouth.

A

B

Figure 12-43 A, Anterior view of the right zygomaticus minor (Z Min). The orbicularis oris (OOr) and zygomaticus major (Z Maj) have been ghosted in. **B**, Palpation of the right zygomaticus minor as the client elevates her upper lip. The zygomaticus major has been ghosted in.

MUSCLES OF FACIAL EXPRESSION—SEATED—cont'd

Zygomaticus Major:

❏ **ATTACHMENTS:**

o Zygomatic bone *to the* fascia at the corner (angle) of the mouth* (Figure 12-44, A)

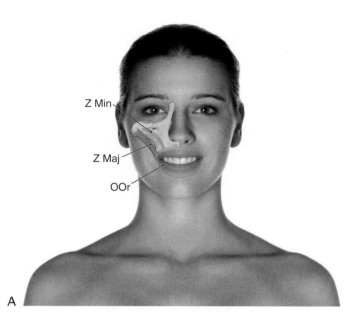

Figure 12-44 A, Anterior view of the right zygomaticus major (Z Maj). The orbicularis oris (OOr) and zygomaticus minor (Z Min) have been ghosted in. **B**, Anterolateral view illustrating a common zygomaticus major TrP and its corresponding referral zone. **C**, Palpation of the right zygomaticus major as the client smiles. The zygomaticus minor has been ghosted in.

❏ **ACTIONS:**

o Elevates and draws the corner of the mouth laterally

Palpation steps:
1. Gently place palpating finger(s) immediately superolateral to the corner of the mouth.
2. Ask the client to smile by drawing the corner of the mouth both superiorly and laterally, and feel for the contraction of the zygomaticus major (Figure 12-44, C).
3. Once felt, palpate the entire muscle toward the zygomatic bone as the client alternately contracts and relaxes it. Note: It can be difficult to distinguish the zygomaticus major from the nearby levator anguli oris, which also elevates the corner of the mouth. Also, be sure to distinguish the zygomaticus major from the nearby zygomaticus minor, which contracts with elevation of the upper lip.

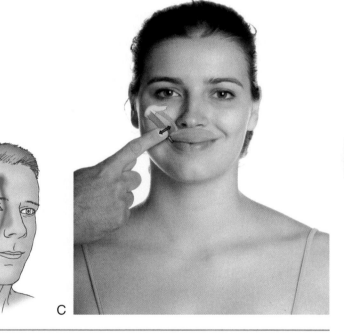

TRIGGER POINTS

1. Trigger points (TrPs) in the zygomaticus major often result from or are perpetuated by acute or chronic overuse of the muscle (e.g., habitual smiling).
2. TrPs in the zygomaticus major may produce allergy symptoms (sneezing, itchy eyes) and apparent sinus pain.
3. The referral patterns of zygomaticus major TrPs must be distinguished from the referral patterns of TrPs in the other muscles of facial expression, sternocleidomastoid (SCM), temporalis, masseter, and frontalis.
4. TrPs in the zygomaticus major are often incorrectly assessed as sinusitis, a cold, or headache.
5. Associated TrPs often occur in the other muscles of facial expression, muscles of mastication (temporalis, masseter, and the lateral and medial pterygoids), SCM, and upper trapezius.

---

*The term *modiolus* is used to describe the fascia at the corner of the mouth that is the common attachment for the zygomaticus major, levator anguli oris, risorius, depressor anguli oris, buccinator, and orbicularis oris. The modiolus can be easily palpated. Wearing either a glove or a finger cot, place the index finger of your palpating hand inside the client's mouth just lateral to the corner of the mouth, and your thumb outside the client's mouth in a similar location. Compress the skin and mucosa of the cheek just lateral to the corner of the mouth between your index finger and thumb and feel for the modiolus.

MUSCLES OF FACIAL EXPRESSION—SEATED—cont'd

Levator Anguli Oris:

❑ **ATTACHMENTS:**

o Maxilla *to the* fascia at the corner (angle) of the mouth (Figure 12-45, A)

❑ **ACTIONS:**

o Elevates the corner of the mouth

Palpation steps:

1. Gently place palpating finger(s) immediately superior to the corner of the mouth.
2. Ask the client to elevate the corner of the mouth directly superiorly as if to show you the canine tooth (making what could be described as a Dracula-like expression), and feel for the contraction of the levator anguli oris (Figure 12-45, B).
3. Once felt, palpate the entire muscle as the client alternately contracts and relaxes it. Note: The most superior aspect of this muscle is deep to the zygomaticus minor and levator labii superioris and can be difficult to palpate and discern from these muscles. Furthermore, try to distinguish the levator anguli oris from the zygomaticus major, which also elevates the corner of the mouth.

A

B

Figure 12-45 A, Anterior view of the right levator anguli oris. The orbicularis oris has been ghosted in. **B,** Palpation of the right levator anguli oris as the client elevates the corner of the mouth (making a Dracula-like expression).

MUSCLES OF FACIAL EXPRESSION—SEATED—cont'd

Risorius:

❑ **ATTACHMENTS:**

o Fascia superficial to the masseter *to the* fascia at the corner (angle) of the mouth (Figure 12-46, A)

❑ **ACTIONS:**

o Draws the corner of the mouth laterally

Palpation steps:

1. Gently place palpating finger(s) immediately lateral to the corner of the mouth.
2. Ask the client to draw the corner of the mouth directly laterally, and feel for the contraction of the risorius (Figure 12-46, B).
3. Once felt, palpate the entire muscle as the client alternately contracts and relaxes it. Note: Make sure that you are not palpating too far superiorly on the zygomaticus major, which can also draw the corner of the mouth laterally.

A

B

Figure 12-46 A, Anterior view of the right risorius. The orbicularis oris has been ghosted in. **B**, Palpation of the right risorius as the client draws the corner of the mouth laterally.

12

MUSCLES OF FACIAL EXPRESSION—SEATED—cont'd

Depressor Anguli Oris:

❏ **ATTACHMENTS:**

o Mandible *to the* fascia at the corner (angle) of the mouth (Figure 12-47, A)

❏ **ACTIONS:**

o Depresses and draws the corner of the mouth laterally

Palpation steps:

1. Gently place palpating finger(s) slightly lateral and inferior to the corner of the mouth.
2. Ask the client to frown by depressing and drawing the corner of the mouth laterally and feel for the contraction of the depressor anguli oris (Figure 12-47, B).
3. Once felt, palpate the entire muscle as the client alternately contracts and relaxes it. Note: It can be very difficult to distinguish the depressor anguli oris from the nearby depressor labii inferioris, because both muscles engage with depressing and drawing laterally the lower lip/corner of the mouth.

A

B

Figure 12-47 A, Anterior view of the right depressor anguli oris. The orbicularis oris has been ghosted in. **B**, Palpation of the right depressor anguli oris as the client frowns. The orbicularis oris has been ghosted in.

12

MUSCLES OF FACIAL EXPRESSION—SEATED—cont'd

Depressor Labii Inferioris:

❏ **ATTACHMENTS:**

o Mandible *to the* fascia of the lower lip (Figure 12-48, A)

❏ **ACTIONS:**

o Depresses, everts, and draws the lower lip laterally

Palpation steps:

1. Gently place palpating finger(s) inferior to the lower lip and slightly lateral to the midline.
2. Ask the client to depress and draw the lower lip laterally, and feel for the contraction of the depressor labii inferioris (Figure 12-48, B).
3. Once felt, palpate the entire muscle as the client alternately contracts and relaxes it. Note: It can be very difficult to distinguish the depressor labii inferioris from the nearby depressor anguli oris, because both muscles engage with depressing and drawing laterally the lower lip/corner of the mouth.

A

B

Figure 12-48 A, Anterior view of the right depressor labii inferioris. The orbicularis oris has been ghosted in. **B**, Palpation of the right depressor labii inferioris as the client depresses and draws the lower lip laterally. The orbicularis oris has been ghosted in.

12

MUSCLES OF FACIAL EXPRESSION—SEATED—cont'd

Mentalis:

❑ **ATTACHMENTS:**

o Mandible *to the* fascia and skin of the chin (Figure 12-49, A)

❑ **ACTIONS:**

o Elevates, protracts, and everts the lower lip; wrinkles the skin of the chin

Palpation steps:

1. Gently place palpating finger(s) approximately 1 inch (2.5 cm) inferior to the lower lip and slightly lateral to the midline.
2. Ask the client to depress and stick out the lower lip as if pouting, and feel for the contraction of the mentalis (Figure 12-49, B).
3. Once felt, palpate the entire muscle as the client alternately contracts and relaxes it. Note: The inferior aspect of the mentalis is superficial and easy to palpate. The superior aspect of the mentalis is more challenging to palpate and discern because it is deep to the depressor labii inferioris.

A

B

Figure 12-49 A, Lateral view of the right mentalis. **B**, Palpation of the right mentalis as the client sticks out the lower lip as if pouting.

12

MUSCLES OF FACIAL EXPRESSION—SEATED—cont'd

Buccinator:

❏ **ATTACHMENTS:**

o Maxilla and the mandible *to the* fascia at the corner of the mouth and the muscular tissue of the lips (Figure 12-50, A)

❏ **ACTIONS:**

o Compresses the cheek against the teeth

Palpation steps:

1. Gently place palpating finger(s) lateral and slightly superior to the corner of the mouth.
2. Ask the client to take in a deep breath, purse the lips, and press the lips against the teeth as if expelling air while playing the trumpet, and feel for the contraction of the buccinator (Figure 12-50, C).
3. Once felt, palpate the entire muscle as the client alternately contracts and relaxes it. Note: Much of the buccinator is deep to the masseter and other muscles of facial expression, making its palpation and discernment more difficult.

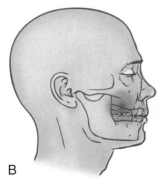

Buccinator
Masseter

A

B

C

Figure 12-50 A, Lateral view of the right buccinator. The masseter has been ghosted in. **B**, Lateral view illustrating a common buccinator TrP and its corresponding referral zone. **C**, Palpation of the right buccinator as the client takes in a deep breath, purses the lips, and presses the lips against the teeth as if playing the trumpet.

12

TRIGGER POINTS

1. Trigger points (TrPs) in the buccinator often result from or are perpetuated by acute or chronic overuse of the muscle (e.g., playing a brass or woodwind instrument or repeatedly blowing up balloons) or poor-fitting dental appliances (e.g., braces, night guards).
2. TrPs in the buccinator tend to produce a deep aching in the jaw and difficulty chewing and swallowing.
3. The referral patterns of buccinator TrPs must be distinguished from the referral patterns of TrPs in the other muscles of facial expression, the temporalis, and the masseter.
4. TrPs in the buccinator are often incorrectly assessed as a headache or temporomandibular joint (TMJ) dysfunction.
5. Associated TrPs often occur in the other muscles of facial expression, muscles of mastication (temporalis, masseter, and lateral and medial pterygoids), sternocleidomastoid, and upper trapezius.

MUSCLES OF FACIAL EXPRESSION—SEATED—cont'd

Orbicularis Oris:

❏ **ATTACHMENTS:**

o The orbicularis oris encircles the mouth (Figure 12-51, A).

❏ **ACTIONS:**

o Closes the mouth and protracts the lips

Palpation steps:

1. Wearing a finger cot or glove, gently place palpating finger(s) on the tissue of the lips.
2. Ask the client to pucker up the lips, and feel for the contraction of the orbicularis oris (Figure 12-51, B).
3. Once felt, palpate the entire muscle as the client alternately contracts and relaxes it. Note: Be careful to distinguish the inferior aspect of the orbicularis oris from the mentalis, because both muscles elevate and protract the lower lip.

12

A

B

Figure 12-51 A, Anterior view of the orbicularis oris (bilaterally). **B,** Palpation of the orbicularis oris on the right side as the client puckers the lips.

Muscles of the Head

For all palpations of the muscles of the head, the client is supine; you are seated at the head of the table.

Scalp Muscle(s):

1. **Occipitofrontalis:** First place palpating hands over the frontal bone, then over the occipital bone, each time feeling for the contraction of the occipitofrontalis as the client contracts the muscle by elevating the eyebrows. Once felt, palpate the entire muscle. Note: This muscle is often palpated just as well when it is relaxed.
2. **Detour to other scalp muscles (temporoparietalis and auricularis anterior, superior, and posterior):** For the temporoparietalis, palpate approximately 1 to 2 inches (2.5 to 5 cm) superior and slightly anterior to the ear; feel for the contraction of the temporoparietalis as the client elevates the ear. For the auricularis anterior, superior, and posterior, palpate immediately anterior, superior, and posterior to the ear, respectively, as the client tries to move the ear in that direction. Note: Most people are unable to control the contraction of these muscles, so they must usually be palpated when relaxed.

Muscles of Mastication:

3. **Temporalis:** Place palpating fingers over the temporal fossa and feel for the contraction of the temporalis as the client elevates the mandible at the TMJs by clenching the teeth. Once felt, palpate the entire muscle as the client alternately contracts and relaxes it.
4. **Masseter:** Place palpating fingers between the zygomatic arch and the angle of the mandible and feel for the contraction of the masseter as the client elevates the mandible at the TMJs by clenching the teeth. Once felt, palpate from the zygomatic arch to the angle of the mandible as the client alternately contracts and relaxes the muscle.
5. **Lateral pterygoid:** Wearing a finger cot or glove, run a palpating finger along the external surface of the upper teeth until you reach the back molars. Then press posteriorly and superiorly and feel for a little pocket. Palpate here for the lateral pterygoid between the condyle of the mandible and the gum above the upper teeth. To contract the lateral pterygoid, ask the client to either protract or slowly and carefully contralaterally deviate the mandible at the TMJs.
6. **Medial pterygoid:** Curl palpating fingers around the angle of the mandible to the internal surface and palpate for the contraction of the medial pterygoid's inferior attachment as the client elevates the mandible at the TMJs by clenching the teeth. Once felt, try to palpate it as superiorly as possible. Note: The medial pterygoid can be palpated inside the mouth. Wearing a finger cot or glove, run an index finger along the internal surfaces of the bottom teeth until you reach the back molars. Then press

posterolaterally against the inside wall of the mouth and feel for the contraction of the medial pterygoid as the client protracts the mandible at the TMJs.

Muscles of Facial Expression of the Eye:

7. **Orbicularis oculi:** Gently place palpating fingers on the tissue around the client's eye. Ask the client to somewhat forcefully close the eye as if to squint, and feel for the contraction of the orbicularis oculi. Once felt, palpate the entire muscle as the client alternately contracts and relaxes it.
8. **Levator palpebrae superioris:** Gently place palpating fingers on the client's upper eyelid. Ask the client to elevate the upper eyelid, and feel for the contraction of the levator palpebrae superioris. Once felt, palpate as much of the muscle as possible as the client alternately contracts and relaxes it.
9. **Corrugator supercilii:** Gently place palpating fingers on the medial portion of the client's eyebrow. Ask the client to frown, bringing the eyebrows down, and feel for the contraction of the corrugator supercilii. Once felt, palpate the entire muscle as the client alternately contracts and relaxes it.

Muscles of Facial Expression of the Nose:

10. **Procerus:** Gently place palpating fingers on the bridge of the client's nose. Ask the client to make a look of disdain, bringing the eyebrows down and/or wrinkling the skin of the nose upward, and feel for the contraction of the procerus. Once felt, palpate the entire muscle as the client alternately contracts and relaxes it.
11. **Nasalis:** Gently place palpating fingers on the inferolateral aspect of the client's nose. Ask the client to flare the nostril (as when taking in a deep breath), and feel for the contraction of the nasalis. Once felt, palpate the entire muscle as the client alternately contracts and relaxes it.
12. **Depressor septi nasi:** Gently place palpating fingers directly inferior to the client's nose. Ask the client to constrict the nostril (as if pulling the middle of the nose down toward the mouth), and feel for the contraction of the depressor septi nasi. Once felt, palpate the entire muscle as the client alternately contracts and relaxes it.

Muscles of Facial Expression of the Mouth:

13. **Levator labii superioris alaeque nasi:** Gently place palpating fingers just lateral to the client's nose. Ask the client to either elevate the upper lip to show you the upper gum or flare the nostril, and feel for the contraction of the levator

12

labii superioris alaeque nasi. Once felt, palpate the entire muscle as the client alternately contracts and relaxes it.

14. **Levator labii superioris:** Gently place palpating fingers approximately $1/2$ inch (1 cm) lateral to the center of the upper lip at its superior margin. Ask the client to elevate the upper lip to show you the upper gum, and feel for the contraction of the levator labii superioris. Once felt, palpate the entire muscle toward the eye as the client alternately contracts and relaxes it.

15. **Zygomaticus minor:** Gently place palpating fingers approximately $1/2$ to $3/4$ inch (1 to 2 cm) lateral to the center of the upper lip at its superior margin. Ask the client to elevate the upper lip to show you the upper gum, and feel for the contraction of the zygomaticus minor. Once felt, palpate the entire muscle toward the zygomatic bone as the client alternately contracts and relaxes it.

16. **Zygomaticus major:** Gently place palpating fingers immediately superolateral to the corner of the mouth. Ask the client to smile by drawing the corner of the mouth both superiorly and laterally, and feel for the contraction of the zygomaticus major. Once felt, palpate the entire muscle toward the zygomatic bone as the client alternately contracts and relaxes it.

17. **Levator anguli oris:** Gently place palpating fingers immediately superior to the corner of the mouth. Ask the client to elevate the corner of the mouth directly superiorly as if to show you the canine tooth (making what could be described as a Dracula-like expression), and feel for the contraction of the levator anguli oris. Once felt, palpate the entire muscle as the client alternately contracts and relaxes it.

18. **Risorius:** Gently place palpating fingers immediately lateral to the corner of the mouth. Ask the client to draw the corner of the mouth directly laterally, and feel for the contraction of the risorius. Once felt, palpate the entire muscle as the client alternately contracts and relaxes it.

19. **Depressor anguli oris:** Gently place palpating fingers slightly lateral and inferior to the corner of the mouth. Ask the client to depress and draw the corner of the mouth laterally, and feel for the contraction of the depressor anguli oris. Once felt, palpate the entire muscle as the client alternately contracts and relaxes it.

20. **Depressor labii inferioris:** Gently place palpating fingers inferior to the lower lip and slightly lateral to the midline. Ask the client to depress and draw the lower lip laterally, and feel for the contraction of the depressor labii inferioris. Once felt, palpate the entire muscle as the client alternately contracts and relaxes it.

21. **Mentalis:** Gently place palpating fingers approximately 1 inch (2.5 cm) inferior to the lower lip and slightly lateral to the midline. Ask the client to depress and stick out the lower lip as if pouting, and feel for the contraction of the mentalis. Once felt, palpate the entire muscle as the client alternately contracts and relaxes it.

22. **Buccinator:** Gently place palpating finger(s) lateral and slightly superior to the corner of the mouth. Ask the client to take in a deep breath, purse the lips, and press the lips against the teeth as if playing a trumpet, and feel for the contraction of the buccinator. Once felt, palpate the entire muscle as the client alternately contracts and relaxes it.

23. **Orbicularis oris:** Wearing a finger cot or glove, place palpating finger(s) on the tissue of the lips. Ask the client to pucker up the lips, and feel for the contraction of the orbicularis oris. Once felt, palpate the entire muscle as the client alternately contracts and relaxes it.

Chapter 13

Tour #4—Palpation of the Muscles of the Arm

Overview

This chapter is a palpation tour of the muscles of the arm. The tour begins with the deltoid, then covers the muscles of the anterior arm, and finishes with palpation of the posterior arm. Palpation for each of the muscles is shown in the seated position, but alternate palpation positions are also described. The major muscles of the region are each given a separate layout; there are also a number of detours to other muscles of the region. Trigger point (TrP) information and stretching are given for each of the muscles covered in this chapter. The chapter closes with an advanced *Whirlwind Tour* that describes the sequential palpation of all of the muscles of the chapter.

Chapter Outline

Chapter Objectives

After completing this chapter, the student should be able to perform the following for each of the muscles covered in this chapter:

1. State the attachments.
2. State the actions.
3. Describe the starting position for palpation.
4. Describe and explain the purpose of each of the palpation steps.
5. Palpate each muscle.
6. State the "Palpation Key."
7. Describe alternate palpation positions.
8. State the locations of the most common TrP(s).
9. Describe the TrP referral zones.
10. State the most common factors that create and/or perpetuate TrPs.
11. State the symptoms most commonly caused by TrPs.
12. Describe and perform a stretch.

Video demonstrations of the muscle palpations in this chapter are presented in Chapter 13 on DVD 1.

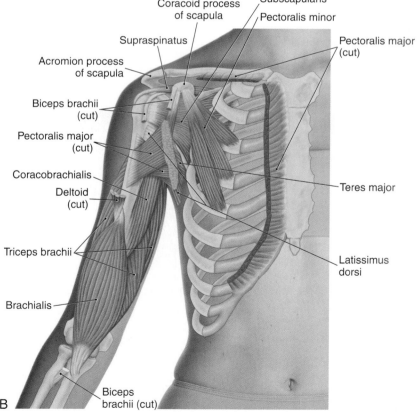

Figure 13-1 Anterior views of the right arm region. **A**, Superficial view. **B**, Deep view with the pectoralis major and deltoid cut and/or removed.

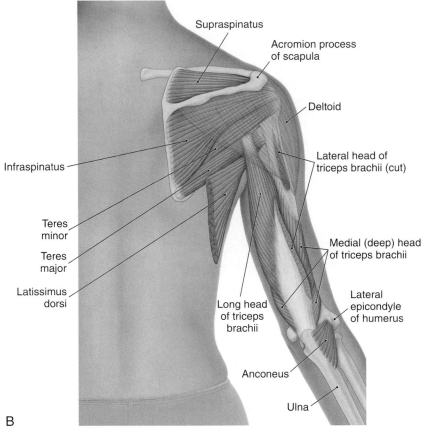

Figure 13-2 Posterior views of the right arm region. **A**, Superficial view. **B**, Deep view with the deltoid ghosted in.

13

Acromion process of scapula

Clavicle

Deltoid

Biceps brachii

Lateral intermuscular septum

Brachialis

Brachioradialis

Extensor carpi radialis longus

Triceps brachii

Lateral epicondyle of humerus

Extensor carpi radialis brevis

Anconeus

Extensor digitorum

Extensor carpi ulnaris

Extensor digiti minimi

Figure 13-3 Lateral view of the right arm region.

Figure 13-4 Medial view of the right arm region.

Upper trapezius

Clavicle

Deltoid

Coracobrachialis

Biceps brachii

Brachialis

Bicipital aponeurosis

Pronator teres

Flexor carpi radialis

Palmaris longus

Flexor carpi ulnaris

Flexor digitorum superficialis

Pectoralis major

Median nerve

Brachial artery

Ulnar nerve

Triceps brachii

Medial epicondyle

Extensor digitorum

Extensor digiti minimi

Extensor carpi ulnaris

Ulna

13

DELTOID—SEATED

❏ ATTACHMENTS:

o Lateral ⅓ of the clavicle and the acromion process and spine of the scapula *to the* deltoid tuberosity of the humerus

❏ ACTIONS:

o The entire deltoid abducts the arm at the shoulder joint and downwardly rotates the scapula at the shoulder (glenohumeral) and scapulocostal joints.

o The anterior deltoid also flexes, medially rotates, and horizontally flexes the arm at the shoulder joint.

o The posterior deltoid also extends, laterally rotates, and horizontally extends the arm at the shoulder joint.

Starting position (Figure 13-6):

o Client seated

o Therapist standing behind the client

o Palpating hand placed on the lateral arm immediately distal to the acromion process of the scapula

o Support hand placed on the distal arm, just proximal to the elbow joint

Palpation steps:

1. To palpate the entire deltoid, resist the client from abducting the arm at the shoulder joint and feel for the contraction of the deltoid.

2. Continue palpating the deltoid toward its distal attachment by strumming perpendicular to its fibers (Figure 13-7).

3. To isolate the anterior deltoid, place palpating hand just inferior to the lateral clavicle, resist the client from horizontally flexing the arm at the shoulder joint, and feel for the contraction of the anterior deltoid; palpate to the distal attachment by strumming perpendicular to its fibers (Figure 13-8, A).

4. To isolate the posterior deltoid, place palpating hand just inferior to the spine of the scapula, resist the client from horizontally extending the arm at the shoulder joint, and feel for the contraction of the posterior deltoid; palpate to the distal attachment by strumming perpendicular to its fibers (Figure 13-8, B).

5. Once the entire deltoid has been located, have the client relax it and palpate to assess its baseline tone.

A   B   C

Figure 13-5 The right deltoid. **A**, Lateral view. The proximal end of the brachialis has been ghosted in. **B**, Anterior view. The proximal ends of the pectoralis major and brachialis have been ghosted in. **C**, Posterior view. The proximal end of the triceps brachii has been ghosted in.

13

DELTOID—SEATED—cont'd

Figure 13-6 Starting position for seated palpation of the right deltoid.

Figure 13-7 Close-up strumming of the right middle deltoid as the client abducts the arm against resistance.

A

B

Figure 13-8 Palpation of the anterior and posterior deltoid. **A**, Palpation of the anterior deltoid as the client horizontally flexes the arm against resistance. **B**, Palpation of the posterior deltoid as the client horizontally extends the arm against resistance.

Palpation Notes:
1. The posterior deltoid attaches on the spine of the scapula much further medially than most people realize. The attachment extends nearly to the root of the spine of the scapula.
2. When horizontally flexing the arm at the shoulder joint to palpate the anterior deltoid, the clavicular head of the pectoralis major will also contract. It is usually not difficult to discern the border between these two muscles, because there is usually a visible and palpable small groove located between them.

Alternate Palpation Position—Supine
The anterior deltoid can be palpated with the client supine. See Palpation of the Anterior Deltoid in Tour #1, page 163.

The posterior deltoid can be palpated with the client prone. See Palpation of the Posterior Deltoid in Tour #1, page 152.

Palpation Key:
Resist abduction for the entire muscle.

DELTOID—SEATED—cont'd

TRIGGER POINTS

1. Trigger points (TrPs) in the deltoid often result from or are perpetuated by acute overuse, chronic overuse (e.g., holding the arm up in abduction for prolonged periods), direct trauma (e.g., impact during sports), injections, and TrPs in the supraspinatus or infraspinatus.
2. TrPs in the deltoid may produce weakness when performing abduction of the arm at the shoulder joint.
3. The referral patterns of deltoid TrPs must be distinguished from the referral patterns of TrPs in the scalenes, supraspinatus, infraspinatus, teres minor, teres major, sub-

scapularis, pectoralis major and minor, coracobrachialis, biceps brachii, and triceps brachii.
4. TrPs in the deltoid are often incorrectly assessed as a rotator cuff tear, bicipital tendinitis, subdeltoid/subacromial bursitis, glenohumeral or acromioclavicular joint arthritis, or C5 nerve compression.
5. Associated TrPs often occur in the clavicular head of the pectoralis major, supraspinatus, biceps brachii, teres major, infraspinatus, triceps brachii, and latissimus dorsi.

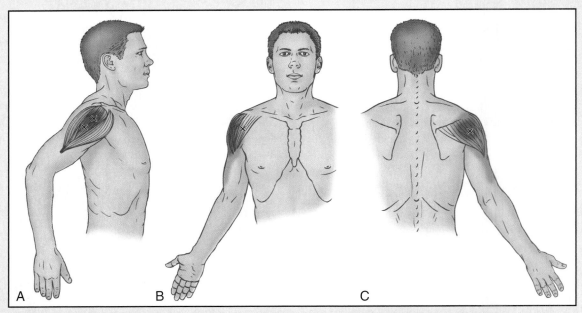

Figure 13-9 Common deltoid TrPs and their corresponding referral zones. **A**, Middle deltoid. **B**, Anterior deltoid. **C**, Posterior deltoid.

STRETCHING THE DELTOID

Figure 13-10 Stretches of the right deltoid. **A**, Stretch of the anterior deltoid. **B**, Stretch of the posterior deltoid. **C**, Stretch of the middle deltoid. Note: See also Figure 10-50 for another middle deltoid stretch.

13

BICEPS BRACHII—SEATED

❑ **ATTACHMENTS:**

o Supraglenoid tubercle (long head) and coracoid process (short head) of the scapula *to the* radial tuberosity and the deep fascia overlying the common flexor tendon

❑ **ACTIONS:**

o Flexes the forearm at the elbow joint; supinates the forearm at the radioulnar joints
o Flexes the arm at the shoulder joint
o Long head abducts the arm at the shoulder joint; short head adducts the arm at the shoulder joint

Starting position (Figure 13-12):

o Client seated with the arm relaxed and the forearm fully supinated and resting on the client's thigh
o Therapist seated to the side and facing the client
o Palpating hand placed in the middle of the anterior arm
o Support hand placed on the client's anterior distal forearm, just proximal to the wrist joint

Palpation steps:

1. With mild to moderate force, resist the client from flexing the forearm at the elbow joint and feel for the contraction of the biceps brachii (Figure 13-13).
2. Strumming perpendicular to the fibers, first palpate to the distal tendon on the radius; then palpate toward the proximal attachments as far as possible.
3. Once the biceps brachii has been located, have the client relax it and palpate to assess its baseline tone.

Figure 13-11 Anterior view of the right biceps brachii. The coracobrachialis and distal end of the brachialis have been ghosted in.

Figure 13-12 Starting position for seated palpation of the right biceps brachii.

Figure 13-13 Palpation of the right biceps brachii as the client flexes the forearm at the elbow joint against resistance.

13

BICEPS BRACHII—SEATED—cont'd

Palpation Notes:

1. Because the biceps brachii is a flexor and supinator of the forearm, it is best to resist the client's forearm flexion when the forearm is fully supinated.
2. It is important that the client's arm is fully relaxed and hanging vertically. Otherwise, flexors of the arm at the shoulder joint will have to contract to hold it in flexion, and the contractions of these muscles will make it more difficult to discern the biceps brachii from other muscles in the proximal arm.
3. In addition to palpating the biceps brachii when it is contracted, it is easy to palpate it when it is relaxed. When relaxed, the biceps brachii can usually be gently pinched away from the underlying muscles. Also, with the arm muscles relaxed, feel for the groove between the biceps brachii and the brachialis on the lateral side of the arm (Figure 13-14, A).
4. The biceps brachii is not as wide as most people think. It does not cover the entire anterior arm. Much of the antero-

lateral arm is composed of the brachialis muscle. See Figure 13-1.
5. The distal aponeurosis of the biceps brachii that attaches into soft tissue overlying the common flexor tendon (near the medial epicondyle of the humerus) can often be palpated and discerned from adjacent soft tissue.
6. The proximal attachment of the biceps brachii on the coracoid process of the scapula can be palpated through the axilla by reaching deep to the pectoralis major and anterior deltoid. To do this, the pectoralis major and anterior deltoid must be slackened and relaxed; this can be accomplished by passively flexing the arm and supporting it in this position (Figure 13-14, B), and slowly reaching toward the coracoid process with the palpating fingers. The proximal tendon of the long head of the biceps brachii can also be accessed in this manner (see Figure 13-14, B); the supraglenoid tubercle attachment on the scapula is usually not palpable.

Figure 13-14 Palpation of the lateral border and proximal tendons of the right biceps brachii. **A,** Palpation of the border between the biceps brachii and the brachialis when they are relaxed. **B,** Palpation of the proximal tendons in the axilla deep to the pectoralis major (ghosted in) and anterior deltoid (not shown).

BICEPS BRACHII—SEATED—cont'd

TRIGGER POINTS

1. Trigger points (TrPs) in the biceps brachii often result from or are perpetuated by acute or chronic overuse of the muscle (e.g., lifting a heavy object with the forearm fully supinated at the radioulnar joints, prolonged use of a manual screwdriver) or TrPs in the infraspinatus.
2. TrPs in the biceps brachii may produce a pain that is superficial and dull, or restrict elbow joint extension.
3. The referral patterns of biceps brachii TrPs must be distinguished from the referral patterns of TrPs in the deltoid, coracobrachialis, brachialis, supinator, pectoralis major and minor, subclavius, infraspinatus, subscapularis, and scalenes.
4. TrPs in the biceps brachii are often incorrectly assessed as bicipital tendinitis, subdeltoid/subacromial bursitis, glenohumeral joint arthritis, or C5 nerve compression.
5. Associated TrPs often occur in the brachialis, coracobrachialis, supinator, triceps brachii, anterior deltoid, supraspinatus, upper trapezius, and coracobrachialis.

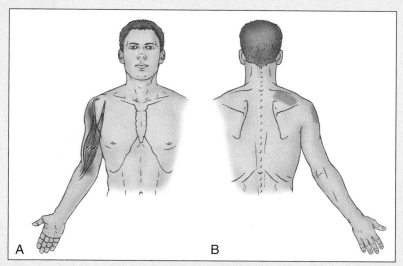

Figure 13-15 A, Anterior view illustrating common biceps brachii TrPs and their corresponding referral zone. **B**, Posterior view showing the remainder of the referral zone.

13

STRETCHING THE BICEPS BRACHII

Figure 13-16 A stretch of the right biceps brachii. The elbow and shoulder joints are fully extended with the forearm fully pronated as the client holds onto a doorframe and leans away.

Alternate Palpation Position—Supine
The biceps brachii can also be easily palpated with the client supine. Follow the seated directions.

Palpation Key:
Resist forearm flexion with the forearm fully supinated.

BRACHIALIS—SEATED

❏ ATTACHMENTS:

o Distal ½ of the anterior shaft of the humerus (beginning just distal to the deltoid tuberosity) *to the* tuberosity and coronoid process of the ulna

❏ ACTIONS:

o Flexes the forearm at the elbow joint

Starting position (Figure 13-18):

o Client seated with the arm relaxed and the forearm fully pronated and resting on the client's thigh
o Therapist seated to the side and facing the client
o Palpating hand placed on the anterolateral arm (immediately posterior to the biceps brachii)
o Supporting hand placed on the client's anterior distal forearm, just proximal to the wrist joint

Palpation steps:

1. With gentle force, resist the client from flexing the forearm at the elbow joint (with the forearm fully pronated), and feel for the contraction of the brachialis (Figure 13-19).
2. Strumming perpendicular to the fibers, palpate the lateral side of the brachialis to its proximal attachment and then to its distal attachment.
3. The preceding two steps can also be used to palpate the anterior aspect of the brachialis through the relaxed biceps brachii, as the brachialis is contracting.
4. Once the brachialis has been located, have the client relax it and palpate to assess its baseline tone.

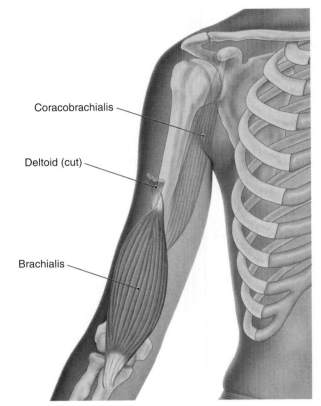

Coracobrachialis

Deltoid (cut)

Brachialis

Figure 13-17 Anterior view of the right brachialis; the coracobrachialis and distal end of the deltoid have been ghosted in.

13

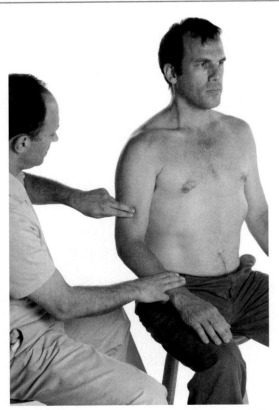

Figure 13-18 Starting position for seated palpation of the right brachialis.

Figure 13-19 Palpation of the right brachialis as the client is gently resisted from flexing the forearm at the elbow joint, with the forearm in a fully pronated position.

BRACHIALIS—SEATED—cont'd

Palpation Notes:

1. The brachialis can flex the forearm at the elbow joint whether the forearm is pronated or supinated. The reason that it is important to palpate the brachialis (the lateral or anterior aspect) with the forearm pronated is that it relaxes the biceps brachii via reciprocal inhibition (the biceps brachii is a supinator of the forearm). However, resistance to the client's forearm flexion must be gentle, or reciprocal inhibition will be overridden and the biceps brachii will be recruited to contract, making palpation of the brachialis more difficult.

2. The proximal attachment of the brachialis is located around the deltoid tuberosity of the humerus; therefore this landmark is useful to help locate the brachialis.

3. The anterior aspect of the brachialis does not have to be palpated through the biceps brachii; rather, it can also be palpated directly. Passively flex the client's fully supinated forearm approximately 45 degrees to relax and slacken the biceps brachii. Locate the border between these two muscles and push the biceps brachii medially out of the way. Now palpate posteriorly toward the shaft of the humerus to palpate directly the anterior aspect of the brachialis (Figure 13-20).

4. **The medial aspect of the brachialis is partially superficial and palpable in the distal half of the medial arm. Palpation here must be done prudently due to the presence of the brachial artery and the median and ulnar nerves (see Figure 13-4).**

5. It is difficult to palpate the brachialis all the way to its ulnar attachment.

Figure 13-20 Pushing the biceps brachii out of the way medially to access the anterior aspect of the right brachialis.

Alternate Palpation Position—Supine

The brachialis can also be easily palpated with the client supine. Follow the seated directions.

TRIGGER POINTS

1. Trigger points (TrPs) in the brachialis often result from or are perpetuated by acute or chronic overuse of the muscle (e.g., heavy lifting, especially with forearms fully pronated) or prolonged shortening of the muscle (e.g., sleeping with elbow joint fully flexed).

2. TrPs in the brachialis may produce soreness of the thumb or radial nerve entrapment.

3. The referral patterns of brachialis TrPs must be distinguished from the referral patterns of TrPs in the brachioradialis, subclavius, extensor carpi radialis longus, pronator teres, supinator, adductor pollicis, opponens pollicis, and scalenes.

4. TrPs in the brachialis are often incorrectly assessed as bicipital tendinitis, supraspinatus tendinitis, C5 or C6 nerve compression, or carpal tunnel syndrome.

5. Associated TrPs often occur in the biceps brachii, brachioradialis, supinator, and adductor pollicis.

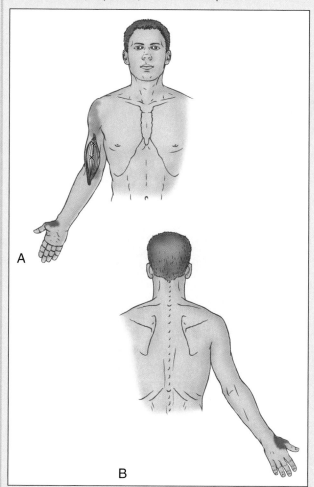

A

B

Figure 13-21 A, Anterior view illustrating common brachialis TrPs and their corresponding referral zone. **B**, Posterior view showing the remainder of the referral zone.

13

BRACHIALIS—SEATED—cont'd

STRETCHING THE BRACHIALIS

Figure 13-22 A stretch of the right brachialis. The client's elbow joint is fully extended with the forearm in a position that is halfway between full supination and full pronation.

🔑

Palpation Key:

Gently resist forearm flexion with the forearm fully pronated.

DETOUR ▶

Brachioradialis: The three major flexors of the forearm at the elbow joint—the biceps brachii, brachialis, and brachioradialis—are all palpated by resisting flexion of the forearm at the elbow joint. The difference is that the biceps brachii is palpated with the forearm in full supination; the brachialis is palpated with the forearm in full pronation; and the brachioradialis is palpated with the forearm in a position that is halfway between full supination and full pronation.

Figure 13-23 Palpation of the right biceps brachii and brachioradialis. **A**, Palpation of the biceps brachii with the client's forearm in full supination. **B**, Palpation of the brachioradialis with the client's forearm positioned halfway between full supination and full pronation.

CORACOBRACHIALIS—SEATED

❑ **ATTACHMENTS:**

o Coracoid process of the scapula *to the* middle ¹/₃ of the medial shaft of the humerus

❑ **ACTIONS:**

o Flexes, adducts, and horizontally flexes the arm at the shoulder joint

Starting position (Figure 13-25):

o Client seated with the arm abducted to 90 degrees and laterally rotated at the shoulder joint, and the forearm flexed at the elbow joint approximately 90 degrees
o Therapist seated or standing in front of the client
o Palpating hand placed on the medial aspect of the proximal half of the client's arm
o Support hand placed on the distal end of the client's arm, just proximal to the elbow joint

Palpation steps:

1. Resist the client's horizontal flexion of the arm at the shoulder joint and feel for the contraction of the coracobrachialis (Figure 13-26).
2. Strumming perpendicular to the fibers, palpate from attachment to attachment.
3. Once the coracobrachialis has been located, have the client relax it and palpate to assess its baseline tone.

Figure 13-24 Anterior view of the right coracobrachialis. The deltoid and proximal end of the pectoralis minor have been ghosted in.

Figure 13-25 Starting position for seated palpation of the right coracobrachialis.

Figure 13-26 Palpation of the right coracobrachialis as the client horizontally flexes the arm at the shoulder joint against resistance. Note: The deltoid has been ghosted in.

Palpation Notes:

1. To easily discern the coracobrachialis from the short head of the biceps brachii, it is important for the forearm to be passively flexed 90 degrees or more so that the biceps brachii stays relaxed.
2. If there is doubt as to whether you are on the coracobrachialis or the short head of the biceps brachii, resist the client from performing flexion of the forearm at the elbow joint. This will cause the short head of the biceps brachii to contract, but not the coracobrachialis. Where these two muscles overlap, the coracobrachialis is deep (posterior) to the short head of the biceps brachii.
3. **Palpation of the coracobrachialis must be done prudently because of the presence of the brachial artery and the median, ulnar, and musculocutaneous nerves (see Figure 13-4).**

Alternate Palpation Position—Supine
The coracobrachialis can be palpated with the client supine. Follow the seated directions.

CORACOBRACHIALIS—SEATED—cont'd

TRIGGER POINTS

1. Trigger points (TrPs) in the coracobrachialis often result from or are perpetuated by acute or chronic overuse of the muscle (e.g., lifting heavy objects in front of the body) or TrPs in synergistic muscles.
2. TrPs in the coracobrachialis may produce severe pain, restricted shoulder joint motion (abduction and extension), and entrapment of the musculocutaneous nerve.
3. The referral patterns of coracobrachialis TrPs must be distinguished from the referral patterns of TrPs in the biceps brachii, triceps brachii, scalenes, supraspinatus, in-

fraspinatus, anterior deltoid, pectoralis major and minor, extensor carpi radialis longus, extensor digitorum, extensor indicis, and second dorsal interosseus manus.
4. TrPs in the coracobrachialis are often incorrectly assessed as carpal tunnel syndrome, subdeltoid/subacromial bursitis, acromioclavicular joint arthritis, supraspinatus tendinitis, or C5, C6, or C7 nerve compression.
5. Associated TrPs often occur in the anterior deltoid, biceps brachii, pectoralis major, and triceps brachii long head.

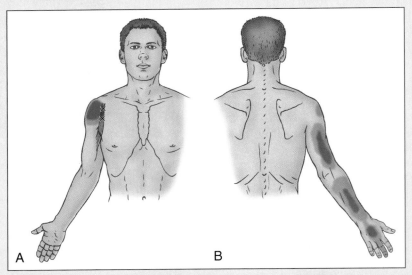

Figure 13-27 A, Anterior view illustrating common coracobrachialis TrPs and their corresponding referral zone. **B**, Posterior view showing the remainder of the referral zone.

STRETCHING THE CORACOBRACHIALIS

Palpation Key:
Resist horizontal flexion of the arm with the elbow joint flexed.

Figure 13-28 A stretch of the right coracobrachialis. The client's arm is extended and adducted behind the body.

13

CORACOBRACHIALIS—SEATED—cont'd

DETOUR

Humeral Attachments of the Subscapularis, Latissimus Dorsi, and Teres Major: If the humeral attachment of the coracobrachialis has been found, the humeral attachments of the latissimus dorsi, teres major, and subscapularis are close by. The latissimus dorsi and teres major are on the medial lip of the bicipital groove, just proximal to the humeral attachment of the coracobrachialis. Just proximal to the bicipital groove attachments of these two muscles is the humeral attachment of the subscapularis on the lesser tu-

bercle of the humerus. To locate all three of these muscular attachments, palpate more proximally into the axilla against the humerus while resisting extension and adduction of the arm for the latissimus dorsi and teres major; then palpate further proximally onto the lesser tubercle while resisting medial rotation of the arm for the subscapularis. See page 353 for palpation of the latissimus dorsi, page 158 for palpation of the teres major, and page 165 for palpation of the subscapularis.

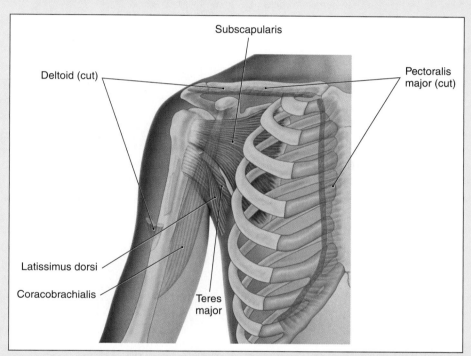

Figure 13-29 The humeral attachments of the right latissimus dorsi, teres major, and subscapularis are shown. The coracobrachialis and cut ends of the pectoralis major and deltoid are ghosted in.

TRICEPS BRACHII—SEATED

❏ ATTACHMENTS:

o Infraglenoid tubercle of the scapula (long head) and the posterior shaft of the humerus (lateral and medial heads) *to the* olecranon process of the ulna

❏ ACTIONS:

o Entire muscle extends the forearm at the elbow joint
o Long head adducts and extends the arm at the shoulder joint

Starting position (Figure 13-31):

o Client seated with the arm relaxed and hanging vertically, and the posterior forearm resting on the client's or therapist's thigh
o Therapist seated in front of or to the side of the client
o Palpating hand placed on the posterior surface of the arm

Palpation steps:

1. Ask the client to extend the forearm at the elbow joint by pressing the forearm against the thigh, and feel for the contraction of the triceps brachii (Figure 13-32).
2. Palpate from attachment to attachment by strumming perpendicular to the fibers.
3. Once the triceps brachii has been located, have the client relax it and palpate to assess its baseline tone.

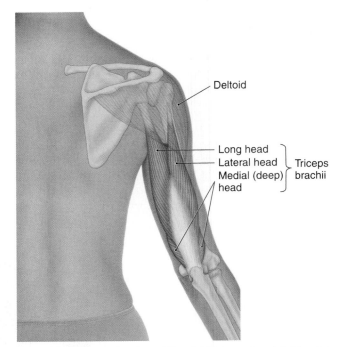

Figure 13-30 Posterior view of the right triceps brachii. The deltoid has been ghosted in.

Figure 13-31 Starting position for seated palpation of the right triceps brachii.

Figure 13-32 Palpation of the belly of the right triceps brachii as the client extends the forearm against resistance.

TRICEPS BRACHII—SEATED—cont'd

Palpation Notes:

1. The proximal attachment of the triceps brachii on the scapula can be difficult to palpate and discern, because it is deep to the posterior deltoid and teres minor muscles (Figure 13-33). To palpate it, follow the triceps brachii proximally with baby steps as the client alternately contracts and relaxes the triceps brachii (extending the forearm at the elbow joint by pressing the forearm against the thigh and then relaxing it). It is important that the musculature across the shoulder joint stays relaxed. If the posterior deltoid and teres minor can be slackened by holding the client's shoulder joint in a small degree of passive extension and lateral rotation, greater access to the triceps brachii is usually allowed.

2. The lateral and medial borders of the triceps brachii can be discerned from the brachialis by asking the client to alternately perform forearm extension against resistance (by pressing the forearm against the thigh) and forearm flexion against resistance (you provide the resistance to forearm flexion with your support hand). The triceps brachii contraction will be felt with forearm extension; the brachialis contraction will be felt with forearm flexion.

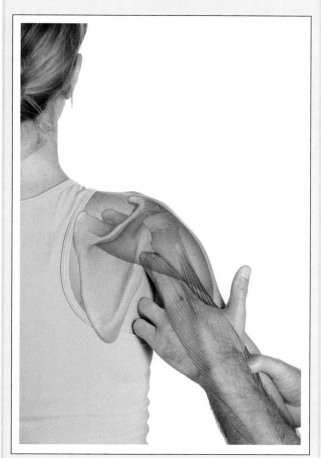

Figure 13-33 Palpation of the proximal attachment of the triceps brachii deep to the posterior deltoid (and teres minor, not shown).

Alternate Palpation Position—Prone

Figure 13-34 The triceps brachii can be easily palpated with the client prone. Position the client prone with the arm abducted 90 degrees at the shoulder joint and resting on the table, and the forearm flexed 90 degrees at the elbow joint and hanging off the table. In this position, ask the client to extend the forearm at the elbow joint against gravity and feel for the contraction of the triceps brachii (added resistance to forearm extension with your support hand can be given).

Palpation Key:
Client presses the forearm against the thigh.

13

TRIGGER POINTS

1. Trigger points (TrPs) in the triceps brachii often result from or are perpetuated by acute or chronic overuse of the muscle (e.g., using the backhand stroke in tennis, doing push-ups, shifting gears manually when driving, using crutches).
2. TrPs in the triceps brachii may produce vague diffuse pain in its referral zone and radial nerve entrapment (resulting in paresthesia of the posterior distal forearm and posterior hand).
3. The referral patterns of triceps brachii TrPs must be distinguished from the referral patterns of TrPs in the anconeus, extensor carpi radialis longus, brachioradialis, extensor digitorum, supinator, scalenes, pectoralis minor, supraspi-

natus, infraspinatus, teres minor, teres major, subscapularis, deltoid, coracobrachialis, latissimus dorsi, flexor digitorum superficialis, flexor digitorum profundus, abductor digiti minimi manus, and first dorsal interosseus manus.
4. TrPs in the triceps brachii are often incorrectly assessed as lateral or medial epicondylitis/epicondylosis, olecranon bursitis, thoracic outlet syndrome, cubital tunnel syndrome, C7 nerve compression, or elbow joint arthritis.
5. Associated TrPs often occur in the biceps brachii, brachialis, brachioradialis, anconeus, supinator, extensor carpi radialis longus, latissimus dorsi, teres major, teres minor, and serratus posterior superior.

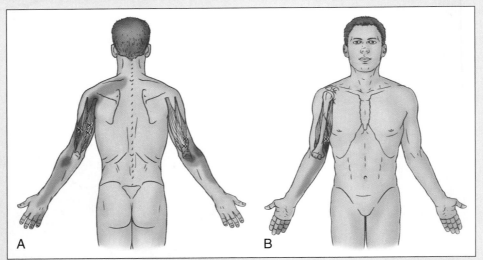

Figure 13-35 Common triceps brachii TrPs and their corresponding referral zones. **A**, Posterior view showing long and lateral head TrPs on the left and a medial head TrP and an attachment TrP on the right. **B**, Anterior view of another medial head TrP.

STRETCHING THE TRICEPS BRACHII

Figure 13-36 A stretch of the right triceps brachii. The client pulls the arm behind the head with the forearm fully flexed at the elbow joint.

TRICEPS BRACHII—SEATED—cont'd

DETOUR

Anconeus: The anconeus is superficial and easily palpated on the posterior side of the proximal forearm. It attaches from the lateral epicondyle of the humerus to the posterior proximal ulna (Figure 13-37, B) and extends the forearm at the elbow joint. To palpate the anconeus, first place your palpating finger directly between the olecranon process of the ulna and the lateral epicondyle of the humerus. Then palpate the anconeus toward its distal attachment by strumming perpendicular to its fibers while the client performs extension of the forearm at the elbow joint against resistance (Figure 13-37, B).

Triceps brachii

Anconeus

A

B

C

Figure 13-37 The right anconeus. **A**, Posterior view of the anconeus. The distal end of the triceps brachii has been ghosted in. **B**, Palpation of the anconeus, strumming perpendicular to the fibers as the client extends the forearm against resistance. **C**, Posterior view illustrating a common anconeus TrP and its corresponding referral zone. Note: A TrP in the anconeus might be incorrectly assessed as tennis elbow.

13

Client Seated:

1. **Deltoid:** The client is seated; you are standing behind the client. To palpate the entire deltoid, palpate proximally on the lateral arm immediately distal to the acromion process of the scapula, and feel for the contraction of the deltoid as the client abducts the arm at the shoulder joint (resistance may be added if needed). Palpate the deltoid toward its distal attachment by strumming perpendicular to the fibers as the client alternately contracts and relaxes the muscle. To isolate the anterior deltoid, resist the client's horizontal flexion of the arm at the shoulder joint and feel for its contraction. Strum perpendicular to the fibers from attachment to attachment. To isolate the posterior deltoid, resist the client's horizontal extension of the arm at the shoulder joint and feel for its contraction. Strum perpendicular to the fibers from attachment to attachment.

2. **Biceps brachii:** The client is seated; you are seated to the side and facing the client. Palpate in the middle of the anterior arm and feel for the contraction as you resist the client's forearm flexion at the elbow joint, with the forearm in full supination. (Note: Be sure that the support hand that gives resistance is on the distal forearm and not on the client's hand.) Once felt, continue palpating to the distal tendon and then continue palpating proximally as far as possible, by strumming perpendicular to the fibers as the client alternately contracts and relaxes the muscle. The proximal tendons can be palpated in the axilla, deep to the pectoralis major and anterior deltoid. The short head's tendon can be palpated all the way to the coracoid process; the supraglenoid tubercle attachment of the long head cannot usually be palpated. (Note: To distinguish the short head from the coracobrachialis, the short head of the biceps brachii will contract with elbow joint flexion; the coracobrachialis will not.) To distinguish the lateral border of the biceps brachii from the brachialis, ask the client to alternately flex the forearm with the forearm supinated and then pronated. The biceps brachii contraction will be more easily felt when the forearm is fully supinated; the brachialis contraction will be more easily felt when the forearm is fully pronated.

3. **Brachialis:** The client is seated; you are seated to the side and facing the client. Feel for the contraction of the brachialis in the anterolateral arm as the client flexes the forearm at the elbow joint with the forearm fully pronated. If resistance is given, apply only a gentle force to the client's forearm flexion. Once felt, continue palpating the brachialis in the anterolateral arm, both proximally toward the deltoid tuberosity and distally as far as possible. Then palpate the brachialis deep to the biceps brachii as the client flexes the forearm, with the forearm fully pronated, against gentle resistance. To distinguish the border between the brachialis and biceps brachii in the anterolateral arm, ask the client to alternately flex the forearm with it pronated and then supinated. The brachialis contraction will be more easily felt when the forearm is fully pronated; the biceps brachii contraction will be more easily felt when the forearm is fully supinated. To distinguish the border between the brachialis and the triceps brachii, have the client alternately flex and extend the forearm against moderate to strong resistance; the brachialis contraction will be felt with forearm flexion; the triceps brachii contraction will be felt with forearm extension.

4. **Coracobrachialis:** Have the client seated with the arm abducted 90 degrees and laterally rotated at the shoulder joint, and the forearm flexed at the elbow joint approximately 90 degrees; you are seated or standing in front of the client. Place palpating hand on the medial aspect of the proximal half of the client's arm and feel for the contraction of the coracobrachialis as you resist the client's horizontal flexion of the arm at the shoulder joint. Once felt, strum perpendicular to the fibers from attachment to attachment. Note: To distinguish the coracobrachialis from the short head of the biceps brachii, use flexion of the forearm at the elbow joint; the biceps brachii short head will contract with elbow joint flexion; the coracobrachialis will not.

5. **Triceps brachii:** The client is seated with the arm relaxed and hanging vertically, and the posterior forearm resting on the client's or therapist's thigh; you are seated facing the client. Place palpating hand on the posterior arm and feel for the contraction of the triceps brachii as the client extends the forearm against the resistance of the thigh. Once felt, palpate to the olecranon process attachment and then as far proximally as possible by strumming perpendicular to the fibers as the client alternately contracts and relaxes the muscle. Following the long head to its scapular attachment deep to the deltoid and teres minor is challenging but can be done if the deltoid is sufficiently relaxed. To distinguish the border between the triceps brachii and the brachialis, have the client alternately extend and flex the forearm against moderate to strong resistance; the triceps brachii contraction will be felt with forearm extension; the brachialis contraction will be felt with forearm flexion.

Chapter 14

Tour #5—Palpation of the Muscles of the Forearm

Overview

This chapter is a palpation tour of the muscles of the forearm. The tour begins with the muscles of the anterior forearm from superficial to deep, then describes palpation of the radial group, and finishes with palpation of the muscles of the posterior forearm from superficial to deep. Palpation for each of the muscles is shown in the seated position, but alternate palpation positions are also described. The major muscles or muscle groups of the region are each given a separate layout; there is also a detour to the pronator quadratus. Trigger point (TrP) information and stretching is given for each of the muscles covered in this chapter. The chapter closes with an advanced *Whirlwind Tour* that describes the sequential palpation of all of the muscles of the chapter.

Chapter Outline

Chapter Objectives

After completing this chapter, the student should be able to perform the following for each of the muscles covered in this chapter:

1. State the attachments.
2. State the actions.
3. Describe the starting position for palpation.
4. Describe and explain the purpose of each of the palpation steps.
5. Palpate each muscle.
6. State the "Palpation Key."
7. Describe alternate palpation positions.
8. State the locations of the most common TrP(s).
9. Describe the TrP referral zones.
10. State the most common factors that create and/or perpetuate TrPs.
11. State the symptoms most commonly caused by TrPs.
12. Describe and perform a stretch.

 Video demonstrations of the muscle palpations in this chapter are presented in Chapter 14 on DVD 1.

Biceps brachii

Brachialis

Triceps brachii

Medial epicondyle
of humerus

Pronator teres

Brachioradialis

Flexor carpi radialis

Palmaris longus — Wrist flexor
group

Flexor carpi ulnaris

Flexor digitorum superficialis

Extensor carpi
radialis longus

Flexor pollicis
longus

Abductor
pollicis longus

Flexor digitorum profundus

Pronator
quadratus

Palmar carpal ligament

Radial
styloid

Transverse carpal ligament
(flexor retinaculum)

Flexor digitorum superficialis

Flexor digitorum profundus

Flexor pollicis
longus

A

Figure 14-1 Views of the anterior forearm. **A,** Superficial view.

B

Figure 14-1, cont'd B, Intermediate view.

Continued

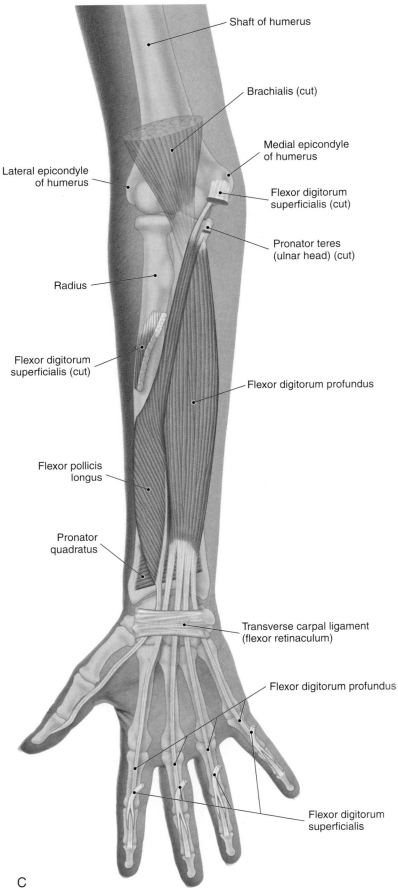

Shaft of humerus

Brachialis (cut)

Medial epicondyle
of humerus

Lateral epicondyle
of humerus

Flexor digitorum
superficialis (cut)

Pronator teres
(ulnar head) (cut)

Radius

Flexor digitorum
superficialis (cut)

Flexor digitorum profundus

Flexor pollicis
longus

Pronator
quadratus

Transverse carpal ligament
(flexor retinaculum)

Flexor digitorum profundus

Flexor digitorum
superficialis

C

Figure 14-1, cont'd C, Deep view.

14

Triceps brachii

Brachioradialis

Medial epicondyle of humerus

Lateral epicondyle of humerus

Olecranon process of ulna

Extensor carpi radialis longus (ECRL)

Anconeus

Extensor carpi radialis brevis (ECRB)

Flexor carpi ulnaris

Extensor digitorum

Extensor digiti minimi

Extensor carpi ulnaris

Abductor pollicis longus

Extensor pollicis brevis

Extensor pollicis longus

Extensor indicis

ECRL tendon

ECRB tendon

A

Figure 14-2 Views of the posterior forearm. **A,** Superficial view.

14

Brachioradialis

Extensor carpi radialis longus (ECRL) (cut)

Medial epicondyle
of humerus

Lateral epicondyle
of humerus

Olecranon process
of ulna

Supinator

Extensor carpi radialis
brevis (ECRB)
(cut)

ECRL (cut)

Extensor pollicis
longus (EPL)

Abductor pollicis longus (APL)

Extensor pollicis brevis

Extensor indicis

Ulnar styloid

Extensor digitorum
tendon to index finger
(cut)

ECRL tendon

ECRB tendon

Ulna

Radius

APL

EPL

C

B

Figure 14-2, cont'd B, Deep view. **C**, Close-up of two of the deep muscles.

14

Figure 14-2, cont'd B, Deep view. **C**, Close-up of two of the deep muscles.

Figure 14-3 A, Lateral view of the forearm. **B**, Medial view of the forearm.

BRACHIORADIALIS—SEATED

❏ ATTACHMENTS:

o Proximal ²/₃ of the lateral supracondylar ridge of the humerus *to the* styloid process of the radius

❏ ACTIONS:

o Flexes the forearm at the elbow joint
o Pronates the supinated forearm at the radioulnar joints to a position halfway between full pronation and supination, or supinates the pronated forearm at the radioulnar joints to a position halfway between full pronation and supination

Starting position (Figure 14-5):

o Client seated with the arm relaxed and the forearm flexed at the elbow joint and in a position that is halfway between full pronation and full supination, and resting on the client's thigh
o Therapist seated to the side and facing the client
o Palpating hand placed on the proximal anterolateral forearm
o Support hand placed on the client's anterior distal forearm, just proximal to the wrist joint

Palpation steps:

1. With moderate force, resist the client from flexing the forearm at the elbow joint and feel for the contraction of the brachioradialis (Figure 14-6).
2. Strumming perpendicular to the fibers, palpate from attachment to attachment.
3. Once the brachioradialis has been located, have the client relax it and palpate to assess its baseline tone.

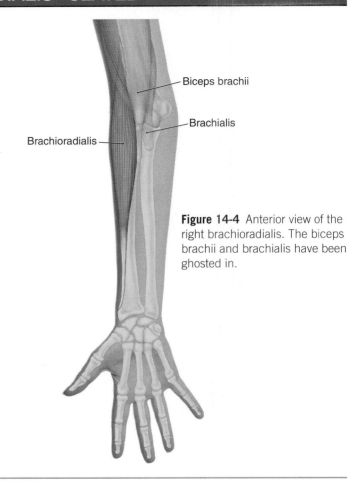

Biceps brachii

Brachialis

Brachioradialis

Figure 14-4 Anterior view of the right brachioradialis. The biceps brachii and brachialis have been ghosted in.

14

Figure 14-5 Starting position for seated palpation of the right brachioradialis.

Figure 14-6 Palpation of the right brachioradialis as the client's forearm flexion at the elbow joint is resisted while the forearm is positioned halfway between full pronation and full supination. Note: The extensor carpi radialis longus has been ghosted in.

BRACHIORADIALIS—SEATED—cont'd

Palpation Notes:

1. The brachioradialis is superficial for its entire path except where the abductor pollicis longus and extensor pollicis brevis cross superficial to it in the distal forearm.

2. The three major flexors of the elbow joint are the biceps brachii, the brachialis, and the brachioradialis. They are all palpated by resisting flexion of the forearm at the elbow joint; the difference is the position of the forearm. For palpation of the biceps brachii, the forearm is fully supinated; for the brachialis, the forearm is fully pronated; for the brachioradialis, the forearm is halfway between full pronation and full supination (Figure 14-7).

3. The "key" to recall the palpation position for the brachioradialis is to think of the position of the upper extremity when hitchhiking: the forearm is flexed and halfway between full pronation and full supination. However, the thumb should be relaxed; if it is extended as in hitchhiking, the abductor pollicis longus and extensor pollicis brevis will contract, making it more difficult to palpate the distal end of the brachioradialis.

Figure 14-7 Palpation of the three major elbow joint flexors as forearm flexion at the elbow joint is resisted. Note that the difference between the three palpations lies in the degree of pronation or supination of the forearm at the radioulnar joints. **A,** Palpation of the biceps brachii with the forearm fully supinated. **B,** Palpation of the brachialis with the forearm fully pronated. **C,** Palpation of the brachioradialis with the forearm halfway between full supination and full pronation.

14

BRACHIORADIALIS—SEATED—cont'd

TRIGGER POINTS

1. Trigger points (TrPs) in the brachioradialis often result from or are perpetuated by acute or chronic overuse of the muscle (e.g., lifting objects with the forearm halfway between full pronation and full supination, digging with a shovel, extensive handshaking).
2. TrPs in the brachioradialis may produce weakness of forearm flexion at the elbow joint and limited forearm pronation when coupled with forearm extension.
3. The referral patterns of brachioradialis TrPs must be distinguished from the referral patterns of TrPs in the supinator, extensor carpi radialis longus and brevis, extensor digitorum, subclavius, scalenes, supraspinatus, coracobrachialis, brachialis, triceps brachii, and 1st dorsal interosseus manus.
4. TrPs in the brachioradialis are often incorrectly assessed as lateral epicondylitis/epicondylosis, C5 or C6 nerve compression, or de Quervain's stenosing tenosynovitis.
5. Associated TrPs often occur in the extensor carpi radialis longus and brevis, extensor digitorum, extensor digiti minimi, supinator, and triceps brachii.

Figure 14-8 Right lateral view illustrating a common brachioradialis TrP and its corresponding referral zone.

STRETCHING THE BRACHIORADIALIS

Figure 14-9 A stretch of the right brachioradialis. The client's forearm is fully extended; the client then uses the other hand to fully pronate the forearm.

Palpation Key:
Place forearm in the hitchhiking position.

PRONATOR TERES—SEATED

❏ **ATTACHMENTS:**

o Medial epicondyle of the humerus (via the common flexor tendon), the medial supracondylar ridge of the humerus, and the coronoid process of the ulna *to the middle* ¹/₃ of the lateral radius

❏ **ACTIONS:**

o Pronates the forearm at the radioulnar joints and flexes the forearm at the elbow joint

Starting position (Figure 14-11):

o Client seated with the arm relaxed and the forearm flexed at the elbow joint and in a position that is halfway between full pronation and full supination, and resting on the client's thigh
o Therapist seated facing the client
o Palpating hand placed on the proximal anterior forearm
o Support hand placed on the client's anterior distal forearm, just proximal to the wrist joint

Palpation steps:

1. With moderate force, resist the client from pronating the forearm at the radioulnar joints and feel for the contraction of the pronator teres (Figure 14-12).
2. Strumming perpendicular to the fibers, palpate from attachment to attachment. Be sure to strum across the entire muscle belly.
3. Once the pronator teres has been located, have the client relax it and palpate to assess its baseline tone.

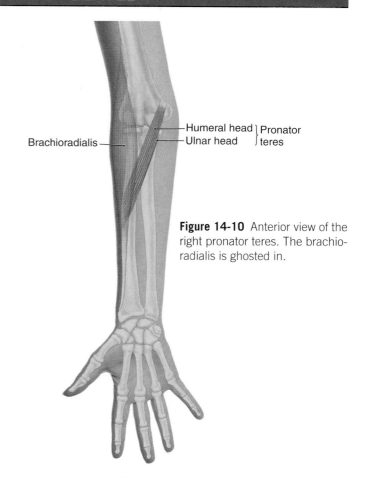

Brachioradialis ⎯ — Humeral head ⎤ Pronator
— Ulnar head ⎦ teres

Figure 14-10 Anterior view of the right pronator teres. The brachioradialis is ghosted in.

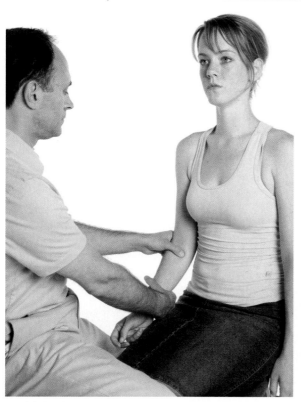

Figure 14-11 Starting position for seated palpation of the right pronator teres.

Figure 14-12 Palpation of the right pronator teres as the client pronates the forearm at the radioulnar joints against resistance.

14

PRONATOR TERES—SEATED—cont'd

Palpation Notes:

1. When resisting the client's forearm pronation, a gentle but firm grasp is needed by the support hand. Otherwise only the client's skin will be held and the underlying forearm bones will be allowed to move. This will result in unsuccessful resistance to forearm pronation and will be uncomfortable for the client.
2. The belly of the pronator teres is superficial and should be easily palpable.
3. The distal end of the pronator teres runs deep to the brachioradialis and can be challenging to palpate. To palpate the distal attachment on the radius, passively flex the client's elbow joint to slacken the brachioradialis; then push the brachioradialis laterally and press deep to it, feeling for the pronator teres attachment on the radius (Figure 14-13).
4. Most of the pronator teres can be palpated if the client is resisted from pronating the forearm with the forearm starting in anatomic position. However, in this position, the brachioradialis may be recruited for pronation, blocking our ability to palpate the distal attachment of the pronator teres. To better palpate the distal attachment of the pronator teres through the brachioradialis, relax the brachioradialis by having the client begin with the forearm halfway between full pronation and full supination.
5. The pronator teres can also be palpated by resisting the client's forearm flexion at the elbow joint. However, this will cause every elbow joint flexor to contract, making it difficult to discern the pronator teres from adjacent muscles.
6. It is difficult to discern the humeral head of the pronator teres from its ulnar head.
7. **The median nerve runs between the humeral and ulnar heads of the pronator teres, therefore, deep work should be done prudently.**

Figure 14-13 Close-up showing palpation of the radial attachment of the right pronator teres by slackening and pushing the brachioradialis out of the way (see Palpation Note #3).

Alternate Palpation Position—Supine

The pronator teres can also be palpated with the client supine. Follow the palpation steps indicated for the seated palpation.

TRIGGER POINTS

1. Trigger points (TrPs) in the pronator teres often result from or are perpetuated by acute or chronic overuse of the muscle (e.g., using a screwdriver, hitting a forehand in tennis with poor form).
2. TrPs in the pronator teres may entrap the median nerve.
3. The referral patterns of pronator teres TrPs must be distinguished from the referral patterns of TrPs in the flexor carpi radialis, brachialis, subscapularis, supraspinatus, infraspinatus, subclavius, scalenes, and adductor pollicis.
4. TrPs in the pronator teres are often incorrectly assessed as medial epicondylitis/epicondylosis, thoracic outlet syndrome, carpal tunnel syndrome, or wrist joint dysfunction.
5. Associated TrPs often occur in the biceps brachii, brachialis, and pronator quadratus.

Figure 14-14 Anterior view illustrating a common pronator teres TrP and its corresponding referral zone.

14

PRONATOR TERES—SEATED—cont'd

STRETCHING THE PRONATOR TERES

Palpation Key:
Resist forearm pronation from a midway position of pronation and supination.

Figure 14-15 A stretch of the right pronator teres. The client's forearm is fully extended; the client then uses the other hand to fully supinate the forearm.

14

WRIST FLEXOR GROUP—SEATED

o The wrist flexor group is composed of the flexor carpi radialis (FCR), palmaris longus (PL), and flexor carpi ulnaris (FCU).

❏ ATTACHMENTS:
o Proximal attachments:
  o All three wrist flexors attach to the medial epicondyle of the humerus via the common flexor tendon.
  o The flexor carpi ulnaris also attaches to the proximal $^2/_3$ of the ulna.
o Distal attachments:
  o The flexor carpi radialis attaches to the radial side of the anterior hand at the bases of the second and third metacarpals.
  o The palmaris longus attaches into the palmar aponeurosis of the palm of the hand.
  o The flexor carpi ulnaris attaches to the ulnar side of the anterior hand at the base of the fifth metacarpal, the pisiform, and the hook of the hamate.

❏ ACTIONS:
o All three wrist flexors flex the hand at the wrist joint.
o The flexor carpi radialis also radially deviates the hand at the wrist joint.
o The flexor carpi ulnaris also ulnar deviates the hand at the wrist joint.

Starting position (Figure 14-17):
o Client seated with the arm relaxed and the forearm flexed at the elbow joint and fully supinated, and resting on the client's thigh
o Therapist seated to the side and facing the client
o Palpating hand placed on the distal anterior forearm (after visualizing the distal tendons)
o Support hand placed on the client's hand, just proximal to the fingers

Palpation steps:
1. Resist the client from flexing the hand at the wrist joint and look for the distal tendons of all three wrist flexors to become visible (be sure that you do not contact the fingers when offering resistance because that will cause finger flexor muscles to be engaged also, making it more difficult to discern the muscles of the wrist flexor group) (Figure 14-18).
2. If they do not become visible, they should be palpable by strumming perpendicularly across them.
3. Continue palpating the flexor carpi radialis proximally to the medial epicondyle by strumming across its fibers. Repeat this for the other two wrist flexors.
4. Once the wrist flexors have been located, have the client relax them and palpate to assess their baseline tone.

Pronator teres

Flexor carpi radialis

Palmaris longus

Flexor carpi ulnaris

Figure 14-16 Anterior view of the right wrist flexor group of muscles. The pronator teres has been ghosted in.

14

WRIST FLEXOR GROUP—SEATED—cont'd

Figure 14-17 Starting position for seated palpation of the right wrist flexor group.

Figure 14-18 All three muscles of the right wrist flexor group are engaged with flexion of the hand against resistance. The distal tendons are often visible, as seen here; the tendon of the flexor carpi radialis is being palpated.

Palpation Notes:
1. The palmaris longus is often missing (unilaterally or bilaterally).
2. The distal tendon of the flexor carpi radialis is much closer to the palmaris longus' distal tendon near the wrist than is the flexor carpi ulnaris' distal tendon.
3. All wrist flexors contract with wrist joint flexion, so to engage and isolate only one muscle in the group,

Figure 14-19 Palpation of the muscles of the right wrist flexor group. **A**, Palpation of the flexor carpi radialis as the client radially deviates the hand against resistance. The palmaris longus has been ghosted in. **B**, Palpation of the flexor carpi ulnaris as the client ulnar deviates the hand against resistance (the palmaris longus has been ghosted in). **C**, The palmaris longus is engaged when the client cups his hand.

(Continued)

WRIST FLEXOR GROUP—SEATED—cont'd

which is especially important because their muscle bellies merge proximally, a different action must be used. Resist radial deviation of the hand at the wrist joint to engage the flexor carpi radialis (Figure 14-19, A), and resist ulnar deviation of the hand at the wrist joint to engage the flexor carpi ulnaris (Figure 14-19, B). The palmaris longus will stay relaxed and soft when both radial and ulnar deviations are done (if the client starts in anatomic position).

4. The palmaris longus can often be made visible and palpable by asking the client to cup the hand (Figure 14-19, C).
5. It is especially important to not cross the finger joints when resisting the client's wrist joint flexion, because doing so would engage the flexor muscles of the fingers (flexors digitorum superficialis and profundus and flexor pollicis longus). This would make distinguishing the superficial wrist flexor muscles from these deeper muscles difficult.
6. Another method to engage and palpate the flexor carpi ulnaris is to ask the client to actively perform abduction of the little finger at the metacarpophalangeal joint. This will require the flexor carpi ulnaris to contract to stabilize the pisiform (Figure 14-20).

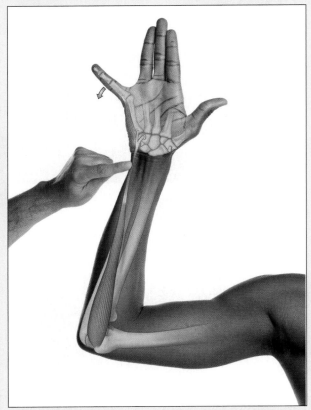

Figure 14-20 Abduction of the little finger at the metacarpophalangeal joint causes the flexor carpi ulnaris to engage as a stabilizer of the pisiform bone.

Alternate Palpation Position—Supine

The wrist flexor muscles can also be palpated with the client supine. Follow the palpation steps indicated for the seated palpation.

TRIGGER POINTS

1. Trigger points (TrPs) in the wrist flexors often result from or are perpetuated by acute or chronic overuse of the muscle (e.g., gripping objects, painting, playing tennis), trauma to the forearm/wrist/hand, or TrPs in the pectoralis minor (for the FCR and FCU), triceps brachii (for the PL), latissimus dorsi, and serratus posterior superior (for the FCU).
2. TrPs in the PL usually produce a sharp needlelike referral pain, which is different in quality than the usual deeper aching pain typical of TrPs; they also typically result in tenderness in the palm when gripping and handling objects (e.g., gardening and power tools). TrPs in the FCU may cause entrapment of the ulnar nerve.
3. The referral pattern of a TrP in a wrist flexor must be distinguished from the referral patterns of TrPs in the other wrist flexors, pronator teres, subclavius, subscapularis, infraspinatus, latissimus dorsi, brachialis, and opponens pollicis.
4. TrPs in the wrist flexors are often incorrectly assessed as medial epicondylitis/epicondylosis, pathologic cervical disk, thoracic outlet syndrome, carpal tunnel syndrome, wrist joint dysfunction (for the FCR and FCU), or ulnar nerve compression (for the FCU).
5. Associated TrPs often occur in the other wrist joint flexors, flexor digitorum superficialis, and flexor digitorum profundus.

Figure 14-21 Common TrPs and their corresponding referral zones for the muscles of the wrist flexor group. **A**, Flexor carpi radialis (FCR). **B**, Palmaris longus (PL). **C**, Flexor carpi ulnaris (FCU).

WRIST FLEXOR GROUP—SEATED—cont'd

STRETCHING THE WRIST FLEXOR GROUP

Palpation Key:
For wrist flexors, resist wrist flexion.

Figure 14-22 A stretch of the right wrist flexor group. With the forearm fully extended, the client uses the other hand to extend the right hand. If ulnar deviation is added to the extension, the stretch of the flexor carpi radialis will be enhanced (but the flexor carpi ulnaris will slacken). If radial deviation is added to the extension, the stretch of the flexor carpi ulnaris will be enhanced (but the flexor carpi radialis will slacken).

14

FLEXORS DIGITORUM SUPERFICIALIS AND PROFUNDUS—SEATED

Flexor Digitorum Superficialis (Figure 14-23, A):

❑ ATTACHMENTS:
o Medial epicondyle of the humerus (via the common flexor tendon) and the coronoid process of the ulna, and the proximal ½ of the anterior shaft of the radius *to the* anterior surfaces of the middle phalanges of fingers two through five

❑ ACTIONS:
o Flexes fingers two through five at the metacarpophalangeal (MCP) and proximal interphalangeal (IP) joints
o Flexes the hand at the wrist joint; flexes the forearm at the elbow joint

Flexor Digitorum Profundus (Figure 14-23, B):

❑ ATTACHMENTS:
o Proximal ½ of the anterior surface of the ulna (and the interosseus membrane) *to the* anterior surfaces of the distal phalanges of fingers two through five

❑ ACTIONS:
o Flexes fingers two through five at the MCP and the proximal and distal IP joints
o Flexes the hand at the wrist joint

Starting position (Figure 14-24):
o Client seated with the arm relaxed and the forearm flexed at the elbow joint and fully supinated, and resting on the client's thigh
o Therapist seated to the side and facing the client
o Begin palpating the flexor digitorum superficialis by placing your palpating fingers on the proximal medial forearm (slightly anterior and distal to the medial epicondyle of the humerus)

Palpation steps:
1. For the flexor digitorum superficialis, ask the client to flex the proximal phalanges of fingers two through five at the MCP joints, and feel for the contraction of the flexor digitorum superficialis (Figure 14-25, A). If resistance is added with your support hand, be sure to isolate your pressure against the proximal phalanges (i.e., do not cross the proximal IP joints to contact either the middle or distal phalanges).
2. Palpate the flexor digitorum superficialis by strumming perpendicular to the fibers from the proximal attachment at the medial epicondyle of the humerus to the distal tendons at the anterior wrist.
3. For the flexor digitorum profundus, begin palpation more medially and posteriorly on the forearm against the shaft of the ulna. Ask the client to flex the distal phalanges of fingers two through five at the distal IP joints and feel for the contraction of the flexor digitorum profundus (Figure 14-25, B).
4. Palpate the flexor digitorum profundus as far distally as possible by strumming perpendicular to the fibers.
5. Once the flexors digitorum superficialis and profundus have been located, have the client relax them and palpate to assess their baseline tone.

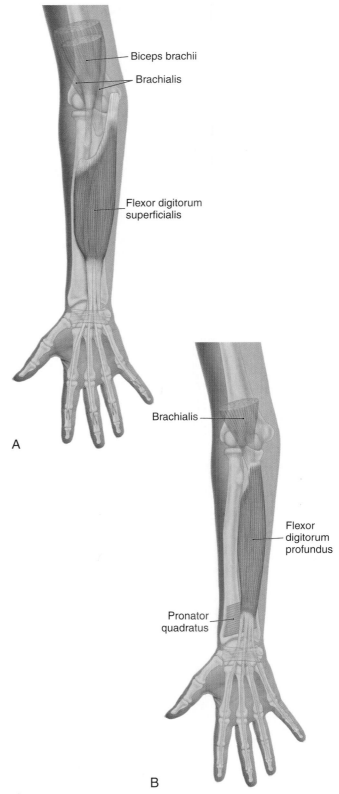

A

B

Figure 14-23 Anterior views of the right flexors digitorum superficialis and profundus. **A,** Anterior view of the right flexor digitorum superficialis. The distal ends of the biceps brachii and brachialis have been ghosted in. **B,** Anterior view of the right flexor digitorum profundus. The pronator quadratus and distal end of the brachialis have been ghosted in.

FLEXORS DIGITORUM SUPERFICIALIS AND PROFUNDUS—SEATED—cont'd

Figure 14-24 Starting position for seated palpation of the right flexor digitorum superficialis.

Figure 14-25 Palpation of the flexors digitorum superficialis and profundus. **A**, Palpation of the right flexor digitorum superficialis, starting distal and anterior to the medial epicondyle of the humerus. **B**, Palpation of the right flexor digitorum profundus, starting against the shaft of the ulna. Note the difference in the type of finger flexion that is performed by the client against resistance.

Palpation Notes:

1. Although most clients are able to isolate flexion of the fingers at the MCP joints for the flexor digitorum superficialis palpation, it is usually difficult for them to isolate flexion of the fingers at the distal IP joints for palpation of the flexor digitorum profundus. However, even if the proximal IP joints flex somewhat with this palpation, it is usually still possible to discern the flexor digitorum profundus.

2. To palpate the flexor digitorum profundus, it is important to use the ulnar border of the shaft of the ulna as a landmark. Once this landmark has been found, drop just off it anteriorly and you will be on the flexor digitorum profundus. (You will actually be palpating through the ulnar head of the flexor carpi ulnaris, but the flexor carpi ulnaris is very thin here and does not obstruct palpation of the flexor digitorum profundus.)

3. Sometimes the flexors digitorum superficialis and profundus can be discerned from each other by changing the position of the wrist joint. For the flexor digitorum superficialis, have the client's wrist joint in slight flexion; for the flexor digitorum profundus, have the client's wrist joint in extension. In both cases, ask for a gentle contraction of finger flexion.

4. Once the flexors digitorum superficialis and profundus split distally to form separate tendons, isolating flexion of an individual finger allows for individual palpation of the tendons. For example, have the client flex only the index finger and feel for the tendon to that finger to tense and the associated muscle belly fibers to contract. This can be done for the flexor digitorum superficialis and the flexor digitorum profundus.

Alternate Palpation Position—Supine

The two flexor digitorum muscles can also be palpated with the client supine. Follow the palpation steps indicated for the seated palpation.

14

FLEXORS DIGITORUM SUPERFICIALIS AND PROFUNDUS—SEATED—cont'd

TRIGGER POINTS

1. Trigger points (TrPs) in the flexors digitorum superficialis and profundus often result from or are perpetuated by acute or chronic overuse of the muscle (e.g., repetitive or forceful gripping of a steering wheel, tennis racquet, golf club, or gardening or work tools).
2. TrPs in the flexors digitorum superficialis and profundus may produce sharp referral pain that is felt not only throughout the anterior aspect of the finger that it flexes, but also phantom pain that is felt beyond the tip of the finger, entrapment of the median and/or ulnar nerve, and restriction of extension of the finger joints and wrist joint.
3. The referral patterns of flexors digitorum superficialis and profundus TrPs must be distinguished from the referral patterns of TrPs in the triceps brachii, subclavius, pectoralis minor, latissimus dorsi, and first dorsal interosseus manus.
4. TrPs in the flexors digitorum superficialis and profundus are often incorrectly assessed as a pathologic cervical disc, thoracic outlet syndrome, carpal tunnel syndrome, pronator teres syndrome, or joint dysfunction or arthritis of the metacarpophalangeal and interphalangeal joints.

5. Associated TrPs often occur in the flexor carpi radialis, flexor carpi ulnaris, pectoralis minor, and scalenes.
6. Note: No distinction has been made between TrPs within the flexor digitorum superficialis and the flexor digitorum profundus.

Figure 14-26 Anterior view illustrating common flexor digitorum superficialis and flexor digitorum profundus TrPs and their corresponding referral zones.

STRETCHING THE FLEXORS DIGITORUM SUPERFICIALIS AND PROFUNDUS

Figure 14-27 A stretch of the right flexors digitorum superficialis and profundus. With the forearm and hand fully extended, the client uses the other hand to extend the fingers at the metacarpophalangeal and interphalangeal joints.

Palpation Key:

Flex MCP joints for the flexor digitorum superficialis. Flex distal IP joints and palpate against the shaft of the ulna for the flexor digitorum profundus.

14

FLEXOR POLLICIS LONGUS—SEATED

❑ **ATTACHMENTS:**

o Anterior surface of the distal radius and the interosseus membrane, the coronoid process of the ulna, and the medial epicondyle of the humerus *to the* anterior surface of the base of the distal phalanx of the thumb

❑ **ACTIONS:**

o Flexes the thumb at the carpometacarpal (CMC), metacarpophalangeal (MCP), and interphalangeal (IP) joints
o Flexes the hand at the wrist joint; flexes the forearm at the elbow joint

Starting position (Figure 14-29):

o Client seated with the arm relaxed and the forearm flexed at the elbow joint and fully supinated, and resting on the client's thigh
o Therapist seated to the side and facing the client
o Palpating fingers placed on the distal anterior forearm (near the tendon of the flexor carpi radialis)

Palpation steps:

1. Ask the client to flex the distal phalanx of the thumb at the IP joint, and feel for the contraction of the flexor pollicis longus near the wrist (Figure 14-30).
2. Continue palpating the flexor pollicis longus as far proximal as possible as the client alternately contracts and relaxes it by flexing the thumb at the IP joint. Because this muscle is so deep, it is usually not helpful to try to strum perpendicular to its fibers.
3. Once the flexor pollicis longus has been located, have the client relax it and palpate to assess its baseline tone.

Figure 14-28 Anterior view of the right flexor pollicis longus. The pronator quadratus and distal end of the brachialis have been ghosted in.

Figure 14-29 Starting position for seated palpation of the right flexor pollicis longus.

Figure 14-30 Palpation of the belly of the right flexor pollicis longus as the thumb flexes at the interphalangeal joint. The pronator quadratus has been ghosted in.

14

FLEXOR POLLICIS LONGUS—SEATED—cont'd

Palpation Notes:

1. The flexor pollicis longus is often missing the ulnar and humeral attachments proximally. In these individuals, the muscle usually stops approximately halfway up the forearm. Furthermore, when present, the humeroulnar head is usually small and therefore difficult to palpate.
2. Even though this muscle is deep, it is usually not necessary to use much pressure to feel its contraction when the client flexes the thumb at the IP joint.
3. **The radial artery is near the flexor pollicis longus, so if you feel a pulse, move off the artery.**
4. It is best to palpate the flexor pollicis longus by asking the client to isolate flexion of the thumb at the IP joint. If the client also flexes the thumb at the CMC and/or MCP joints, other muscles of the thumb will be engaged, lessening the strength of the flexor pollicis longus contraction. Furthermore, these other muscles are located in the thenar eminence of the hand, and their contraction makes it more difficult to palpate and discern the distal tendon of the flexor pollicis longus.

Alternate Palpation Position—Supine

The flexor pollicis longus can also be palpated with the client supine. Follow the palpation steps indicated for the seated palpation.

Palpation Key:
Think of clicking a lighter with your thumb.

TRIGGER POINTS

1. Trigger points (TrPs) in the flexor pollicis longus often result from or are perpetuated by acute or chronic overuse of the muscle (e.g., repetitive or forceful gripping of a steering wheel, tennis racquet, golf club, or gardening or work tools).
2. TrPs in the flexor pollicis longus may produce sharp referral pain that is felt not only throughout the anterior aspect of the thumb but also beyond the tip of the thumb (phantom pain). In addition, extension of the thumb joints and wrist joint may be restricted.
3. The referral patterns of flexor pollicis longus TrPs must be distinguished from the referral patterns of TrPs in the opponens pollicis, adductor pollicis, brachialis, and subclavius.
4. TrPs in the flexor pollicis longus are often incorrectly assessed as medial epicondylitis/epicondylosis, carpal tunnel syndrome, thoracic outlet syndrome, pathologic cervical disc, thoracic outlet syndrome, or osteoarthritis of the thumb.
5. Associated TrPs often occur in the flexor digitorum superficialis and flexor digitorum profundus.

Figure 14-31 Anterior view illustrating a common flexor pollicis longus TrP and its corresponding referral zone.

STRETCHING THE FLEXOR POLLICIS LONGUS

Figure 14-32 A stretch of the right flexor pollicis longus. With the forearm and hand fully extended, the client uses the other hand to extend the thumb at the carpometacarpal, metacarpophalangeal, and interphalangeal joints.

14

FLEXOR POLLICIS LONGUS—SEATED—cont'd

DETOUR

Pronator Quadratus: The pronator quadratus is deep and difficult to palpate and discern. It attaches from the distal anterior ulna to the distal anterior radius and pronates the forearm at the radioulnar joints. Palpate with firm pressure in the anterior distal forearm on the radial side while resisting the client's forearm pronation at the radioulnar joints; be sure to apply resistance to the client's forearm, not the hand (Figure 14-33, B). If you are successful in feeling the pronator quadratus, follow it toward its ulnar attachment. Note: The median and ulnar nerves and the radial and ulnar arteries are all located in the anterior wrist; therefore, prudence must be exercised when palpating deeply here.

Trigger Points:
1. The same factors that create and/or perpetuate TrPs in the pronator teres are likely to create and/or perpetuate TrPs in the pronator quadratus.
2. TrPs in the pronator quadratus are associated with TrPs in the pronator teres.
3. TrP referral patterns have not been established for the pronator quadratus.

Pronator teres

Pronator quadratus

A

B

Figure 14-33 A, Anterior view of the right pronator quadratus. The pronator teres has been ghosted in. **B,** View of the pronator quadratus being palpated as pronation of the forearm at the radioulnar joints is resisted.

14

The radial group is composed of the brachioradialis, the extensor carpi radialis longus, and the extensor carpi radialis brevis. Palpation of the brachioradialis has already been covered (see page 286). Here we will discuss palpation of the other two radial group muscles.

❏ ATTACHMENTS:

o Extensor carpi radialis longus (ECRL): Distal $\frac{1}{3}$ of the lateral supracondylar ridge of the humerus *to the* radial side of the posterior hand at the base of the second metacarpal

o Extensor carpi radialis brevis (ECRB): Lateral epicondyle of the humerus (via the common extensor tendon) *to the* radial side of the posterior hand at the base of the third metacarpal

❏ ACTIONS:

o Both extensor carpi radialis muscles radially deviate (abduct) and extend the hand at the wrist joint, and flex the forearm at the elbow joint.

Starting position (Figure 14-35):

o Client seated with the arm relaxed and the forearm flexed at the elbow joint and in a position that is halfway between full pronation and full supination, and resting on the client's thigh

o Therapist seated to the side and facing the client

o The radial group is pinched with the palpating fingers

Palpation steps:

1. The radial group of muscles can usually be pinched and separated from the rest of the musculature of the forearm. Pinch the radial group of muscles between your thumb on one side and your index finger (or index and middle fingers) on the other side, and gently pull them away from the forearm (Figure 14-35).

2. Move your palpating fingers onto the extensors carpi radialis longus and brevis (posterior to the brachioradialis) and feel for their contraction as the client radially deviates the hand at the wrist joint (Figure 14-36, A). Resistance to radial deviation can be added with your support hand if desired.

3. Continue palpating the extensor carpi radialis muscles toward their distal attachments by strumming perpendicularly across them.

4. Once the extensors carpi radialis longus and brevis have been located, have the client relax them and palpate to assess their baseline tone.

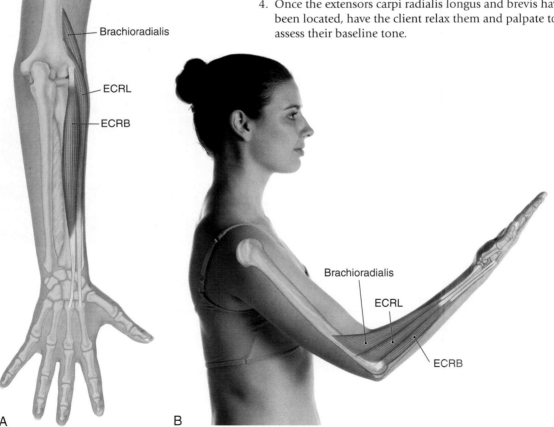

A   B

Figure 14-34 Views of the right radial group of muscles. **A,** Posterior view. **B,** Lateral view. *ECRL,* Extensor carpi radialis longus; *ECRB,* extensor carpi radialis brevis.

Figure 14-35 The right radial group of muscles is being pinched between the thumb and index finger of the therapist.

Figure 14-36 Palpation of the right extensors carpi radialis longus and brevis. **A**, Palpation of the extensors carpi radialis longus and brevis as the client radially deviates the hand at the wrist joint. **B**, Palpation of the distal tendon of the extensor carpi radialis brevis as it engages to stabilize the hand from flexing at the wrist joint when the hand makes a fist (see Palpation Note #5).

14

Palpation Notes:
1. The brachioradialis is the most anterior of the three muscles of the radial group; the extensor carpi radialis brevis is the most posterior; the extensor carpi radialis longus is in the middle.
2. Immediately posterior to the radial group (i.e., posterior to the extensor carpi radialis brevis) is the extensor digitorum.
3. To distinguish the border between the extensor carpi radialis brevis and extensor digitorum, have the client alternately perform radial deviation of the hand at the wrist joint and extension of the fingers at the metacarpophalangeal and interphalangeal joints. The extensor carpi radialis brevis will contract with radial deviation of the hand, and the extensor digitorum will contract with finger extension.
4. To distinguish the border between the extensor carpi radialis longus and brachioradialis, have the client alternately

perform radial deviation of the hand at the wrist joint and flexion of the forearm at the elbow joint. The extensor carpi radialis longus will contract with radial deviation of the hand, and the brachioradialis will contract with forearm flexion.
5. Distinguishing between the bellies of the two extensor carpi radialis muscles is challenging. One way is by location. Another method is to ask the client to perform gentle to moderate flexion of the fingers (i.e., make a fist). This will tend to engage the extensor carpi radialis brevis to act to stabilize the wrist joint from flexing (because of the pull of the finger flexor muscles), but not the extensor carpi radialis longus. Flexion of the fingers will usually cause palpable and often visible tensing of the distal tendon of the extensor carpi radialis brevis (Figure 14-36, B).

Alternate Palpation Position—Supine
The extensor carpi radialis muscles can also be palpated with the client supine. Follow the palpation steps indicated for the seated palpation.

RADIAL GROUP—SEATED—cont'd

TRIGGER POINTS

1. Trigger points (TrPs) in the extensor carpi radialis longus (ECRL) and extensor carpi radialis brevis (ECRB) often result from or are perpetuated by acute or chronic over-use of the muscle (e.g., forceful or repetitive gripping of the hand, hitting a one-handed backhand in tennis) and TrPs in the scalenes or supraspinatus.
2. TrPs in the extensors carpi radialis may produce a weak or painful grip (e.g., when shaking hands), restricted ulnar deviation of the hand at the wrist joint, and entrapment of the radial nerve (the ECRB only).
3. The referral patterns of extensors carpi radialis TrPs must be distinguished from the referral patterns of TrPs in the brachioradialis, extensor digitorum, extensor indicis, supinator, triceps brachii, subclavius, scalenes, supraspinatus, infraspinatus, subscapularis, coracobrachialis, brachialis, latissimus dorsi, adductor pollicis, and first dorsal interosseus manus.
4. TrPs in the extensors carpi radialis are often incorrectly assessed as lateral epicondylitis/epicondylosis, C7 or C8 nerve compression, carpal tunnel syndrome, wrist joint dysfunction or arthritis, or de Quervain's stenosing tenosynovitis.
5. Associated TrPs of the extensors carpi radialis often occur in the brachioradialis, extensor digitorum, supinator, scalenes, and supraspinatus.

Figure 14-37 A, **B**, Posterior views illustrating common extensor carpi radialis longus and brevis TrPs and their corresponding referral zones. **A**, Extensor carpi radialis longus. **B**, Extensor carpi radialis brevis.

STRETCHING THE RADIAL GROUP

Figure 14-38 A stretch of the right extensors carpi radialis longus and brevis. The client uses the other hand to flex and ulnar deviate the right hand. Note: See page 288, Figure 14-9, for a stretch of the brachioradialis of the radial group.

Palpation Key:
Pinch the radial group away from the forearm.

14

EXTENSOR DIGITORUM AND EXTENSOR DIGITI MINIMI—SEATED

❏ **ATTACHMENTS:**

o Extensor digitorum: Lateral epicondyle of the humerus (via the common extensor tendon) *to the* posterior surfaces of the middle and distal phalanges of fingers two through five

o Extensor digiti minimi: Lateral epicondyle of the humerus (via the common extensor tendon) *to the* posterior surfaces of the middle and distal phalanges of the little finger (by attaching into the distal tendon of the extensor digitorum to the little finger)

❏ **ACTIONS:**

o Extensor digitorum: extends fingers two through five at the metacarpophalangeal (MCP) and interphalangeal (IP) joints; extends the hand at the wrist joint; extends the forearm at the elbow joint

o Extensor digiti minimi: extends the little finger (#5) at the MCP and IP joints; extends the hand at the wrist joint; extends the forearm at the elbow joint

Starting position (Figure 14-40):

o Client seated with the arm relaxed, and the forearm flexed at the elbow joint, fully pronated at the radioulnar joints, and resting on the client's thigh

o Therapist seated facing the client

o Palpating fingers placed on the middle of the posterior proximal forearm

o Support hand placed on the posterior side of the fingers (if resistance is given)

Palpation steps:

1. Ask the client to fully extend fingers two through five at the MCP and IP joints, and feel for the contraction of the extensor digitorum and extensor digiti minimi (Figure 14-41). Resistance can be given to finger extension with your supporting hand if desired (be sure that the client is not attempting to extend the hand at the wrist joint, or all muscles in the posterior forearm will contract).

Figure 14-39 Posterior view of the right extensor digitorum and extensor digiti minimi. The proximal ends of the extensor carpi ulnaris (ECU) and extensor carpi radialis brevis (ECRB) have been cut and ghosted in.

2. Continue palpating toward the distal attachments by strumming perpendicular to the fibers of these two muscles.

3. The distal tendons of the finger extensors can often be seen on the posterior surface of the hand. If not visible, they are usually easily palpable by strumming perpendicular to them.

4. Once the extensor digitorum and extensor digiti minimi have been located, have the client relax them and palpate to assess their baseline tone.

14

Figure 14-40 Starting position for seated palpation of the right extensor digitorum and extensor digiti minimi.

Figure 14-41 Palpation of the right extensor digitorum and extensor digiti minimi as the client extends fingers two through five against resistance.

EXTENSOR DIGITORUM AND EXTENSOR DIGITI MINIMI—SEATED—cont'd

Palpation Notes:

1. If the client is asked to extend one finger at a time, the tendon and associated muscle belly fibers of the extensor digitorum that go to that finger can be separately palpated.
2. Distinguishing between the extensor digitorum and the extensor carpi radialis brevis is accomplished by asking the client to radially deviate the hand at the wrist joint. This engages the extensor carpi radialis brevis but not the extensor digitorum. Or have the client extend the fingers; this engages the extensor digitorum but not the extensor carpi radialis brevis.
3. Distinguishing between the extensor digiti minimi and the extensor carpi ulnaris is accomplished by asking the client to ulnar deviate the hand at the wrist joint. This engages the extensor carpi ulnaris but not the extensor digiti minimi. Or have the client extend the fingers; this engages the extensor digiti minimi but not the extensor carpi ulnaris.
4. Distinguishing between the extensor digitorum fibers that go to the little finger and the extensor digiti minimi (i.e., locating the border between these two muscles) is extremely difficult because they are next to each other and they are both engaged with the same action (extension of the little finger).

Alternate Palpation Position—Supine

The extensor digitorum and extensor digiti minimi can also be palpated with the client supine. Follow the palpation steps indicated for the seated palpation.

TRIGGER POINTS

1. Trigger points (TrPs) in the extensor digitorum and extensor digiti minimi often result from or are perpetuated by acute or chronic overuse of the muscle (e.g., repetitive finger movements, such as typing or playing piano), keeping the muscle in a chronically lengthened state (e.g., sleeping with the fingers in flexion), or TrPs in the scalenes.
2. TrPs in the extensor digitorum and extensor digiti minimi may produce stiffness of the fingers (i.e., decreased flexion).
3. The referral patterns of extensor digitorum and extensor digiti minimi TrPs must be distinguished from the referral patterns of TrPs in the extensor indicis, dorsal interossei manus, scalenes, subclavius, latissimus dorsi, coracobrachialis, and triceps brachii.
4. TrPs in the extensor digitorum and extensor digiti minimi are often incorrectly assessed as lateral epicondylitis/epicondylosis, arthritis of the fingers, C7 or C6 nerve compression, or carpal joint dysfunction.
5. Associated TrPs often occur in the extensor carpi radialis longus, extensor carpi radialis brevis, supinator, brachioradialis, and extensor carpi ulnaris.
6. Note: A TrP in the extensor digitorum or extensor digiti minimi usually results in referral of pain into the dorsum of the hand and the finger that is controlled by those muscle fibers. TrPs occur most commonly in the fibers of the middle and ring fingers.

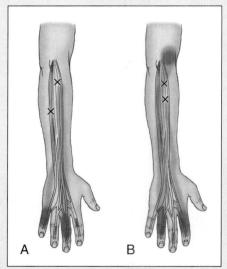

Figure 14-42 Posterior views illustrating common extensor digitorum and extensor digiti minimi TrPs and their corresponding referral zones. **A,** A TrP in the extensor digiti minimi referring into the little finger, and a TrP in the extensor digitorum referring into the middle finger. **B,** TrPs in the extensor digitorum referring into the index and ring fingers.

14

EXTENSOR DIGITORUM AND EXTENSOR DIGITI MINIMI—SEATED—cont'd

STRETCHING THE EXTENSOR DIGITORUM AND EXTENSOR DIGITI MINIMI

Figure 14-43 A stretch of the right extensors digitorum and digiti minimi. With the forearm and hand fully flexed, the client uses the other hand to flex fingers two through five.

Palpation Key:
Extend the fingers and palpate in the middle of the posterior forearm.

14

YOU ARE HERE

EXTENSOR CARPI ULNARIS—SEATED

❏ **ATTACHMENTS:**

o Lateral epicondyle of the humerus (via the common extensor tendon) and the middle ⅓ of the posterior ulna *to the* ulnar side of the posterior hand at the base of the fifth metacarpal

❏ **ACTIONS:**

o Extends and ulnar deviates the hand at the wrist joint
o Extends the forearm at the elbow joint

Starting position (Figure 14-45):

o Client seated with the arm relaxed, and the forearm flexed at the elbow joint, fully pronated at the radioulnar joints, and resting on the client's thigh
o Therapist seated facing the client
o Palpating fingers placed immediately posterior to the shaft of the ulna
o Support hand placed on the ulnar side of the hand, proximal to the fingers (if resistance is given)

Palpation steps:

1. Ask the client to ulnar deviate the hand at the wrist joint and feel for the contraction of the extensor carpi ulnaris (Figure 14-46). Resistance can be given with your support hand if desired.
2. Palpate proximally toward the lateral epicondyle and distally toward the fifth metacarpal by strumming perpendicular to the fibers as the client alternately contracts and relaxes the muscle.
3. Once the extensor carpi ulnaris has been located, have the client relax it and palpate to assess its baseline tone.

Figure 14-44 Posterior view of the right extensor carpi ulnaris. The anconeus has been ghosted in. The proximal tendons of the extensor digitorum (ED) and extensor digiti minimi (EDM) have been cut and ghosted in.

14

Figure 14-45 Starting position for seated palpation of the right extensor carpi ulnaris.

Figure 14-46 Palpation of the right extensor carpi ulnaris immediately posterior to the shaft of the ulna as the client ulnar deviates the hand at the wrist joint against resistance.

EXTENSOR CARPI ULNARIS—SEATED—cont'd

Palpation Notes:

1. The extensor carpi ulnaris is all the way on the ulnar side of the posterior forearm, directly adjacent to the shaft of the ulna.
2. When having the client perform ulnar deviation of the hand at the wrist joint, make sure that the client's fingers are relaxed. If the fingers are extended, the extensor digitorum and extensor digiti minimi will be engaged, making it difficult to discern the extensor carpi ulnaris from these muscles.
3. Distinguishing between the extensor carpi ulnaris and the extensor digiti minimi is accomplished by asking the client to extend the little finger. This engages the extensor digiti minimi but not the extensor carpi ulnaris. Or have the client ulnar deviate the hand at the wrist joint; this engages the extensor carpi ulnaris but not the extensor digiti minimi.

Alternate Palpation Position—Supine
The extensor carpi ulnaris can also be palpated with the client supine. Follow the palpation steps indicated for the seated palpation.

TRIGGER POINTS

1. Trigger points (TrPs) in the extensor carpi ulnaris often result from or are perpetuated by acute or chronic overuse of the muscle (e.g., holding the hands in ulnar deviation when typing), direct trauma, and TrPs in the scalenes or serratus posterior superior.
2. The referral patterns of extensor carpi ulnaris TrPs must be distinguished from the referral patterns of TrPs in the extensor carpi radialis brevis, extensor indicis, supinator, scalenes, subscapularis, and coracobrachialis.
3. TrPs in the extensor carpi ulnaris are often incorrectly assessed as wrist joint dysfunction or arthritis, carpal tunnel syndrome, or C7 or C8 nerve compression.
4. Associated TrPs often occur in the extensor digitorum, extensor digiti minimi, scalenes, and serratus posterior superior.
5. Note: Because the extensor carpi ulnaris does not have to support a weight against gravity as often as the radial deviators of the hand (extensors carpi radialis longus and brevis), it usually does not develop trigger points as often as they do.

Figure 14-47 Posterior view illustrating a common extensor carpi ulnaris TrP and its corresponding referral zone.

STRETCHING THE EXTENSOR CARPI ULNARIS

Figure 14-48 A stretch of the right extensor carpi ulnaris. With the forearm fully flexed, the client uses the other hand to flex and radially deviate the hand.

Palpation Key:
Palpate immediately posterior to the shaft of the ulna.

SUPINATOR—SEATED

❑ ATTACHMENTS:

o   Lateral epicondyle of the humerus and the supinator crest
of the ulna *to the* proximal ⅓ of the radius (posterior,
lateral, and anterior sides)

❑ ACTION:

o   Supinates the forearm at the radioulnar joints

Starting position (Figure 14-50):

o   Client seated with the arm relaxed, and the forearm flexed
at the elbow joint, in a position that is halfway between
full pronation and full supination, and resting on the client's thigh
o   Therapist seated facing the client
o   Palpating fingers pinch the radial group of muscles away
from the forearm
o   Support hand placed on the client's distal forearm, just
proximal to the wrist joint

Palpation steps:

1. The radial group of muscles can usually be pinched and
separated from the rest of the musculature of the forearm.
Pinch the radial group of muscles between your thumb on
one side and your index and middle fingers on the other
side, and gently pull them away from the forearm.
2. Gently but firmly sink in (between the extensor carpi radialis brevis of the radial group and the extensor digitorum)
toward the supinator attachment on the radius; ask the
client to supinate the forearm against resistance, and feel
for the contraction of the supinator (Figure 14-51).

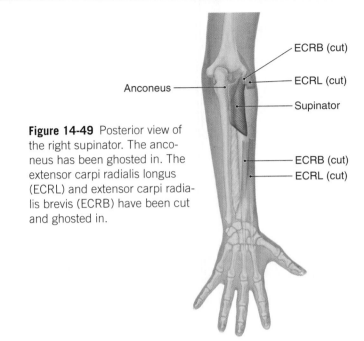

Figure 14-49 Posterior view of
the right supinator. The anconeus has been ghosted in. The
extensor carpi radialis longus
(ECRL) and extensor carpi radialis brevis (ECRB) have been cut
and ghosted in.

Anconeus

ECRB (cut)
ECRL (cut)
Supinator
ECRB (cut)
ECRL (cut)

3. Continue palpating the supinator (through the more
superficial musculature) toward its proximal attachment
and feel for its contraction as the client alternately contracts and relaxes the supinator.
4. Once the supinator has been located, have the client relax
it and palpate to assess its baseline tone.

Figure 14-50 Starting position for seated palpation of the right
supinator.

Figure 14-51 Palpation of the right supinator against the radius between the radial group of muscles and the extensor
digitorum.

14

SUPINATOR—SEATED—cont'd

Palpation Notes:

1. When resisting the client's forearm supination, a gentle but firm grasp is needed by the support hand. Otherwise only the client's skin will be held and the underlying forearm bones will be allowed to move. This will result in unsuccessful resistance to forearm supination and will be uncomfortable for the client.
2. The supinator can also be palpated on the anterior/medial side of the brachioradialis. Have the client's brachioradialis slackened by passively flexing the client's elbow joint (20 to 30 degrees). Push the brachioradialis laterally and then press in deep toward the head and shaft of the radius; you will encounter the supinator (Figure 14-52).
3. **The deep branch of the radial nerve runs through the supinator muscle. Be aware of this when pressing in deeply against the supinator.**

Figure 14-52 Palpation of the right supinator by pushing the brachioradialis laterally and then pressing in toward the radius (see Palpation Note #2).

Alternate Palpation Position—Supine

The supinator can also be palpated with the client supine. Follow the palpation steps indicated for the seated palpation.

TRIGGER POINTS

1. Trigger points (TrPs) in the supinator often result from or are perpetuated by acute or chronic overuse of the muscle (e.g., using a screwdriver, turning tight doorknobs, hitting a backhand in tennis with poor form).
2. TrPs in the supinator may produce entrapment of the deep branch of the radial nerve; supinator TrPs are the most common TrPs that cause lateral epicondylar pain.
3. The referral patterns of supinator TrPs must be distinguished from the referral patterns of TrPs in the extensor carpi radialis longus, brachioradialis, extensor digitorum, biceps brachii, brachialis, triceps brachii, supraspinatus, infraspinatus, subclavius, scalenes, adductor pollicis, and first dorsal interosseus manus.
4. TrPs in the supinator are often incorrectly assessed as lateral epicondylitis/epicondylosis, C5 or C6 nerve compression, or de Quervain's stenosing tenosynovitis.
5. Associated TrPs often occur in the extensor carpi radialis longus, extensor carpi radialis brevis, extensor digitorum, extensor digiti minimi, triceps brachii, anconeus, brachioradialis, biceps brachii, brachialis, and palmaris longus.

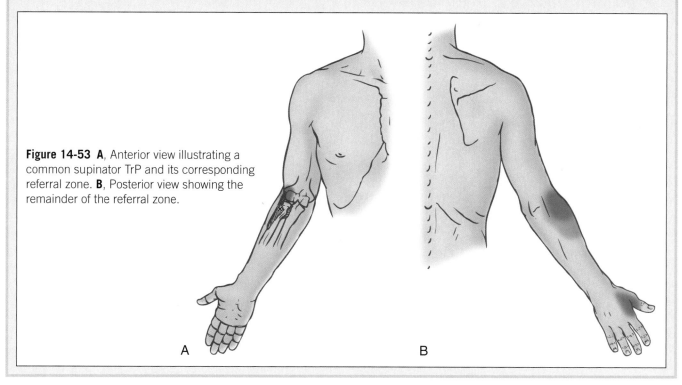

Figure 14-53 A, Anterior view illustrating a common supinator TrP and its corresponding referral zone. **B**, Posterior view showing the remainder of the referral zone.

A   B

14

SUPINATOR—SEATED—cont'd

STRETCHING THE SUPINATOR

Palpation Key:
Pull radial group away and sink into the supinator against the radius.

Figure 14-54 A stretch of the right supinator. The client uses the other hand to fully pronate the right forearm. Note: It is easy to confuse pronation of the forearm at the radioulnar joints with medial rotation of the arm at the shoulder joint. Be sure that forearm pronation is being done.

DEEP DISTAL FOUR GROUP—SEATED

The deep distal four group is composed of the abductor pollicis longus, extensor pollicis brevis, extensor pollicis longus, and extensor indicis.

❑ ATTACHMENTS:

o Abductor pollicis longus: Middle $^1/_3$ of the posterior radius, interosseus membrane, and ulna *to the* base of the metacarpal of the thumb

o Extensor pollicis brevis: Distal $^1/_3$ of the posterior radius and interosseus membrane *to the* base of the proximal phalanx of the thumb

o Extensor pollicis longus: Middle $^1/_3$ of the posterior ulna and interosseus membrane *to the* base of the distal phalanx of the thumb

o Extensor indicis: Distal $^1/_3$ of the posterior ulna and interosseus membrane *to the* posterior surfaces of the middle and distal phalanges of the index finger (by attaching into the ulnar side of the distal tendon of the extensor digitorum to the index finger)

❑ ACTIONS:

o Abductor pollicis longus: abducts and extends the thumb at the carpometacarpal (CMC) joint; radially deviates the hand at the wrist joint

o Extensor pollicis brevis: abducts and extends the thumb at the CMC joint, and extends the thumb at the metacarpophalangeal (MCP) joint; radially deviates the hand at the wrist joint

o Extensor pollicis longus: extends the thumb at the CMC, MCP, and interphalangeal (IP) joints; radially deviates the hand at the wrist joint

o Extensor indicis: extends the index finger at the MCP and IP joints; extends the hand at the wrist joint

Starting position (Figure 14-56):

o Client seated with the arm relaxed and the forearm flexed at the elbow joint and fully pronated at the radioulnar joints, and resting on the client's thigh; client's thumb actively extended (Note: Extension of the thumb at the CMC joint is a frontal plane motion away from the palm of the hand.)

o Therapist seated facing the client

o Palpating fingers placed on the radial side of the posterior wrist (after visualizing the tendons)

Palpation steps:

1. First visualize the distal tendons of the abductor pollicis longus, extensor pollicis brevis, and extensor pollicis longus as they define the anatomic snuffbox (see Palpation Note #1) by asking the client to actively extend the thumb at the CMC joint (Figure 14-56). Note that the tendons of the abductor pollicis longus and extensor pollicis brevis are right next to each other and may appear to be one tendon (see Palpation Note #2).

2. Once located, palpate each of these muscles individually back to its proximal attachment by strumming perpendicular to the fibers as the client alternately contracts and relaxes that muscle by extending the thumb (Figure 14-57).

3. To palpate the extensor indicis, first locate its distal tendon on the posterior side of the hand by asking the client to extend the index finger at the MCP and IP joints (Figure 14-58).

4. Continue palpating the extensor indicis proximally by strumming perpendicular to its fibers as the client alternately contracts and relaxes the muscle.

5. Once the muscles of the deep distal four group have been located, have the client relax them and palpate to assess their baseline tone.

14

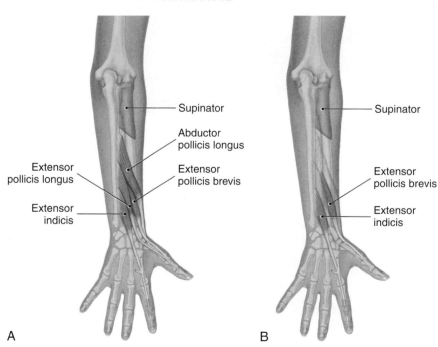

Figure 14-55 Posterior views of the muscles of the right deep distal four group. **A,** All four muscles with the supinator ghosted in. **B,** Same illustration with the abductor pollicis longus and extensor pollicis longus ghosted in.

A   B

DEEP DISTAL FOUR GROUP—SEATED—cont'd

Figure 14-56 Starting position for seated palpation of the right deep distal four muscles. Before beginning their palpation, first visualize the tendons of the anatomic snuffbox by having the client extend the thumb (see Palpation Note #1).

Figure 14-57 Palpation of the three thumb muscles of the right deep distal four group (abductor pollicis longus, and extensors pollicis brevis and longus) as the client extends the thumb at the carpometacarpal (CMC) joint.

Palpation Key:
Visualize the tendons around the anatomic snuffbox (the three "pollicis" muscles).

Figure 14-58 Palpation of the right extensor indicis of the deep distal four group as the client extends the index finger at the metacarpophalangeal joint.

Palpation Notes:

1. The anatomic snuffbox is a depression that is bordered by the three thumb (pollicis) muscles of the deep distal four group. The abductor pollicis longus and extensor pollicis brevis border the anatomic snuffbox on the radial side; the extensor pollicis longus borders the anatomic snuffbox on the ulnar side.

2. The distal tendons of the abductor pollicis longus and extensor pollicis brevis are extremely close to each other and often appear to be one tendon. If so, these two tendons can be separated by gently placing a fingernail between them. These two tendons run superficial to the distal end of the brachioradialis muscle.

3. To engage the thumb muscles of the deep distal four group and make them more readily visible and palpable, a small amount of thumb abduction at the CMC joint in addition to thumb extension can be done.

4. Even though the muscles of the deep distal four group are deep, they are usually easily palpable through the more superficial muscles.

5. It can be difficult to discern the extensor indicis from the portion of the extensor digitorum that goes to the index finger. Perhaps the best way to distinguish these two muscles from each other is to note the different locations of the bellies and therefore the different directions of fibers. The extensor indicis orients much more transversely across the distal forearm from radial to ulnar to reach its proximal attachment on the ulna; whereas the extensor digitorum is oriented much more longitudinally in the forearm, traveling proximally to the lateral epicondyle of the humerus. In the dorsum of the hand, the distal tendon of the extensor indicis is located to the ulnar side of the distal tendon of the extensor digitorum that goes to the index finger.

Alternate Palpation Position—Supine
The muscles of the deep distal four group can also be palpated with the client supine. Follow the palpation steps indicated for the seated palpation.

DEEP DISTAL FOUR GROUP—SEATED—cont'd

TRIGGER POINTS

1. Trigger points (TrPs) in the muscles of the deep distal four group often result from or are perpetuated by acute or chronic overuse of the muscle (e.g., repetitive motions of the index finger or thumb, such as playing a musical instrument or typing).
2. TrPs in the deep distal four group may produce discomfort and difficulty when performing fine motor tasks with the index finger and/or thumb.
3. The referral patterns of extensor indicis TrPs must be distinguished from the referral patterns of TrPs in the extensors carpi radialis brevis and longus, extensor carpi ulnaris, extensor digitorum, coracobrachialis, brachialis, supinator, scalenes, subclavius, and first dorsal interosseus.
4. TrPs in the muscles of the deep distal four group are often incorrectly assessed as wrist joint dysfunction or de Quervain's stenosing tenosynovitis.
5. Associated TrPs often occur in the extensor digitorum and extensor digiti minimi.

6. Note: TrP referral patterns have not yet been established for the deep distal four group muscles that go to the thumb. When assessing these muscles for TrPs, look primarily for central TrPs in the middle of the bellies.

Figure 14-59 Posterior view illustrating a common extensor indicis TrP and its corresponding referral zone.

STRETCHING THE DEEP DISTAL FOUR GROUP

Palpation Key:

Extend the index finger (extensor indicis).

Figure 14-60 A stretch of the three thumb muscles of the deep distal four group. The thumb is curled inside the hand and the hand is then ulnar deviated. Note: To stretch the extensor indicis of the deep distal four group, the hand should be fully flexed at the wrist joint and the index finger should be fully flexed at the metacarpophalangeal and interphalangeal joints, as seen in Figure 14-43.

14

Whirlwind Tour   **Muscles of the Forearm**

For all palpations of the muscles of the forearm, the client is seated with the arm relaxed in neutral position, and the forearm is flexed at the elbow joint to 90 degrees and relaxed on the client's thigh. You are seated to the side or directly in front of the client and facing the client.

1. **Brachioradialis:** The client is seated with the arm relaxed; the forearm is flexed and in a position that is halfway between full pronation and full supination and resting on the client's thigh. Resist further flexion of the forearm at the elbow joint; first look for the brachioradialis to become visible, then palpate for it at the proximal anterolateral forearm. Once felt, continue palpating it to its proximal and distal attachments by strumming perpendicular to its fibers as the client alternately contracts and relaxes it. Note: The brachioradialis is superficial and is easily palpable for its entire length except for a small distal portion that is deep to the abductor pollicis longus and the extensor pollicis brevis.

2. **Pronator teres:** The client is seated with the arm relaxed; the forearm is flexed and in a position that is halfway between full pronation and full supination and resting on the client's thigh. Resist further pronation of the forearm and feel for the contraction of the pronator teres in the proximal anterior forearm. Once felt, continue palpating to the proximal attachment on the medial epicondyle and toward its distal attachment on the radius by strumming perpendicular to its fibers as the client alternately contracts and relaxes the muscle. Note: The pronator teres is superficial for its entire course except at its distal attachment on the radius where it is deep to the brachioradialis. To palpate it there, either palpate through the brachioradialis, or if it is possible to slacken the brachioradialis, try to push the brachioradialis out of the way and palpate directly on the radial attachment of the pronator teres.

3. **Wrist flexor group:** The client is seated with the arm relaxed; the forearm is flexed, fully supinated, and resting on the client's thigh. Resist the client from flexing the hand at the wrist joint and first look for the three wrist flexor tendons to become visible. The palmaris longus (PL) is dead center, the flexor carpi radialis (FCR) is slightly radial to the PL, and the flexor carpi ulnaris (FCU) is far to the ulnar side of the wrist. Then palpate them one at a time. Once a tendon is felt, continue palpating it proximally to its proximal attachment on the medial epicondyle by strumming perpendicular to it as the client alternately contracts and relaxes the muscle. Note: To discern these muscles as their bellies merge proximally, ask the client to do radial deviation to contract the FCR and ulnar deviation to contract the FCU; the PL will be located between the other two and will stay relaxed with radial and ulnar deviation of the hand.

4. **Flexor digitorum superficialis (FDS) and flexor digitorum profundus (FDP):** The client is seated with the arm relaxed; the forearm is flexed, fully supinated, and resting on the client's thigh. Ask the client to flex the proximal phalanges of fingers two through five at the metacarpophalangeal joints, and feel for the contraction of the FDS in the proximal anteromedial forearm, just posterior to the humeral belly of the flexor carpi ulnaris (if resistance is given, be sure to isolate pressure against only the proximal phalanges). Once felt, palpate the FDS proximally to the medial epicondyle and distally as far as possible by strumming perpendicular to its fibers as the client alternately contracts and relaxes the muscle. To palpate the FDP, palpate more medially and posteriorly on the proximal forearm against the shaft of the ulna and feel for its contraction as the client flexes of the distal phalanges of fingers two through five at the distal interphalangeal joints. Once felt, palpate the FDP proximally and distally as far as possible by strumming perpendicular to its fibers as the client alternately contracts and relaxes the muscle.

5. **Flexor pollicis longus (FPL):** The client is seated with the arm relaxed; the forearm is flexed, fully supinated, and resting on the client's thigh. Place your palpating fingers on the distal anterior forearm (just radial to the tendon of the flexor carpi radialis), and feel for the contraction of the FPL as the client flexes the distal phalanx of the thumb at the interphalangeal joint. Once felt, continue palpating the FPL proximally as far as possible as the client alternately contracts and relaxes the muscle. Note: It is usually not helpful to try to strum perpendicular to its fibers.

6. **Detour to pronator quadratus:** The pronator quadratus is deep and difficult to palpate. Palpate with firm pressure in the anterior distal forearm on the radial side while resisting pronation of the forearm at the radioulnar joints. To prevent the more superficial tendons of the wrist and finger flexors from tensing and obscuring the contraction of the pronator teres, be sure when resisting the client's forearm pronation that you apply the resistance to the forearm only. If you apply it to the client's hand, these more superficial muscles and their tendons will contract and tense. If you are successful in feeling the pronator quadratus, follow it toward its ulnar attachment.

7. **Radial group (brachioradialis, extensor carpi radialis longus [ECRL], extensor carpi radialis brevis [ECRB]):** The client is seated with the arm relaxed; the forearm is flexed and in a position that is halfway between full pronation and full supination and resting on the client's thigh. Pinch the radial group of muscles between your thumb and index/middle fingers and lift it away from the forearm, separating it from the rest of the forearm musculature. The brachioradialis is the most anterior; the ECRB is the most posterior; and the ECRL is between the other two. Then palpate for the contraction of the ECRL and ECRB as the client radially deviates the hand at the wrist joint (resistance can be added). Once felt, continue palpating the ECRL and ECRB toward their distal attachments by strumming perpendicular to their fibers as the client alternately contracts and relaxes them. Note: The distal tendon of the ECRB can be palpated and often visualized at the wrist if the client is asked to make a

14

fist with the hand in a neutral position or slight extension at the wrist joint.

8. **Extensor digitorum (ED) and extensor digiti minimi (EDM):** The client is seated with the arm relaxed; the forearm is flexed at the elbow joint, fully pronated at the radioulnar joints, and resting on the client's thigh. Feel for the contraction of the ED and EDM in the middle of the posterior forearm as the client fully extends fingers two through five at the metacarpophalangeal and interphalangeal joints. Once felt, continue palpating the ED and EDM proximally to the lateral epicondyle of the humerus and distally as far as possible by strumming perpendicular to its fibers as the client alternately contracts and relaxes the muscles. The EDM is the most ulnar of the fibers that are felt to contract (discerning the border of the ED and EDM is extremely difficult). Note: The distal tendons of the finger extensors can usually be seen on the posterior surface of the hand. If not visible, they are usually easily palpable by strumming perpendicular to them.

9. **Extensor carpi ulnaris (ECU):** The client is seated with the arm relaxed; the forearm is flexed at the elbow joint, fully pronated at the radioulnar joints, and resting on the client's thigh. Feel for the contraction of the ECU immediately posterior to the shaft of the ulna as the client ulnar deviates the hand at the wrist joint (resistance can be given). Once felt, continue palpating the ECU proximally to the lateral epicondyle of the humerus and distally toward the fifth metacarpal by strumming perpendicular to the fibers as the client contracts and relaxes the muscle.

10. **Supinator:** The client is seated with the arm relaxed; the forearm is flexed and in a position that is halfway between full pronation and full supination and resting on the client's thigh. Pinch the radial group of muscles between your thumb and index/middle fingers; lift it away from the forearm, separating it from the rest of the forearm musculature. Slowly and gently but firmly sink in toward the radius between the extensor carpi radialis brevis and the extensor digitorum and feel for the contraction of the supinator as the client supinates the forearm against your resistance. Once felt, continue palpating the supinator (through the more superficial musculature) toward its proximal attachment as the client alternately contracts and relaxes the muscle.

11. **Deep distal four group (abductor pollicis longus [APL], extensor pollicis brevis [EPB], extensor pollicis longus [EPL], extensor indicis [EI]):** The client is seated with the arm relaxed; the forearm is flexed, fully pronated, and resting on the client's thigh. First visualize the distal tendons of the APL, EPB, and EPL on the radial side of the posterior wrist as they define the anatomic snuffbox, by asking the client to actively extend the thumb at the carpometacarpal joint. (Note: The tendons of the APL and EPB lie next to each other and may appear to be one tendon.) Then palpate each tendon one at a time by strumming perpendicular to it as the client alternately contracts and relaxes the muscle by doing extension of the thumb at the carpometacarpal joint; palpate as far proximally and distally as possible toward the attachments of each muscle. To palpate the EI, first visually locate its distal tendon on the posterior side of the hand as the client extends the index finger at the metacarpophalangeal and interphalangeal joints. Then palpate it distally and proximally by strumming perpendicular to its fibers as the client alternately contracts and relaxes the muscle. Note: The EI can be discerned from the extensor digitorum by the direction of the fibers. The EI travels somewhat transversely across the distal forearm to reach its proximal attachment on the distal ulna. The extensor digitorum travels much more longitudinally in the forearm to reach its proximal attachment on the lateral epicondyle of the humerus. On the dorsum of the hand, the distal tendon of the EI is located to the ulnar side of the distal tendon of the extensor digitorum that goes to the index finger.

14

Chapter 15

Tour #6—Palpation of the Intrinsic Muscles of the Hand

Overview

This chapter is a palpation tour of the intrinsic muscles of the hand. The tour begins with the muscles of the thenar group, then covers the muscles of the hypothenar group, and finishes with palpation of the muscles of the central compartment. Palpation for each of the muscles is shown in the seated position, but alternate palpation positions are also described. The major muscles or muscle groups of the region are each given a separate layout; there is also a detour to the palmaris brevis. Trigger point (TrP) information and stretching is given for each of the major muscles covered in this chapter. The chapter closes with an advanced *Whirlwind Tour* that explains the sequential palpation of all of the muscles of the chapter.

Chapter Outline

Chapter Objectives

After completing this chapter, the student should be able to perform the following for each of the muscles covered in this chapter:

1. State the attachments.
2. State the actions.
3. Describe the starting position for palpation.
4. Describe and explain the purpose of each of the palpation steps.
5. Palpate each muscle.
6. State the "Palpation Key."
7. Describe alternate palpation positions.
8. State the locations of the most common TrP(s).
9. Describe the TrP referral zones.
10. State the most common factors that create and/or perpetuate TrPs.
11. State the symptoms most commonly caused by TrPs.
12. Describe and perform a stretch.

⊖ Go to http://evolve.elsevier.com/Muscolino/palpation for video demonstrations of the muscle palpations presented in this chapter.

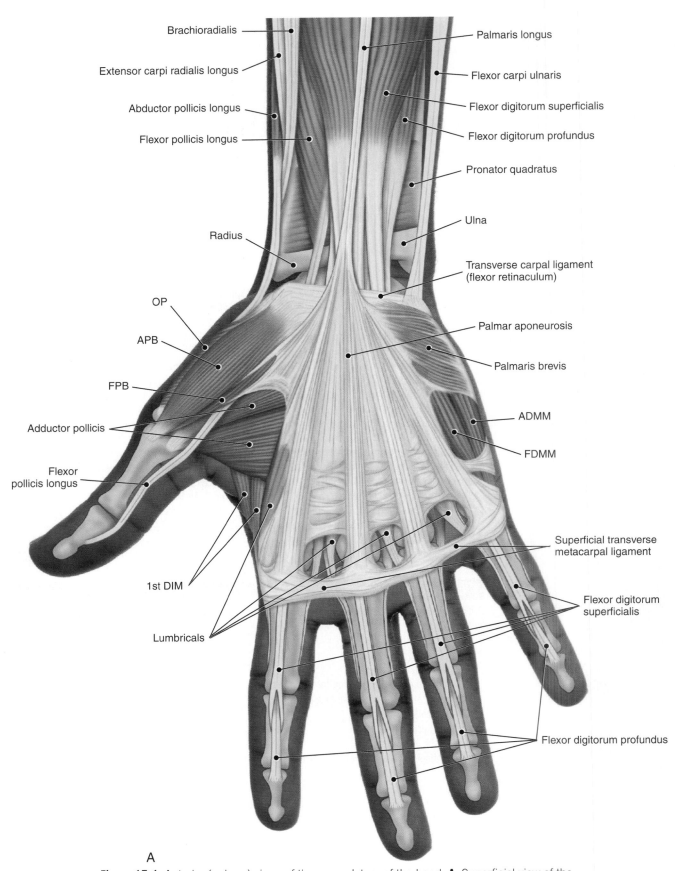

Figure 15-1 Anterior (palmar) views of the musculature of the hand. **A**, Superficial view of the hand with the palmar aponeurosis. *ADMM*, Abductor digiti minimi manus; *APB*, abductor pollicis brevis; *DIM*, dorsal interosseus manus; *FDMM*, flexor digiti minimi manus; *FPB*, flexor pollicis brevis; *ODM*, opponens digiti minimi; *OP*, opponens pollicis; *PI*, palmar interosseus.

Brachioradialis

Extensor carpi radialis longus

Abductor pollicis longus

Flexor pollicis longus

Radius

OP

APB

FPB

Adductor pollicis

Flexor
pollicis longus

1st DIM

Lumbricals

Palmaris longus

Flexor carpi ulnaris

Flexor digitorum superficialis

Flexor digitorum profundus

Pronator quadratus

Ulna

Transverse carpal ligament
(flexor retinaculum)

Palmar aponeurosis

Palmaris brevis

ADMM

FDMM

Superficial transverse
metacarpal ligament

Flexor digitorum
superficialis

Flexor digitorum profundus

A

15

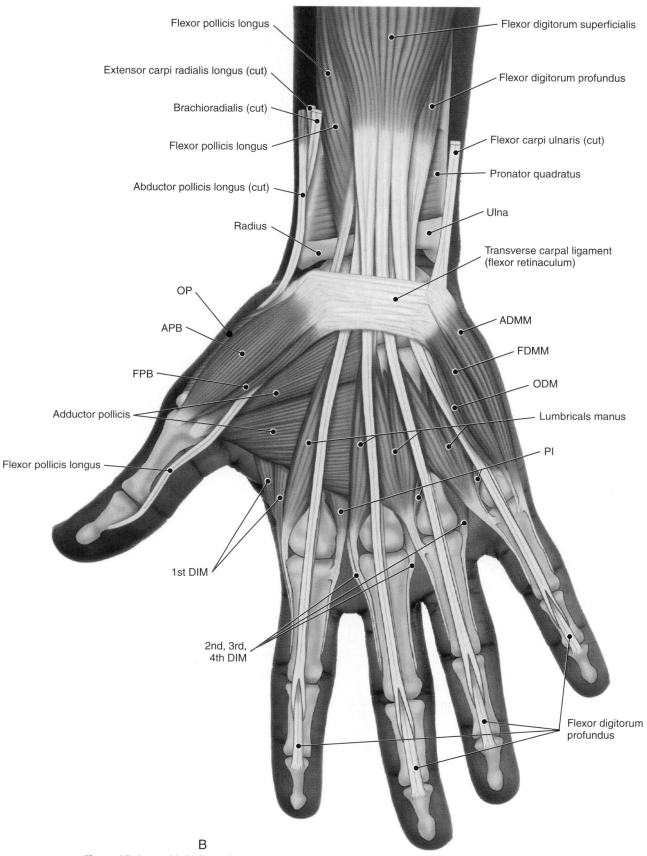

Figure 15-1, cont'd B, Superficial view of the musculature with the palmar aponeurosis removed. *ADMM,* Abductor digiti minimi manus; *APB,* abductor pollicis brevis; *DIM,* dorsal interosseus manus; *FDMM,* flexor digiti minimi manus; *FPB,* flexor pollicis brevis; *ODM,* opponens digiti minimi; *OP,* opponens pollicis; *PI,* palmar interosseus.

Flexor pollicis longus

Flexor digitorum profundus

Extensor carpi radialis longus (cut)

Brachioradialis (cut)

Flexor carpi ulnaris (cut)

Pronator quadratus

Abductor pollicis longus (cut)

Ulna

Radius

Transverse carpal ligament (flexor retinaculum) (cut)

APB (cut)

FPB (cut)

ADMM (cut)

OP

FDMM (cut)

FPB (cut)

ODM

APB (cut)

Lumbricals manus

FDMM (cut)

ADMM (cut)

Adductor pollicis

PI

1st DIM

2nd, 3rd, 4th DIM

C

Figure 15-1, cont'd C, Intermediate view with the more superficial thenar and hypothenar muscles cut. *ADMM*, Abductor digiti minimi manus; *APB*, abductor pollicis brevis; *DIM*, dorsal interosseus manus; *FDMM*, flexor digiti minimi manus; *FPB*, flexor pollicis brevis; *ODM*, opponens digiti minimi; *OP*, opponens pollicis; *PI*, palmar interosseus.

15

YOU ARE HERE

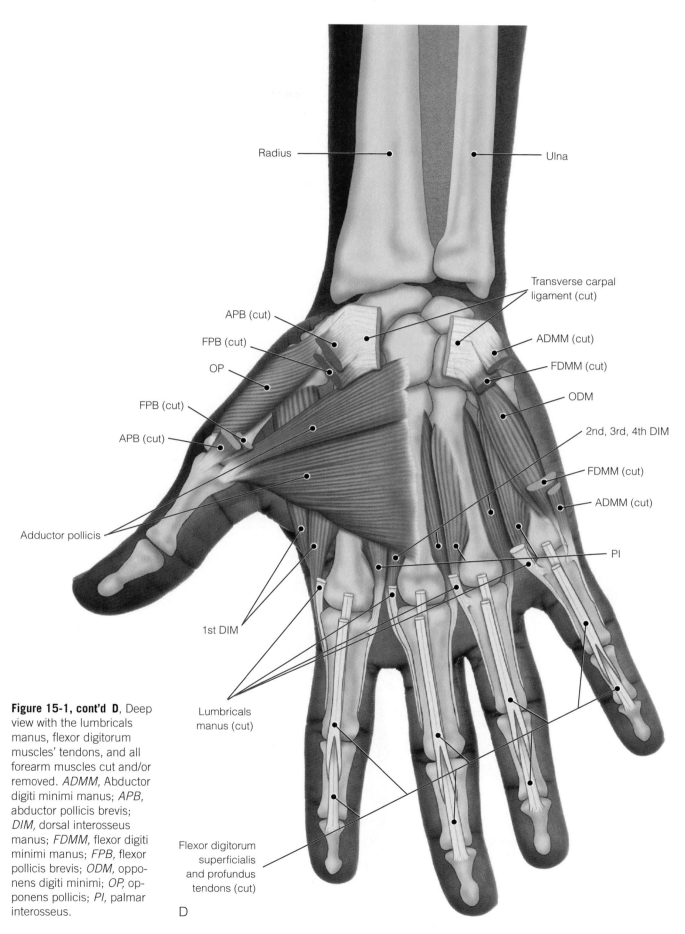

Radius

Ulna

APB (cut)

Transverse carpal ligament (cut)

FPB (cut)

ADMM (cut)

OP

FDMM (cut)

ODM

FPB (cut)

APB (cut)

2nd, 3rd, 4th DIM

FDMM (cut)

ADMM (cut)

Adductor pollicis

PI

1st DIM

Lumbricals manus (cut)

Flexor digitorum superficialis and profundus tendons (cut)

15

Figure 15-1, cont'd D, Deep view with the lumbricals manus, flexor digitorum muscles' tendons, and all forearm muscles cut and/or removed. *ADMM,* Abductor digiti minimi manus; *APB,* abductor pollicis brevis; *DIM,* dorsal interosseus manus; *FDMM,* flexor digiti minimi manus; *FPB,* flexor pollicis brevis; *ODM,* opponens digiti minimi; *OP,* opponens pollicis; *PI,* palmar interosseus.

D

YOU ARE HERE

15

Figure 15-1, cont'd E, Deepest view of the palmar musculature. *ADMM*, Abductor digiti minimi manus; *APB*, abductor pollicis brevis; *DIM*, dorsal interosseus manus; *FDMM*, flexor digiti minimi manus; *FPB*, flexor pollicis brevis; *ODM*, opponens digiti minimi; *OP*, opponens pollicis; *PI*, palmar interosseus.

E

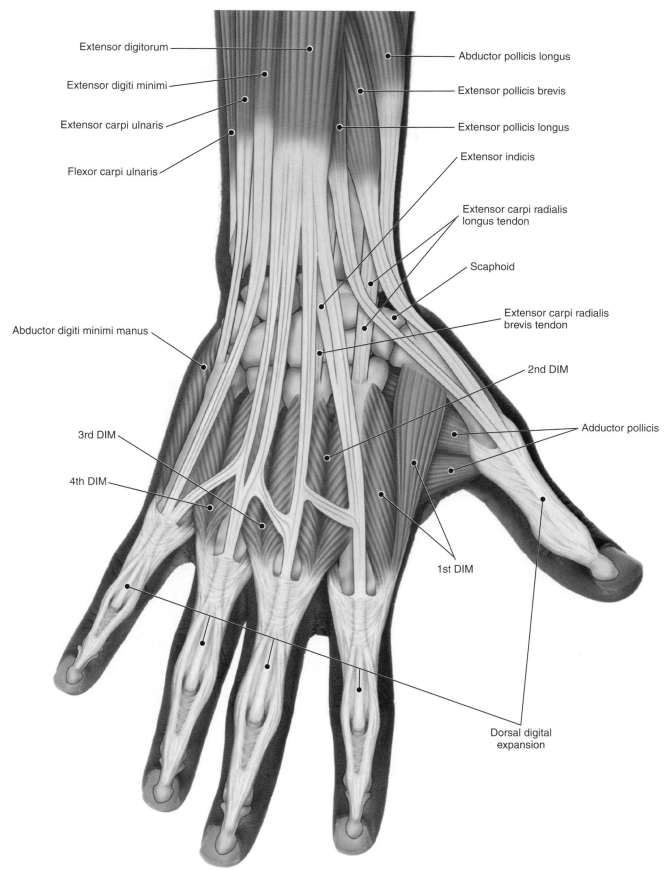

Figure 15-2 Posterior (dorsal) view of the musculature of the hand. *DIM*, Dorsal interosseus manus.

Extensor digitorum

Extensor digiti minimi

Extensor carpi ulnaris

Flexor carpi ulnaris

Abductor digiti minimi manus

3rd DIM

4th DIM

Abductor pollicis longus

Extensor pollicis brevis

Extensor pollicis longus

Extensor indicis

Extensor carpi radialis longus tendon

Scaphoid

Extensor carpi radialis brevis tendon

2nd DIM

Adductor pollicis

1st DIM

Dorsal digital expansion

15

YOU ARE HERE

THENAR GROUP—SEATED

The thenar group is composed of the abductor pollicis brevis (APB), flexor pollicis brevis (FPB), and the opponens pollicis (OP).

Abductor Pollicis Brevis (APB):

❑ ATTACHMENTS:
o Carpals (tubercles of the scaphoid and trapezium) and the flexor retinaculum *to the* lateral side of the base of the proximal phalanx of the thumb (and the dorsal digital expansion)

❑ ACTIONS:
o Abducts and extends the thumb at the carpometacarpal (CMC) joint; flexes the thumb at the metacarpophalangeal (MCP) joint; extends the thumb at the interphalangeal (IP) joint

Flexor Pollicis Brevis (FPB):

❑ ATTACHMENTS:
o Palmar side of the trapezium and the flexor retinaculum *to the* lateral side of the base of the proximal phalanx of the thumb

❑ ACTIONS:
o Flexes and abducts the thumb at the CMC joint; flexes the thumb at the MCP joint

15

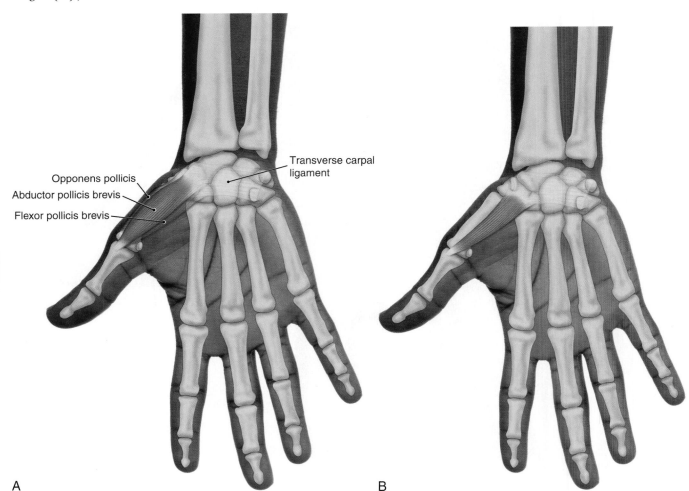

Opponens pollicis
Abductor pollicis brevis
Flexor pollicis brevis

Transverse carpal ligament

A

B

Figure 15-3 Anterior views of the muscles of the right thenar group. **A,** Abductor pollicis brevis. The flexor pollicis brevis and opponens pollicis have been ghosted in. **B,** Flexor pollicis brevis.

THENAR GROUP—SEATED—cont'd

Opponens Pollicis (OP):

❏ ATTACHMENTS:

o Tubercle of the trapezium and the flexor retinaculum *to the* anterior surface and lateral border of the shaft of the first metacarpal (of the thumb)

❏ ACTIONS:

o Opposes (flexes, medially rotates, and abducts) the thumb at the CMC joint

C

Figure 15-3, cont'd C, Opponens pollicis.

Starting position (Figure 15-4):
o Client seated
o Therapist seated facing the client
o Palpating fingers placed on the lateral side of the thenar eminence of the client
o Support hand placed on the anterior surface of the proximal phalanx of the client's thumb

Palpation steps:
1. APB: Palpating the lateral side of the thenar eminence, gently to moderately resist thumb abduction at the carpometacarpal (saddle) joint and feel for the contraction of the APB. It can be helpful to pinch the muscle between your thumb and index finger, as seen in Figure 15-5, A.
2. Once felt, palpate proximally and distally to the attachments of the abductor pollicis brevis (APB). Also try to discern the medial border of the APB from the flexor pollicis brevis (FPB).
3. FPB: Now place palpating fingers at the most medial aspect of the thenar eminence, gently to moderately resist thumb flexion at the CMC (saddle) joint, and feel for the contraction of the FPB (Figure 15-5, B).
4. Once the FPB's contraction is felt in the medial thenar eminence, try to palpate it deep to the ABP as the client alternately contracts the muscle against gentle resistance and relaxes it.
5. OP: To palpate the OP, curl your palpating finger(s) around the shaft of the metacarpal of the thumb as seen in Figure 15-5, C. Ask the client to oppose the thumb against the little finger, exerting gentle pressure against the pad of the little finger, and feel for the OP to contract.
6. Once the OP's contraction is felt against the metacarpal, attempt to palpate the rest of this muscle deep to the other thenar muscles. It can be very difficult to discern the OP from the other thenar muscles. For this reason, it is usually more effective to palpate for tight spots in this muscle with the thenar musculature relaxed.
7. Once the thenar muscles have been located, have the client relax them and palpate to assess their baseline tone.

15

THENAR GROUP—SEATED—cont'd

Figure 15-4 Starting position for seated palpation of the right thenar group.

A

B

C

Figure 15-5 Palpation of the right thenar group. **A**, Palpation of the abductor pollicis brevis as the client abducts the thumb at the carpometacarpal (CMC) joint against resistance. **B**, Palpation of the flexor pollicis brevis as the client flexes the thumb at the CMC joint against resistance. **C**, Palpation of the opponens pollicis by curling around the metacarpal of the thumb as the client opposes the thumb at the CMC joint to the little finger.

Palpation Key:

APB: Palpate the lateral aspect of the thenar eminence.
FPB: Palpate at the most medial aspect of the thenar eminence.
OP: Curl your fingers around the shaft of the metacarpal of the thumb.

15

THENAR GROUP—SEATED—cont'd

Palpation Notes:

1. Movements of the thumb at the saddle are unusual in their direction. Flexion and extension occur within the frontal plane; and abduction and adduction occur within the sagittal plane. Furthermore, opposition is a combination of flexion, abduction, and medial rotation. It is important to know these motions so that the client can be asked to do the proper joint actions to engage the correct muscles to contract for palpation.

2. The abductor pollicis brevis (APB) is superficial in the thenar eminence and easily palpable.

3. Only a small part of the flexor pollicis brevis (FPB) is superficial on the medial side of the thenar eminence. The majority of it is deep to the APB.

4. Only a very small part of the opponens pollicis (OP) is accessible superficially in the lateral aspect of the thenar eminence against the shaft of the metacarpal of the thumb. The rest of the OP is deep to the other thenar eminence muscles and difficult to palpate and discern from them.

5. Even though the APB is superficial and easily palpable, sometimes it can be difficult to discern its medial border from the FPB because both of these muscles abduct and flex the thumb at the CMC. So if excessive resistance is given to either joint motion, both muscles will be engaged to contract. However, the APB is preferentially contracted with abduction, and the FPB is preferentially contracted with flexion of the thumb. Therefore, to better palpate these muscles and to discern their border, it is important to offer only mild or moderate resistance or both muscles will contract, making it impossible to discern these two muscles from each other.

6. The OP is the most difficult thenar muscle to palpate and discern because it is mostly deep to other thenar muscles and because its action of opposition incorporates both abduction and flexion of the thumb at the saddle joint. Therefore, when the OP is engaged to contract, the more superficial APB and FPB tend to contract as well.

TRIGGER POINTS

1. Trigger points (TrPs) in the thenar muscles often result from or are perpetuated by acute or chronic overuse of the muscle (e.g., prolonged pincer gripping such as when writing) or trauma (e.g., falling on an outstretched hand).

2. TrPs in the thenar muscles may produce soreness with use of the thumb (especially when gripping objects with the pincer grip), or weakness and difficulty with fine motor skills of the thumb.

3. The referral patterns of opponens pollicis TrPs must be distinguished from the referral patterns of TrPs in the adductor pollicis, flexor carpi radialis, pronator teres, brachialis, subscapularis, subclavius, and scalenes.

4. TrPs in the thenar muscles are often incorrectly assessed as carpal tunnel syndrome, de Quervain's stenosing tenosynovitis, cervical disc syndrome, or first carpometacarpal osteoarthritis.

5. Associated TrPs often occur in the adductor pollicis, first dorsal interosseus manus, APB, and FPB.

6. Note: TrP referral patterns have not yet been established for the APB and FPB; they likely will follow the referral patterns for the OP. When assessing these muscles for TrPs, look primarily for central TrPs located in the middle of the bellies.

Figure 15-6 Anterior view illustrating a common opponens pollicis TrP and its corresponding referral zone.

15

Alternate Palpation Position—Supine or Prone

The thenar muscles of the hand can also be easily palpated with the client supine or prone. Follow the palpation steps indicated for the seated palpation.

STRETCHING THE THENAR GROUP

Figure 15-7 A stretch of the right thenar group of muscles. The client uses the other hand to grip the metacarpal and proximal phalanx of the right thumb, extend and adduct the metacarpal at the carpometacarpal joint, and extend the proximal phalanx at the metacarpophalangeal joint.

HYPOTHENAR GROUP—SEATED

The hypothenar group is composed of the abductor digiti minimi manus (ADMM), flexor digiti minimi manus (FDMM), and opponens digiti minimi (ODM).

Abductor Digiti Minimi Manus (ADMM):

❑ **ATTACHMENTS:**

o Pisiform and the tendon of the flexor carpi ulnaris *to the* medial side of the base of the proximal phalanx of the little finger (and the dorsal digital expansion)

❑ **ACTIONS:**

o Abducts the little finger at the metacarpophalangeal (MCP) and carpometacarpal (CMC) joints; extends the little finger at the proximal and distal interphalangeal (IP) joints

Flexor Digiti Minimi Manus (FDMM):

❑ **ATTACHMENTS:**

o Hook of the hamate and the flexor retinaculum *to the* anteromedial side of the base of the proximal phalanx of the little finger

❑ **ACTIONS:**

o Flexes the little finger at the MCP and CMC joints

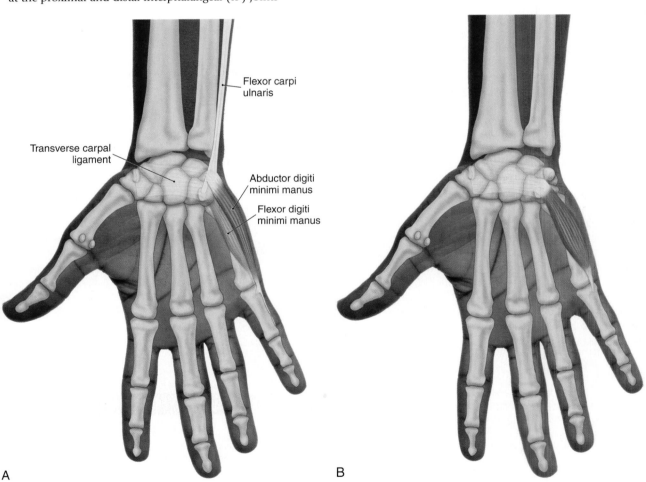

A
B

Figure 15-8 Anterior views of the muscles of the right hypothenar group. **A**, Abductor digiti minimi manus. The flexor digiti minimi manus has been ghosted in. **B**, Flexor digiti minimi manus.

15

Figure 15-8, cont'd C, Opponens digiti minimi.

C

Opponens Digiti Minimi (ODM):

❑ ATTACHMENTS:
o Hook of the hamate and the flexor retinaculum *to the* anterior surface and the medial border of the shaft of the fifth metacarpal

❑ ACTIONS:
o Opposes (flexes, adducts, laterally rotates) the little finger at the CMC joint

Starting position (Figure 15-9):
o Client seated
o Therapist seated facing the client
o Palpating fingers placed on the medial side of the hypothenar eminence of the client
o Support hand placed on the medial surface of the proximal phalanx of the client's little finger

Palpation steps:
1. ADMM: Palpating the medial side of the hypothenar eminence, resist the client from abducting the little finger at the MCP joint and feel for the contraction of the ADMM (Figure 15-10, A).
2. Once felt, palpate distally to the medial side of the base of the proximal phalanx, and proximally to the pisiform.

Also try to discern the lateral border of the ADMM from the FDMM.
3. FDMM: Palpating the lateral side of the hypothenar eminence, ask the client to flex the little finger at the MCP joint (but keep it extended at the interphalangeal joints) and feel for the contraction of the FDMM. If needed, flexion can be gently resisted by placing a finger of your support hand against the anterior surface of the proximal phalanx of the little finger (Figure 15-10, B).
4. Once felt, palpate distally to the anteromedial surface of the base of the proximal phalanx, and proximally to the hook of the hamate. If not previously done, try to discern the border between the FDMM and the ADMM.
5. ODM: Locate the hook of the hamate and palpate immediately distal to it on the most lateral aspect of the hypothenar eminence, and feel for the contraction of the ODM as the client opposes the little finger against the thumb (Figure 15-10, C).
6. Once felt, palpate distally as far as possible deep to the other muscles of the hypothenar eminence.
7. The most distal attachment of the ODM can usually be palpated by curling your palpating finger around to the anterior side of the shaft of the fifth metacarpal (Note: This is similar to how the opponens pollicis was palpated against the first metacarpal.) (Figure 15-10, D).
8. Once the hypothenar muscles have been located, have the client relax them and palpate to assess their baseline tone.

15

HYPOTHENAR GROUP—SEATED—cont'd

Palpation Key:
ADMM: Palpate the medial side of the hypothenar eminence.
FDMM: Flex the little finger at only the MCP joint.
ODM: Find the hook of the hamate and palpate immediately distal to it at the most lateral aspect of the hypothenar eminence.

Figure 15-9 Starting position for seated palpation of the right hypothenar group.

Figure 15-10 Palpation of the right hypothenar group. **A**, Palpation of the abductor digiti minimi manus at the medial side of the hypothenar eminence as the client abducts the little finger against resistance. **B**, Palpation of the flexor digiti minimi manus at the lateral side of the hypothenar eminence as the client flexes the proximal phalanx of the little finger against resistance. **C**, Palpation of the opponens digiti minimi at the far lateral side of the hypothenar eminence as the client opposes the little finger against resistance. **D**, Palpation of the opponens digiti minimi against the metacarpal of the little finger as the client opposes the little finger against resistance.

HYPOTHENAR GROUP—SEATED—cont'd

Palpation Notes:

1. The abductor digiti minimi manus (ADMM) is wholly superficial in the hypothenar eminence and easily palpable.
2. The majority of the flexor digiti minimi manus (FDMM) is superficial on the lateral side of the hypothenar eminence. Its most medial aspect is deep to the ADMM.
3. The majority of the opponens digiti minimi is deep to the other hypothenar muscles. However, its most lateral aspect is superficial on the lateral side of the hypothenar eminence.
4. Sometimes it is difficult to discern the border between the ADMM and the FDMM. When palpating for the ADMM, be sure that the client is not also flexing the little finger. When palpating for the FDMM, be sure that the client is not also abducting the little finger.
5. It is important when palpating for the FDMM that the client only moves the proximal phalanx at the MCP joint. If the IP joints are moved, long finger flexors from the forearm (flexors digitorum superficialis and profundus) will tend to be engaged. For this reason, it is also important that any resistance given is applied only to the proximal phalanx.
6. It is also important when palpating the FDMM that only mild to moderate resistance is given to flexion of the little finger, or the long finger flexors will be engaged.
7. Given the location of the tendons of the long finger flexors next to the ODM, be sure to also discern these structures from each other.
8. The tendons of the long finger flexors to the little finger are located just lateral to the bellies of the FDMM and ODM. To feel the contraction of the tendons of the long finger flexors, have the client flex only the middle and distal phalanges of the little finger at the IP joints. This will engage the long finger flexors but not the FDMM.
9. It can be very difficult to palpate and discern the ODM deep to the FDMM, because flexion of the little finger is a component of opposition of the little finger. For this reason, when opposition of the little finger is done, the FDMM may be engaged, making it difficult to feel the contraction of the deeper ODM.

TRIGGER POINTS

1. Trigger points (TrPs) in the hypothenar muscles often result from or are perpetuated by acute or chronic overuse of the muscle (e.g., prolonged pincer gripping, such as when writing), or trauma (e.g., falling on an outstretched hand).
2. TrPs in the hypothenar muscles may produce weakness or difficulty with fine motor skills of the little finger, or entrapment of the ulnar nerve by the ODM, causing weakness of intrinsic muscles of the hand.
3. The referral patterns of ADMM TrPs must be distinguished from the referral patterns of TrPs in the first dorsal interosseus manus, latissimus dorsi, and triceps brachii.
4. TrPs in the hypothenar muscles are often incorrectly assessed as osteoarthritis of the fingers, cervical disc syndrome, or thoracic outlet syndrome.
5. Associated TrPs often occur in the other hypothenar muscles and the dorsal interossei manus.
6. Note: TrP referral patterns have not yet been established for the FDMM and ADMM. They likely will follow the referral patterns for the ODM. When assessing these muscles for TrPs, look primarily for central TrPs located in the middle of the bellies.

Figure 15-11 Posterior view illustrating a common abductor digiti minimi manus TrP and its corresponding referral zone.

Alternate Palpation Position—Supine or Prone
The hypothenar muscles of the hand can also be easily palpated with the client supine or prone. Follow the palpation steps indicated for the seated palpation.

STRETCHING THE HYPOTHENAR GROUP

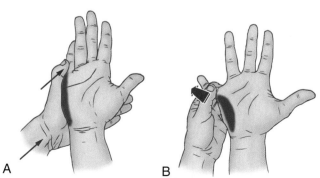

A   B

Figure 15-12 Stretches of the right hypothenar muscles. **A**, Stretch of the abductor digiti minimi manus. The little finger is adducted and extended. **B**, Stretch of the flexor digiti minimi manus and opponens digiti minimi. The little finger and its metacarpal are extended and abducted.

HYPOTHENAR GROUP—SEATED—cont'd

DETOUR

Palmaris Brevis: The palmaris brevis is located in the dermis of the proximal hand on the medial side, over the hypothenar eminence (see Figure 15-13, A). This muscle is extremely thin and difficult to discern from adjacent soft tissue. Given that this muscle's action is to wrinkle the skin of the palm, ask the client to do this by cupping the palm of the hand and feel for this muscle's contraction (this will likely also cause the palmaris longus to contract) (see Figure 15-13, B). Note: Be sure that the little finger is either not moved or moved as little as possible, or you will feel the contraction of the hypothenar muscles.

Palmaris longus

Palmar aponeurosis

Palmaris brevis

Figure 15-13 The palmaris brevis. **A**, Anterior view of the right palmaris brevis. **B**, Palpation of the right palmaris brevis.

A

B

15

ADDUCTOR POLLICIS—SEATED

❏ ATTACHMENTS:

o Capitate, anterior base and shaft of the third metacarpal, and the anterior base of the second metacarpal *to the* anteromedial side of the base of the proximal phalanx of the thumb (and the dorsal digital expansion)

❏ ACTIONS:

o Adducts and flexes the thumb at the carpometacarpal (CMC) joint
o Extends the thumb at the interphalangeal (IP) joint

Starting position (Figure 15-15):

o Client seated
o Therapist seated facing the client
o Palpating fingers placed on the anterior surface of the thumb web of the client's hand
o Fingers of the support hand placed on the posterior surface of the proximal phalanx of the client's thumb

Palpation steps:

1. Palpating the anterior side of the thumb web of the hand, resist the client from adducting the thumb at the CMC (saddle) joint, and feel for the contraction of the adductor pollicis (Figure 15-16).
2. Once felt, palpate the entire adductor pollicis from the proximal phalanx of the thumb to the third metacarpal and capitate.
3. Once the adductor pollicis muscle has been located, have the client relax it and palpate to assess its baseline tone.

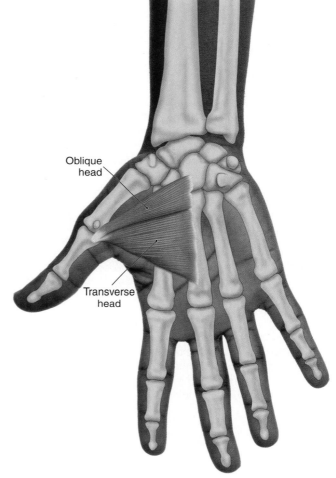

Oblique head

Transverse head

Figure 15-14 Anterior view of the right adductor pollicis.

Figure 15-15 Starting position for seated palpation of the right adductor pollicis.

Figure 15-16 Palpation of the right adductor pollicis as the client adducts the thumb against resistance.

ADDUCTOR POLLICIS—SEATED—cont'd

Palpation Notes:

1. Adduction of the thumb at the saddle joint occurs within the sagittal plane and is a motion toward the palm of the hand.
2. When palpating for the adductor pollicis in the thumb web of the hand, note that other muscles are located within the web (see Figure 15-1). The first dorsal interosseus is located within the thumb web and is attached to both the first and second metacarpals. The flexor pollicis brevis (FPB) is also located within the thumb web close to the first metacarpal, and the first lumbrical manus is located within the thumb web close to the second metacarpal. Of these other muscles, only the FPB also moves the thumb and might engage when asking the client to move the thumb. To be sure that you are not engaging the FPB, make sure that the client is doing pure adduction of the thumb (i.e., is not flexing the thumb as well).

Alternate Palpation Position—Supine or Prone

The adductor pollicis of the hand can also be easily palpated with the client supine or prone. Follow the palpation steps indicated for the seated palpation.

Palpation Key:

Palpate the thumb web of the hand.

TRIGGER POINTS

1. Trigger points (TrPs) in the adductor pollicis often result from or are perpetuated by acute or chronic overuse of the muscle (e.g., prolonged pincer gripping, such as when writing) or trauma (e.g., falling on an outstretched hand).
2. TrPs in the adductor pollicis may produce pain in the thumb web, soreness with use of the thumb (especially when gripping objects with the pincer grip), or weakness and difficulty coordinating the thumb for fine motor activities.
3. The referral patterns of adductor pollicis TrPs must be distinguished from the referral patterns of TrPs in the opponens pollicis, supinator, extensor carpi radialis longus, brachioradialis, brachialis, scalenes, pronator teres, and subclavius.
4. TrPs in the adductor pollicis are often incorrectly assessed as de Quervain's stenosing tenosynovitis, carpal tunnel syndrome, cervical disc syndrome, thoracic outlet syndrome, or joint dysfunction or osteoarthritis of the first carpometacarpal or metacarpophalangeal joint.
5. Associated TrPs often occur in the opponens pollicis, first dorsal interosseus manus, abductor pollicis brevis, or flexor pollicis brevis.

Figure 15-17 A, Anterior view illustrating a common adductor pollicis TrP and its corresponding referral zone. **B**, Posterior view showing the remainder of the referral zone.

STRETCHING THE ADDUCTOR POLLICIS

Figure 15-18 A stretch of the right adductor pollicis. The thumb is moved into abduction and extension.

15

LUMBRICALS MANUS—SEATED

There are four lumbricals manus muscles, numbered one to four from lateral to medial, respectively.

❏ ATTACHMENTS:

o Distal tendons of the flexor digitorum profundus *to the* distal tendons of the extensor digitorum (the dorsal digital expansion).

o Proximally, each lumbrical manus attaches to a tendon or tendons of the flexor digitorum profundus muscle and is located between metacarpals on the lateral side of the finger to which it attaches distally. Distally, each lumbrical manus muscle attaches to the lateral side of the distal tendon of the extensor digitorum (dorsal digital expansion) of a finger. Overall, the lumbricals manus muscles attach to fingers two through five.

❏ ACTIONS:

o Flex fingers two through five at the metacarpophalangeal (MCP) joint

o Extend fingers two through five at the proximal and distal interphalangeal (IP) joints

Starting position (Figure 15-20):

o Client seated

o Therapist seated facing the client

o Place palpating finger(s) over the anterolateral surface of the shaft of the 2nd metacarpal of the client's hand

o If resistance is given, place fingers of the support hand on the anterior surface of the proximal phalanx of the finger of the lumbrical manus being palpated (not seen in Figure 15-20)

Palpation steps:

1. First lumbrical manus: Palpating over the anterolateral surface of the shaft of the second metacarpal, ask the client to flex the index finger at the MCP joint while keeping the interphalangeal (IP) joints completely extended, and feel for the contraction of the first lumbrical manus muscle (Figure 15-21, A). Once located, palpate from attachment to attachment.

2. Once felt, follow the first lumbrical manus proximally and distally from attachment to attachment while the client alternately contracts and relaxes the muscle, as indicated in Step 1.

3. Second lumbrical manus: Follow the same procedure as used for the first lumbrical manus muscle. Palpate over the antero-lateral surface of the third metacarpal, and feel for its contraction as the client flexes the third finger at the MCP joint (with the IP joints fully extended) (see Figure 15-21, B). Once located, palpate from attachment to attachment.

Figure 15-19 Anterior view of the right lumbricals manus. The adductor pollicis has been ghosted in.

Flexor digitorum profundus

Adductor pollicis

Lumbricals manus

15

4. Third and fourth lumbricals manus: Palpating the third and fourth lumbrical manus muscles is similar to the palpation of the first and second lumbricals manus. The only difference is that the placement of the palpating fingers must be more centered between the adjacent metacarpals because of the broader proximal attachments of these lumbricals. For the third lumbrical manus, palpate between the third and fourth metacarpals. For the fourth lumbrical manus, palpate between the fourth and fifth metacarpals.

5. Once each lumbrical manus has been located, have the client relax it and palpate to assess its baseline tone.

LUMBRICALS MANUS—SEATED—cont'd

Figure 15-20 Starting position for seated palpation of the right lumbricals manus.

A

B

Figure 15-21 Palpation of the right lumbricals manus. **A**, Palpation of the first lumbrical manus on the radial side of the metacarpal of the index finger. **B**, Palpation of the second lumbrical manus on the radial side of the metacarpal of the middle finger. The third and fourth lumbricals manus are palpated in a similar manner against the radial side of the metacarpals of the ring and little fingers, respectively.

15

Palpation Notes:
1. The lumbricals manus muscles are actually quite superficial in the hand (for the most part, they are only deep to the palmar fascia) and therefore fairly easy to palpate.
2. To engage a lumbrical manus muscle, be sure that the middle and distal phalanges stay completely extended at the IP joints when the proximal phalanx of the finger is flexed at the MCP joint. Otherwise, the long flexors of the fingers (flexor digitorum superficialis [FDS] and the flexor digitorum profundus [FDP]) will tend to be engaged, making it more difficult to palpate and discern the lumbricals manus.
3. To be sure that you are palpating the lumbrical manus muscle and not the tendon of either the FDS or the FDP, ask the client to flex the finger at the proximal and distal IP joints. If what you are palpating engages with this motion, you are on the tendon of one or both of the long finger flexors (FDS or FDP). If what you are palpating does not engage, then you are on the lumbrical manus muscle to that finger.
4. Because the dorsal interosseus manus and palmar interosseus muscles can also flex the MCP joint of a finger and extend the IP joints of a finger, it is important that the client does not also abduct or adduct the finger at the MCP joint when flexing it. Otherwise, an interosseus muscle to that finger will also be engaged, making it difficult to palpate and discern the lumbrical manus muscle that is being palpated.
5. Perhaps the most difficult lumbrical manus muscle to palpate and discern is the fourth, because it lies adjacent to the flexor digiti minimi manus, which also engages with flexion of the little finger at the MCP joint.

Alternate Palpation Position—Supine or Prone
The lumbricals manus of the hand can also be easily palpated with the client supine or prone. Follow the palpation steps indicated for the seated palpation.

Palpation Key:
Flex the MCP joint, but keep the IP joints extended.

LUMBRICALS MANUS—SEATED—cont'd

TRIGGER POINTS

1. Trigger points (TrPs) in the lumbricals manus often result from or are perpetuated by acute or chronic overuse of the muscle (e.g., typing, prolonged pincer gripping, such as when writing) or altered biomechanics of the fingers (often due to arthritic changes).
2. TrPs in a lumbrical manus muscle generally produce pain along the radial side of the finger to which it attaches. Lumbricals manus TrPs may also produce weakness or difficulty with fine motor skills of the fingers.
3. The referral patterns of lumbricals manus TrPs must be distinguished from the referral patterns of TrPs in the palmar or dorsal interossei muscles of the hand, extensor digitorum, extensor digiti minimi, flexors digitorum superficialis and profundus, pectoralis minor, scalenes, latissimus dorsi, subclavius, and triceps brachii.
4. TrPs in the lumbricals manus are often incorrectly assessed as osteoarthritis of the fingers, cervical disc syndrome, thoracic outlet syndrome, or carpal tunnel syndrome.
5. Associated TrPs often occur in the palmar interossei, the dorsal interossei manus, and the thenar muscles of the thumb.
6. Note: Pain referral patterns from TrPs in the lumbricals manus muscles are not distinguished from the referral patterns of the palmar interossei and dorsal interossei manus muscles of the hand.

Figure 15-22 Posterior (dorsal) view illustrating common lumbricals manus TrPs and their corresponding referral zone. Note: These TrPs are located and therefore palpated anteriorly.

STRETCHING THE LUMBRICALS MANUS

Figure 15-23 A stretch of the right lumbricals manus. The fingers are extended at the metacarpophalangeal joints and flexed at the interphalangeal joints.

15

PALMAR INTEROSSEI (PI)—SEATED

There are three palmar interossei (PI) muscles, numbered one to three from lateral to medial, respectively.

❏ ATTACHMENTS:

o   From the "middle finger side" of the anterior surface of the metacarpals of fingers two, four, and five *to the* base of the proximal phalanx on the middle finger side of fingers two, four, and five (and the dorsal digital expansion)

❏ ACTIONS:

o   Adduct fingers two, four, and five at the metacarpophalangeal (MCP) joints
o   Flex fingers two, four, and five at the MCP joints
o   Extend fingers two, four, and five at the proximal and distal interphalangeal (IP) joints

Starting position (Figure 15-25):

o   Client seated with a pencil or highlighter placed between the index and middle fingers
o   Therapist seated facing the client
o   Palpating finger(s) placed on the palm of the client's hand, between the second and third metacarpals

Palpation steps:

1.   First PI: Palpating in the palm against the second metacarpal between the second and third metacarpals, ask the client to squeeze the highlighter between the index and middle fingers and feel for the contraction of the first PI muscle (Figure 15-26, A).
2.   Once felt, try to follow the first PI proximally and distally from attachment to attachment while the client alternately contracts and relaxes the muscle as indicated in Step 1.
3.   Second PI: Follow the same procedure as used for the first PI muscle. Palpate in the palm against the fourth metacarpal between the fourth and third metacarpals, and feel for the contraction of the second PI as the client squeezes the highlighter between the ring and middle fingers. Once located, palpate from attachment to attachment (Figure 15-26, B).
4.   Third PI: Following the same procedure, palpate in the palm against the fifth metacarpal between the fifth and fourth metacarpals, and feel for the contraction of the

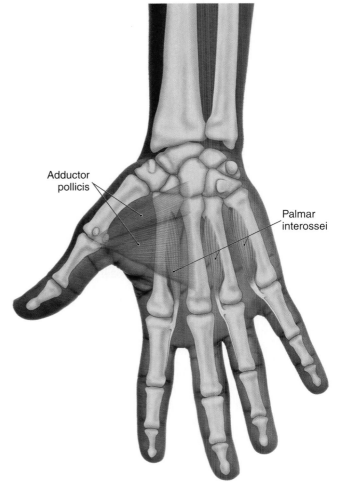

Figure 15-24 Anterior view of the right palmar interossei. The adductor pollicis has been ghosted in.

third PI as the client squeezes the highlighter between the little and ring fingers. Once located, palpate from attachment to attachment (Figure 15-26, C).
5.   Once each PI has been located, have the client relax it and palpate to assess its baseline tone.

15

PALMAR INTEROSSEI (PI)—SEATED—cont'd

Figure 15-25 Starting position for seated palpation of the right palmar interossei.

Palpation Key:

Squeeze a pencil or highlighter between two fingers.

Figure 15-26 Palpation of the right palmar interossei (PI). **A**, Palpation of the first PI as the client adducts the index finger against resistance (provided by a highlighter). **B**, Palpation of the second PI as the client adducts the ring finger against resistance. **C**, Palpation of the third PI as the client adducts the little finger against resistance.

15

PALMAR INTEROSSEI (PI)—SEATED—cont'd

Palpation Notes:

1. Adduction of the index, ring, and little fingers is a frontal plane motion that is toward the middle finger.
2. The palmar interossei (PI) are deep within the palm of the hand, but can be fairly easily palpated and discerned.
3. Squeezing a pencil or highlighter between the index and middle fingers requires adduction of the index finger, thereby engaging the first PI. Similarly, squeezing the pencil or highlighter can be used to engage the other two PI.
4. To isolate a PI, it is important that the client does not attempt to flex the finger at the MCP or IP joints when squeezing (ad-

ducting), or the lumbricals and/or long finger flexors (flexors digitorum superficialis and profundus) will be engaged, making it more difficult to palpate and discern the PI muscle.

5. Careful palpation must be done to discern a PI muscle from the nearby long finger flexor tendons to that finger, because they may engage with adduction of the finger. To determine if you are palpating a long finger flexor tendon, ask the client to flex the finger at the IP joints, being sure to keep the MCP joint completely extended. If what you are palpating tenses, then it is a long finger flexor.

Alternate Palpation Position—Supine or Prone

The palmar interossei can also be easily palpated with the client supine or prone. Follow the palpation steps indicated for the seated palpation.

TRIGGER POINTS

1. Trigger points (TrPs) in the PI often result from or are perpetuated by acute or chronic overuse of the muscle (e.g., prolonged regular gripping, such as holding a tennis racquet or tool; or pincer gripping, such as when writing) or altered biomechanics of the fingers (often due to arthritic changes).
2. TrPs in a PI muscle usually produce pain along the side of the finger where it attaches. PI TrPs may also produce weakness or difficulty with fine motor skills of the associated finger, entrapment of the median or ulnar nerve, or restriction of finger abduction at the metacarpophalangeal joint.
3. The referral patterns of PI TrPs must be distinguished from the referral patterns of TrPs in the lumbricals manus, extensor digitorum, extensor digiti minimi, flexors digitorum superficialis and profundus, scalenes, pectoralis minor, subclavius, latissimus dorsi, and triceps brachii.
4. TrPs in the PI are often incorrectly assessed as osteoarthritis or joint dysfunction of the fingers, cervical disc syndrome, thoracic outlet syndrome, or carpal tunnel syndrome.

5. Associated TrPs often occur in the dorsal interossei manus, lumbricals manus, thenar muscles, and adductor pollicis.
6. Note: Pain referral patterns from TrPs in the PI muscles are not distinguished from the referral patterns of the lumbricals manus muscles (and dorsal interossei manus muscles).

Figure 15-27 Posterior view illustrating common palmar interossei TrPs and their corresponding referral zones. Note: These TrPs are located and therefore palpated anteriorly.

STRETCHING THE PALMER INTEROSSEI

Figure 15-28 Stretches of the three palmar interossei muscles of the right hand. The index, ring, and little fingers are abducted away from the middle finger.

DORSAL INTEROSSEI MANUS (DIM)—SEATED

There are four dorsal interossei manus (DIM) muscles, numbered one to four from lateral to medial, respectively.

❑ ATTACHMENTS:

o Proximally, each dorsal interosseus manus (DIM) muscle attaches proximally to both sides of adjacent metacarpals of fingers one through five.

o Distally, each one attaches to one side of the proximal phalanx of a finger (on the side away from the center of the third finger), and to the tendon of the extensor digitorum (dorsal digital expansion) to that finger.

❑ ACTIONS:

o Abduct fingers two through four at the metacarpophalangeal (MCP) joints

o Flex fingers two through four at the MCP joints

o Extend fingers two through four at the proximal and distal interphalangeal (IP) joints

Starting position (Figure 15-30):

o Client seated

o Therapist seated facing the client

o Palpating finger(s) placed on the dorsal side of the client's hand, between the fourth and fifth metacarpals

o Fingers of the support hand placed on the medial side of the proximal phalanx of the fourth finger

Palpation steps:

1. Fourth DIM: Palpating on the dorsal side of the hand between the fourth and fifth metacarpals, ask the client to abduct the ring finger against your resistance, and feel for the contraction of the fourth DIM (Figure 15-31, A).

2. Once felt, try to follow the fourth DIM proximally and distally from attachment to attachment while the client alternately contracts and relaxes the muscle as indicated in Step 1.

3. Third DIM: Following the same procedure, palpate between the third and fourth metacarpals while resisting ulnar abduction of the middle finger, and feel for the contraction of the third DIM (Figure 15-31, B). Once felt, palpate from attachment to attachment as the client alternately contracts and relaxes the muscle.

4. Second DIM: Following the same procedure, palpate between the third and second metacarpals while resisting radial abduction of the middle finger, and feel for the contraction of the second DIM (Figure 15-31, C). Once felt,

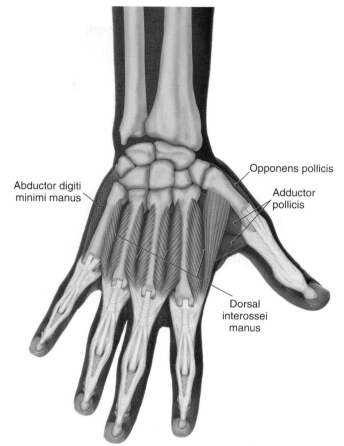

Figure 15-29 Posterior view of the right dorsal interossei manus. The adductor pollicis, opponens pollicis, and abductor digiti minimi manus have been ghosted in.

palpate from attachment to attachment as the client alternately contracts and relaxes the muscle.

5. First DIM: Palpate in the thumb web of the hand on the dorsal side, especially against the second metacarpal, and feel for the contraction of the first DIM as the client abducts the index finger. Resistance may be added if needed (Figure 15-31, D). Once felt, palpate from attachment to attachment as the client alternately contracts and relaxes the muscle.

6. Once each DIM has been located, have the client relax it and palpate to assess its baseline tone.

15

DORSAL INTEROSSEI MANUS (DIM)—SEATED—cont'd

Palpation Key:
Palpate between metacarpals on the dorsal side.

Figure 15-30 Starting position for seated palpation of the right dorsal interossei manus.

Figure 15-31 Palpation of the right dorsal interossei manus (DIM). **A**, Palpation of the fourth DIM as the client abducts the ring finger against resistance. **B**, Palpation of the third DIM as the client ulnar abducts the middle finger against resistance. **C**, Palpation of the second DIM as the client radially abducts the middle finger against resistance. **D**, Palpation of the first DIM as the client abducts the index finger against resistance.

DORSAL INTEROSSEI MANUS (DIM)—SEATED—cont'd

Palpation Notes:

1. Finger abduction is a frontal plane motion away from an imaginary line through the center of the middle finger when it is in anatomic position.
2. The middle finger abducts in two directions, ulnar abduction when moving medially (in the ulnar direction) and radial abduction when moving laterally (in the radial direction).
3. Many people have difficulty isolating abduction motions of their fingers.

4. The DIM muscles are superficial and easy to palpate between the metacarpal bones on the dorsal side of the hand. The only musculoskeletal structures located superficial to them are the extensor tendons of the fingers (extensor digitorum and extensor indicis). To be sure that these other muscles are not contracting, resulting in a tensing of their tendons (which might make palpation and discernment of the DIM more difficult), make sure that the client is not also extending the finger as it is abducted.

Alternate Palpation Position—Supine or Prone

The DIM can also be easily palpated with the client supine or prone. Follow the palpation steps indicated for the seated palpation.

TRIGGER POINTS

1. Trigger points (TrPs) in the DIM often result from or are perpetuated by acute or chronic overuse of the muscle (e.g., typing, prolonged pincer gripping, such as when writing) or altered biomechanics of the fingers (often due to arthritic changes).
2. TrPs in a DIM usually produce pain along the side of the finger where it attaches, weakness or difficulty with fine motor skills of the finger, or entrapment of the median or ulnar nerve.
3. The referral patterns of DIM TrPs must be distinguished from the referral patterns of TrPs in the lumbricals manus, adductor pollicis, brachioradialis, supinator, scalenes, extensor digitorum, flexors digitorum superficialis and profundus, coracobrachialis, brachialis, triceps brachii, subclavius, pectoralis minor, and latissimus dorsi.
4. TrPs in the DIM are often incorrectly assessed as osteoarthritis or joint dysfunction of the fingers, cervical disc syndrome, thoracic outlet syndrome, or carpal tunnel syndrome.
5. Associated TrPs often occur in the palmar interossei, lumbricals manus, thenar muscles, and adductor pollicis.
6. Note: Pain referral patterns from TrPs in the DIM are not distinguished from the referral patterns of the lumbricals manus muscles (and palmar interossei muscles).

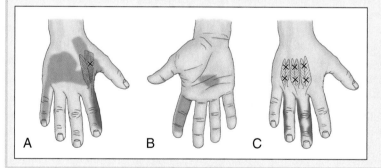

Figure 15-32 Common dorsal interossei manus (DIM) TrPs and their corresponding referral zones. **A**, First DIM TrP and its referral zone; **B**, Remainder of first DIM TrP referral zone. **C**, TrPs and their corresponding referral zones for the second, third, and fourth DIM muscles.

15

STRETCHING THE DORSAL INTEROSSEI MANUS

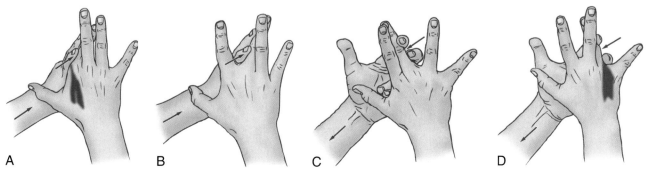

Figure 15-33 Stretches of the four dorsal interossei manus (DIM) muscles of the right hand. **A**, Stretching the first DIM by adducting the index finger toward the middle finger. **B**, Stretching the second DIM by ulnar abducting the middle finger. **C**, Stretching the third DIM by radially abducting the middle finger. **D**, Stretching the fourth DIM by adducting the ring finger toward the middle finger.

Intrinsic Muscles of the Hand

For all palpations of the intrinsic muscles of the hand, the client is seated and the therapist is seated, facing the client.

Thenar Group:

1. **Abductor pollicis brevis (APB):** Palpate on the lateral side of the thenar eminence and feel for the APB as the client abducts the thumb at the CMC joint against gentle resistance. Palpate from the tubercles of the scaphoid and trapezium to the lateral side of the base of the proximal phalanx of the thumb.

2. **Flexor pollicis brevis (FPB):** Now move over to the medial side of the thenar eminence and feel for the FPB as the client flexes the thumb at the CMC joint against gentle resistance. Palpate from attachment to attachment (dorsal surface of the trapezium to the lateral side of the base of the proximal phalanx of the thumb) as best as possible, including the part of the muscle that is deep to the APB.

3. **Opponens pollicis (OP):** Now move over to the shaft of the metacarpal of the thumb. Curl your palpating fingers around from posterior to anterior on the lateral shaft, and feel for the contraction of the OP against the metacarpal as the client gently opposes the thumb against the pad of the little finger. Once felt, try to palpate the rest of this muscle deep to the other two thenar muscles. Because it can be very challenging to feel and discern the contraction of the OP from the contraction of other thenar muscles, it is often advisable to palpate this muscle when the thenar muscles are relaxed.

Hypothenar Group:

4. **Abductor digiti minimi manus (ADMM):** Palpate on the medial side of the hypothenar eminence and feel for the ADMM as the client abducts the little finger at the MCP joint against resistance. Palpate from the pisiform to the medial side of the base of the proximal phalanx of the little finger.

5. **Flexor digiti minimi manus (FDMM):** Now palpate on the lateral side of the hypothenar eminence, and feel for the FDMM as the client flexes the little finger at the MCP joint (with the IP joints extended). Add resistance only if needed. Palpate from the hook of the hamate to the anteromedial side of the base of the proximal phalanx of the little finger.

6. **Opponens digiti minimi (ODM):** Locate the hook of the hamate and then palpate immediately distal to it on the most lateral aspect of the hypothenar eminence. Feel for the contraction of the ODM as the client opposes the little finger against the thumb. Once felt, palpate it deep to the other hypothenar muscles as far as possible. Note: The distal attachment of the ODM can be palpated by curling the palpating the fingers around to the anterior surface of the shaft of the fifth metacarpal.

7. **Detour to the palmaris brevis:** Palpate gently over the proximal hypothenar eminence while asking the client to wrinkle the skin of the hand by cupping the palm. This muscle is difficult to palpate and discern.

Central Compartment Muscles:

8. **Adductor pollicis:** Palpate the thumb web of the hand from the anterior side while resisting the client from adducting the thumb and feel for the contraction of the adductor pollicis. Once felt, palpate from the base of the proximal phalanx of the thumb to the third metacarpal and capitate.

9. **Lumbricals manus:** For the first and second lumbricals manus, palpate on the anterolateral surface of the metacarpal of the index and middle fingers, respectively. For the third and fourth lumbricals manus, palpate between metacarpals on the lateral side of the ring and little fingers respectively. Ask the client to flex the finger at the MCP joint while keeping the IP joints extended, and feel for the contraction of the muscle. Once felt, palpate each one from attachment to attachment as the client alternately contracts and relaxes the muscle.

10. **Palmar interossei (PI):** For PI one, two, and three, palpate on the middle finger side of the metacarpal of fingers two, four, and five, respectively, as the client adducts each of the these fingers at the MCP joint by squeezing a pencil or highlighter. Once each one is felt, follow from attachment to attachment as the client alternately contracts and relaxes the muscle.

11. **Dorsal interossei manus (DIM):** On the dorsal side of the hand, palpate between metacarpals on the side of the finger (fingers two, three, and four) that is away from the center of the middle finger while the client abducts the finger at the MCP joint. Once each DIM is felt, palpate from attachment to attachment.

15

Chapter 16

Tour #7—Palpation of the Trunk Muscles

Overview

This chapter is a palpation tour of the muscles of the trunk. The tour begins with palpation of the posterior trunk muscles and then addresses the muscles of the anterolateral and anterior trunk. Palpation of the posterior trunk muscles is shown in the prone position (except the interspinales, which are shown seated); palpation of the anterolateral musculature is shown with the client side lying; and anterior trunk muscle palpation is shown in the supine position, except the iliopsoas, which is demonstrated with the client seated. Alternate palpation positions are also described. The major muscles or muscle groups of the region are each given a separate layout, and there are also a few detours to other muscles of the region. Trigger point (TrP) information and stretching is given for each of the muscles covered in this chapter. The chapter closes with an advanced *Whirlwind Tour* that explains the sequential palpation of all of the muscles of the chapter.

Chapter Outline

Chapter Objectives

After completing this chapter, the student should be able to perform the following for each of the muscles covered in this chapter:

1. State the attachments.
2. State the actions.
3. Describe the starting position for palpation.
4. Describe and explain the purpose of each of the palpation steps.
5. Palpate each muscle.
6. State the "Palpation Key."
7. Describe alternate palpation positions.
8. State the locations of the most common TrP(s).
9. Describe the TrP referral zones.
10. State the most common factors that create and/or perpetuate TrPs.
11. State the symptoms most commonly caused by TrPs.
12. Describe and perform a stretch.

Video demonstrations of the muscle palpations in this chapter are presented in Chapter 16 on DVD 1.

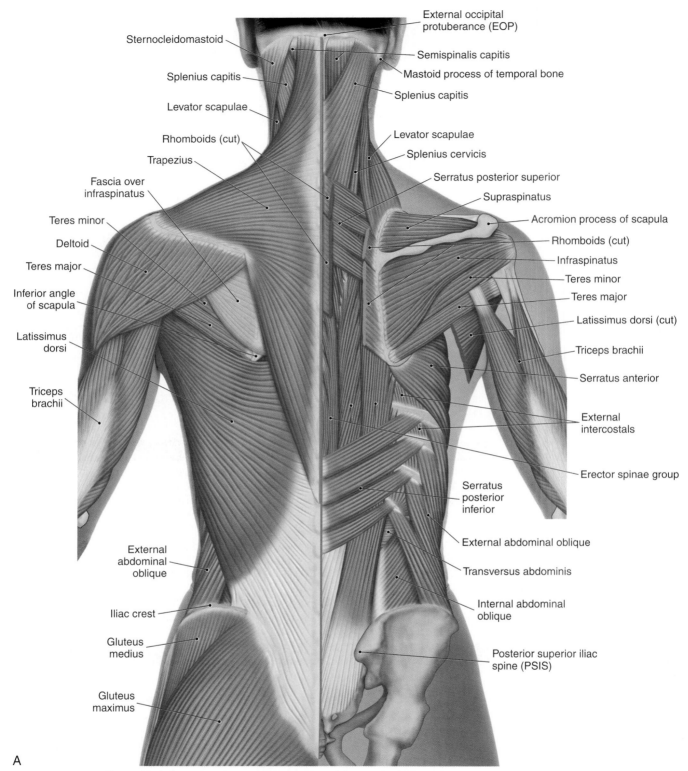

Figure 16-1 Posterior views of the muscles of the trunk. **A,** Superficial view on the left and an intermediate view on the right.

YOU ARE HERE

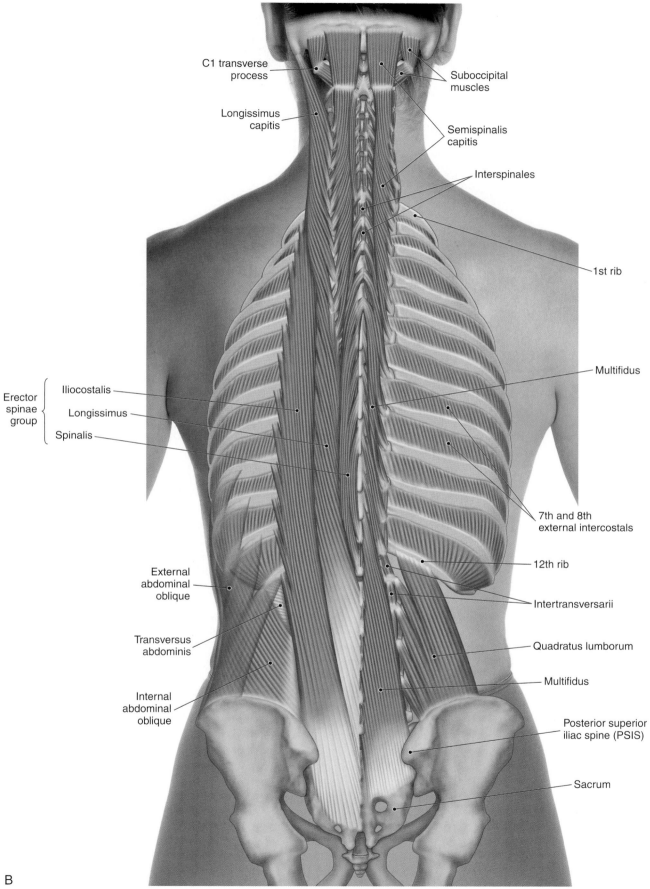

C1 transverse process

Suboccipital muscles

Longissimus capitis

Semispinalis capitis

Interspinales

1st rib

Multifidus

Erector spinae group
Iliocostalis
Longissimus
Spinalis

7th and 8th external intercostals

12th rib

Intertransversarii

External abdominal oblique

Quadratus lumborum

Transversus abdominis

Multifidus

Internal abdominal oblique

Posterior superior iliac spine (PSIS)

Sacrum

B

16

Figure 16-1, cont'd B, Two deeper views, the right side deeper than the left.

Sternocleidomastoid
Upper trapezius
Pectoralis major { Sternocostal head, Clavicular head }
Deltoid
Coracobrachialis
Triceps brachii
Biceps brachii
Latissimus dorsi
Serratus anterior
Rectus abdominis
External abdominal oblique
Iliac crest
Tensor fasciae latae

Subclavius
Clavicle
Coracoid process of scapula
Pectoralis minor
Coracobrachialis
Biceps brachii
Serratus anterior
External intercostals
Internal intercostals
External abdominal oblique (cut)
Internal abdominal oblique
Inguinal ligament
Gluteus medius

A

Figure 16-2 Anterior views of the muscles of the trunk. **A**, Superficial view on the right and an intermediate view on the left.

16

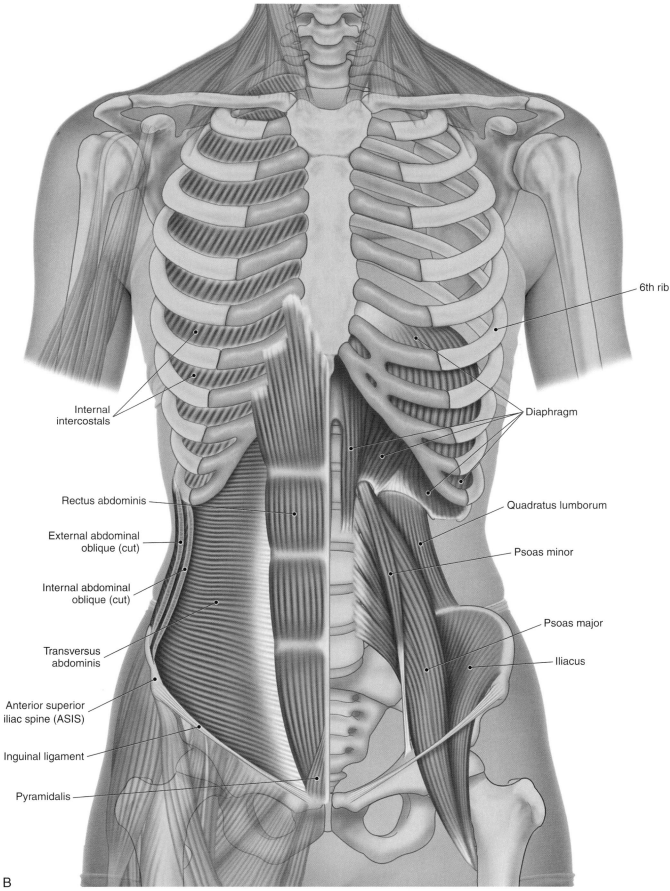

Figure 16-2, cont'd B, Deeper views with the posterior abdominal wall seen on the left.

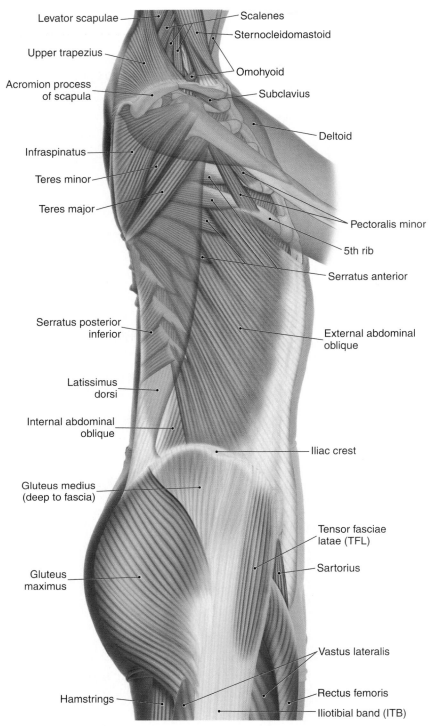

Figure 16-3 Lateral view of the trunk. The latissimus dorsi and deltoid have been ghosted in.

LATISSIMUS DORSI—PRONE

16-1

❑ **ATTACHMENTS:**

o Spinous processes of T7-L5, posterior sacrum, and the posterior iliac crest (all via the thoracolumbar fascia) *to the* lowest three to four ribs and the inferior angle of the scapula *to the* medial lip of the bicipital groove of the humerus

❑ **ACTIONS:**

o Extends, adducts, and medially rotates the arm at the shoulder joint
o Anteriorly tilts the pelvis at the lumbosacral joint via its attachment to the scapula, it also can depress the scapula (shoulder girdle) at the scapulocostal joint

Starting position (Figure 16-5):
o Client prone with the arm relaxed at the side
o Therapist seated to the side of the client
o Palpating fingers placed on the posterior axillary fold of tissue
o Support hand placed on the posterior aspect of the client's arm (just proximal to the elbow joint)

Palpation steps:
1. Ask the client to extend the arm at the shoulder joint and feel for the contraction of the latissimus dorsi in the posterior axillary fold of tissue (Figure 16-6, A).
2. Palpate toward its inferior attachment as the client alternately contracts and relaxes the latissimus dorsi.
3. Beginning again at the posterior axillary fold of tissue, palpate the distal tendon by strumming perpendicularly into the axilla all the way to the humerus (Figure 16-6, B).
4. Once the latissimus dorsi has been located, have the client relax it and palpate to assess its baseline tone.

Figure 16-4 Posterior view of the right latissimus dorsi.

Figure 16-5 Starting position for prone palpation of the right latissimus dorsi.

Palpation Key:

Palpate the posterior axillary fold of tissue.

16

LATISSIMUS DORSI—PRONE—cont'd

Figure 16-6 Palpation of the right latissimus dorsi as the client extends the arm against resistance. **A**, Palpation of the latissimus dorsi in the posterior axillary fold. **B**, Palpation of the humeral attachment at the medial lip of the bicipital groove of the humerus.

Palpation Notes:
1. The posterior axillary fold of tissue is composed of the latissimus dorsi and teres major. If the client lifts the arm into the air and you gently grasp the posterior fold of tissue in your palpating fingers, you are holding the latissimus dorsi and teres major (Figure 16-7).
2. Even though the distal tendon of the latissimus dorsi is up in the axilla, it is quite easy to follow to the humerus. At the humerus, the tendon of the latissimus dorsi is anterior to the tendon of the teres major (see Figure 16-6, B).
3. The teres major is located directly next to (medial to) the distal end of the latissimus dorsi within the posterior axillary fold of tissue. It also attaches onto the medial lip of the bicipital groove of the humerus and has the same three actions upon the arm at the shoulder joint. Distinguishing between these two muscles within the posterior axillary fold of tissue can be challenging. Feel for the rounded contour of the teres major, close to the scapula, medial to the latissimus dorsi. For palpation of the teres major, see Tour #1 (page 158).

Figure 16-7 The posterior axillary fold, which contains the latissimus dorsi and teres major, is being pinched.

LATISSIMUS DORSI—PRONE—cont'd

Alternate Palpation Position—Standing

The latissimus dorsi can be easily palpated with the client standing. The client stands with the arm on the shoulder of the therapist, who is standing to the front and side of the client. Ask the client to push his arm down onto your shoulder in the

direction of extension and adduction of the arm at the shoulder joint and feel for the contraction of the latissimus dorsi. In this position, it is especially easy to follow the latissimus dorsi to its humeral attachment.

Figure 16-8 Standing palpation of the right latissimus dorsi. **A**, The starting position in which the client has his distal arm (just proximal to the elbow joint) on the shoulder of the therapist. **B**, Shows palpation of the humeral attachment as the client tries to move the arm obliquely toward extension and adduction against resistance.

16

LATISSIMUS DORSI—PRONE—cont'd

TRIGGER POINTS

1. Trigger points (TrPs) in the latissimus dorsi often result from or are perpetuated by acute or chronic overuse of the muscle (e.g., rowing, pushing the hand down on a surface to move the body, any activity that requires a forceful motion of pulling the arms down from overhead), overstretching the muscle by hanging from a hand or from both hands, compression of the muscle (e.g., wearing a tight bra) resulting in irritation and ischemia, and TrPs in the serratus posterior superior.

2. TrPs in the latissimus dorsi tend to produce a constant aching pain at rest as well as with contraction of the muscle, difficulty sleeping on the affected side due to pressure on the TrP(s), and joint dysfunction of the vertebrae to which it is attached.

3. The referral patterns of latissimus dorsi TrPs must be distinguished from the referral patterns of TrPs in the scalenes, infraspinatus, subscapularis, erector spinae/transversospinalis of the thoracic region, serratus anterior, serratus posterior superior, rectus abdominis, rhomboids, lower trapezius, teres major, deltoid, and pectoralis minor.

4. TrPs in the latissimus dorsi are often incorrectly assessed as cervical disc syndrome, thoracic outlet syndrome (causing ulnar nerve compression), entrapment of the suprascapular nerve, or bicipital tendinitis.

5. Associated TrPs often occur in the teres major, triceps brachii long head, lower trapezius, erector spinae of the thoracic region, flexor carpi ulnaris, and serratus posterior superior.

Figure 16-9 A, Posterior view illustrating common latissimus dorsi TrPs and their corresponding referral zones. **B,** Anterior view showing another common latissimus dorsi TrP and its referral zone.

16

LATISSIMUS DORSI—PRONE—cont'd

STRETCHING THE LATISSIMUS DORSI

Figure 16-10 A stretch of the right latissimus dorsi. The client uses the other hand to bring the laterally rotated right arm forward and across the body while left laterally flexing the trunk. See also Figure 10-43 for another stretch of the latissimus dorsi.

DETOUR

Serratus Posterior Inferior (SPI): The serratus posterior inferior is a thin respiratory muscle that attaches from the spinous processes of T11-L2 to ribs nine to twelve; its action is to depress ribs nine to twelve. It is located deep to and has the same general direction of fibers as the latissimus dorsi, therefore it can be difficult to palpate and discern the SPI. This muscle may be hypertrophied and easier to palpate in clients who have a chronic obstructive pulmonary disorder. If palpation is attempted, place palpating fingers over the lateral aspect of the muscle (lateral to the erector spinae), ask the client to exhale, and feel for its contraction by strumming perpendicular to its fibers.

Trigger Points:

1. Trigger points (TrPs) in the SPI often result from or are perpetuated by acute or chronic overuse of the muscle (e.g., in clients who have labored breathing due to chronic obstructive respiratory diseases, such as asthma, bronchitis, and emphysema) or trauma (e.g., back strain).
2. TrPs in the SPI tend to produce an aching pain in the lower posterior ribcage and joint dysfunction of T11-L2.
3. The referral patterns of SPI TrPs must be distinguished from the referral patterns of TrPs in the intercostal muscles, latissimus dorsi, and rectus abdominis.
4. TrPs in the SPI are often incorrectly assessed as kidney disease or rib joint dysfunction.
5. Associated TrPs likely occur in the latissimus dorsi and the erector spinae or transversospinalis muscles of the trunk.

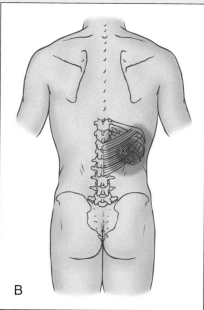

A

B

Figure 16-11 The right serratus posterior inferior (SPI). **A**, Posterior view of the right SPI. **B**, Posterior view showing a common SPI TrP and its corresponding referral zone.

LATISSIMUS DORSI—PRONE—cont'd

DETOUR

Trapezius and Rhomboids: The trapezius and rhomboids were palpated in the palpation tour of the shoulder girdle (Tour #1 in Chapter 10). However, they may also be palpated in this palpation tour of the trunk.

For palpation of the trapezius, have the client prone and ask her to abduct the arm at the shoulder joint to 90 degrees with the elbow joint extended, and to slightly retract the scapula at the scapulocostal joint by pinching the shoulder blade toward the spine. Adding gentle resistance to the client's arm abduction with your support hand might be helpful (Figure 16-12). See page 142 for more information.

For palpation of the rhomboids, have the client prone with the hand in the small of the back. Then ask him to lift the hand up away from the small of the back and feel for the contraction of the rhomboids (Figure 16-13). See page 146 for more information.

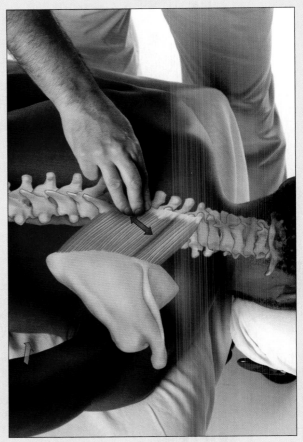

Figure 16-13 Prone palpation of the rhomboids.

Figure 16-12 Prone palpation of the trapezius.

16

ERECTOR SPINAE GROUP—PRONE

❏ **ATTACHMENTS:**

o Onto the pelvis, spine, ribcage, and head

❏ **ACTIONS:**

o Extends, laterally flexes, and ipsilaterally rotates the trunk, neck, and head at the spinal joints
o Anteriorly tilts and elevates the pelvis at the lumbosacral joint

Starting position (Figure 16-15):

o Client prone
o Therapist standing to the side of the client
o Palpating hand placed just lateral to the lumbar spine

Palpation steps:

1. Ask the client to extend the trunk, neck, and head, and feel for the contraction of the erector spinae musculature in the lumbar region (Figure 16-16).
2. Palpate to the inferior attachment on the pelvis and then toward the superior attachment as far as possible by strumming perpendicular to the fibers.
3. Once the erector spinae has been located, have the client relax it and palpate to assess its baseline tone.

Figure 16-14 Posterior view of the right erector spinae group.

Figure 16-15 Starting position for prone palpation of the right erector spinae group.

Figure 16-16 Palpation of the right erector spinae group as the client extends the head, neck, and trunk.

ERECTOR SPINAE GROUP—PRONE—cont'd

Palpation Notes:

1. Even though the erector spinae group is not superficial, it is so thick and massive that it is usually easy to palpate.
2. The erector spinae group is easiest to palpate in the lumbar region.
3. In the thoracic region, the erector spinae spreads out. Most of its fibers are interscapular and easy to palpate. However, some of its fibers run so far lateral that they are located deep to the scapula. To allow for direct access to these fibers, have the client hang the forearm/arm off the table, causing the scapula to protract.
4. In the cervical and upper thoracic region, the majority of the erector spinae is located lateral to the laminar groove.
5. In the neck, it is much more difficult to discern the erector spinae from adjacent musculature.
6. When palpating the erector spinae, keep in mind that the fibers are vertically oriented.
7. The erector spinae group is composed of three muscles: the iliocostalis, longissimus, and spinalis. It may be challenging to discern the border between the iliocostalis and longissimus; it is usually more difficult to discern the border between the longissimus and the spinalis.

TRIGGER POINTS

1. Trigger points (TrPs) in the erector spinae group often result from or are perpetuated by acute or chronic overuse of the muscle (e.g., prolonged standing posture that is stooped or inclined forward; lifting objects, especially with the spine flexed and/or rotated), prolonged immobility (e.g., long car rides), scoliosis (often caused by inequality of lower extremity length or pelvic asymmetry), prolonged sitting, poor seated posture, or carrying a wallet in a back pocket.
2. TrPs in the erector spinae group tend to produce restricted range of motion of the trunk at the spinal joints (specifically restricted flexion and/or contralateral lateral flexion), increased lumbar lordosis, or decreased thoracic kyphosis.
3. The referral patterns of erector spinae group TrPs must be distinguished from the referral patterns of TrPs in the serratus anterior, serratus posterior superior and inferior, rectus abdominis, rhomboids, levator scapulae, scalenes, infraspinatus, latissimus dorsi, quadratus lumborum, psoas major, gluteus maximus, gluteus medius, gluteus minimus, intercostals, and piriformis.
4. TrPs in the erector spinae group are often incorrectly assessed as spinal joint dysfunction, osteoarthritis, pathologic disc conditions, facet syndrome, angina pectoris, pathologic conditions of the lung or abdominal viscera, sacroiliac joint dysfunction, or sciatica.
5. Associated TrPs often occur in the latissimus dorsi, quadratus lumborum, psoas major, transversospinalis group, and serratus posterior superior and inferior.
6. Notes: 1) TrPs can develop at any segmental level; the TrPs shown are examples. 2) TrPs are most likely to develop within the longissimus and iliocostalis; patterns of TrPs and TrP referral zones for the spinalis have not yet been identified. 3) Erector spinae TrPs in the thoracic region usually refer pain both superiorly and inferiorly, whereas erector spinae TrPs in the lumbar region usually refer pain only inferiorly (usually into the buttock). 4) Generally, erector spinae TrPs refer pain more laterally and in a more diffuse pattern than transversospinalis TrPs. 5) Erector spinae TrPs can also refer pain to the anterior thoracic and abdominal wall, usually at the same segmental level.

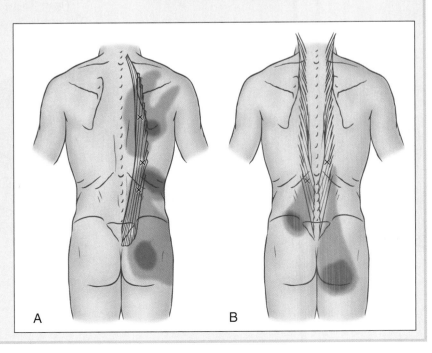

Figure 16-17 Erector spinae (iliocostalis and longissimus) TrPs. **A,** Posterior view showing common iliocostalis TrPs and their referral zones. **B,** Posterior view showing common longissimus TrPs and their referral zones.

A   B

ERECTOR SPINAE GROUP—PRONE—cont'd

STRETCHING THE ERECTOR SPINAE GROUP

Palpation Key:
Extend the trunk
from prone
position.

Figure 16-18 A stretch of the bilateral erector spinae groups. The client sits in a chair and slowly lowers himself into flexion. The stretch for one side can be enhanced by adding some lateral flexion to the opposite side. Note: When returning to the seated position, it is best for the client to place his forearms on the thighs, using them to push himself back up.

16

TRANSVERSOSPINALIS (TS) GROUP—PRONE

❏ ATTACHMENTS:

o Onto the pelvis, spine and head. Generally, each individual transversospinalis muscle attaches from a transverse process inferiorly *to a* spinous process superiorly.

❏ ACTIONS:

o Extends, laterally flexes, and contralaterally rotates the trunk and neck at the spinal joints
o Extends and laterally flexes the head at the atlanto-occipital joint
o Anteriorly tilts and elevates the pelvis at the lumbosacral joint

Starting position (Figure 16-20):

o Client prone
o Therapist standing to the side of the client
o Palpating fingers placed just lateral to the spinous processes of the lumbar spine within the laminar groove

Palpation steps:

1. With palpating finger(s) over the laminar groove of the lumbar spine, ask the client to slightly extend and rotate the lower trunk to the opposite side of the body (contralaterally rotate) at the spinal joints. Feel for the contraction of the transversospinalis musculature of the lumbar spine, particularly the multifidus group (Figure 16-21).
2. Once located, try to strum perpendicular to the direction of fibers and feel for the multifidus deep to the erector spinae.
3. Repeat this procedure superiorly up the spine.
4. To palpate the semispinalis group in the cervical region, have the client prone with the hand in the small of the back (Palpation Note #1). Place palpating fingers over the laminar groove of the cervical spine and ask the client to slightly extend the head and neck at the spinal joints, feeling for the contraction of the semispinalis deep to the upper trapezius (Figure 16-22).
5. Once located, follow the semispinalis up to the attachment on the head by strumming perpendicular to the direction of fibers.
6. Once the transversospinalis musculature has been located, have the client relax it and palpate to assess its baseline tone.

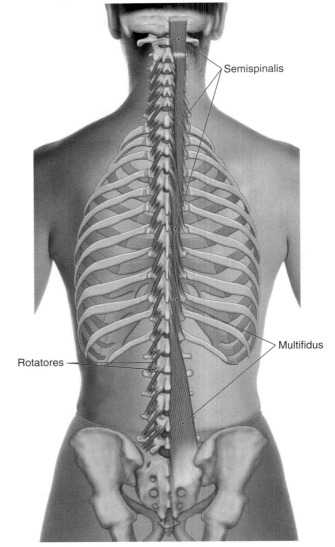

Semispinalis

Multifidus

Rotatores

Figure 16-19 Posterior view of the transversospinalis group. The semispinalis and multifidus are seen on the right; the rotatores are seen on the left.

16

Figure 16-20 Starting position for prone palpation of the right transversospinalis group.

TRANSVERSOSPINALIS (TS) GROUP—PRONE—cont'd

Figure 16-21 Palpation of the right lumbar multifidus as the client extends and contralaterally (left) rotates the trunk.

Figure 16-22 Palpation of the right semispinalis as the client extends the head and neck.

Palpation Notes:

1. The transversospinalis (TS) group is composed of three subgroups: the semispinalis, multifidus, and rotatores. Each subgroup is then composed of smaller individual muscles. The rotatores attach to a vertebra one to two levels above, the multifidus attach to a vertebra three to four levels above, and the semispinales attach to a vertebra five levels above or more.

2. The TS musculature is located deep within the laminar groove of the spine. Although it is quite massive and bulky in the low back (the multifidus is the largest muscle of the lumbar spine) and neck (the semispinalis is the largest muscle of the cervical spine), it can be difficult to clearly discern the TS musculature from more superficial and adjacent musculature.

3. The laminar groove lies within the spinal column between the transverse processes laterally and the spinous processes medially. The TS musculature is located within the laminar groove (except the semispinalis of the neck, which is also located lateral to the laminar groove).

4. When asking the client to extend the trunk to engage the TS of the trunk, the more superficial erector spinae will likely contract at the same time, making it more difficult to discern the TS musculature. Asking the client to also contralaterally rotate is important because it will not only engage the TS musculature but will also reciprocally inhibit the erector spinae musculature.

5. When palpating the semispinalis in the cervical region, the client's hand is placed in the small of the back because this reciprocally inhibits and relaxes the more superficial upper trapezius (placing the hand in the small of the back requires extension and adduction of the arm at the shoulder joint, which requires the coupled action of downward rotation of the scapula at the scapulocostal joint; scapular downward rotation reciprocally inhibits scapular upward rotators; the upper trapezius is a scapular upward rotator).

Alternate Palpation Position—Supine
The semispinalis of the neck can also be palpated with the client supine (see Tour #2, semispinalis capitis palpation, page 210). In the supine position it is more awkward, but the client can still be asked to place the hand in the small of the back.

Palpation Key:
Palpate in the laminar groove.

16

TRANSVERSOSPINALIS (TS) GROUP—PRONE—cont'd

TRIGGER POINTS

1. Trigger points (TrPs) in the transversospinalis (TS) group often result from or are perpetuated by acute or chronic overuse of the muscle (e.g., prolonged standing posture that is stooped or inclined forward; lifting objects, especially with the spine flexed and/or rotated), prolonged immobility (e.g., long car rides), prolonged sitting, poor seated posture, scoliosis (often caused by inequality of lower extremity length or pelvic asymmetry), or carrying a wallet in a back pocket.

2. TrPs in the TS group tend to produce deep pain, restricted range of motion of the trunk at the spinal joints (specifically restricted flexion, extension beyond anatomic position, contralateral lateral flexion, and ipsilateral rotation), increased lumbar lordosis, or decreased thoracic kyphosis.

3. The referral patterns of TS group TrPs must be distinguished from the referral patterns of TrPs in the erector spinae group, rectus abdominis, quadratus lumborum,

psoas major, gluteus maximus, gluteus medius, piriformis, and pelvic floor muscles.

4. TrPs in the TS group are often incorrectly assessed as spinal joint dysfunction, osteoarthritis, pathologic disc conditions, facet syndrome, angina pectoris, pathologic conditions of the lung or abdominal viscera, sacroiliac joint dysfunction, or sciatica.

5. Associated TrPs often occur in the psoas major and erector spinae group.

6. Notes: 1) TrPs can develop at any segmental level; the TrPs shown are examples. 2) Semispinalis TrPs generally refer in the same pattern as longissimus TrPs of the erector spinae group (see Figure 16-17, B). 3) Generally, rotatores TrPs refer pain more medially (usually directly over the spine and slightly lateral to the spine) and in a more circumscribed manner than multifidus TrPs. 4) TS TrPs in the lumbar region can also refer pain to the anterior abdominal wall, usually at the same segmental level.

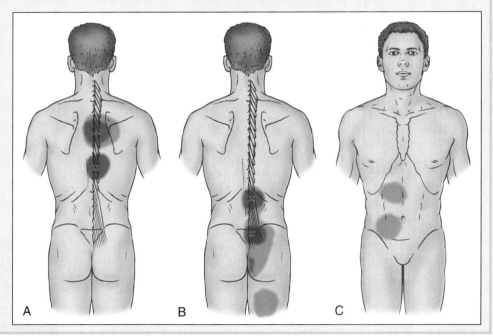

Figure 16-23 Transversospinalis (multifidus and rotatores) TrPs. **A**, Posterior view showing thoracic transversospinalis TrPs and their corresponding referral zones. **B**, Posterior view showing lumbar transversospinalis TrPs and their corresponding referral zones. **C**, The remainder of the lumbar TrP referral zones.

STRETCHING THE TRANSVERSOSPINALIS GROUP

Figure 16-24 A stretch of the right transversospinalis (TS) group. The client flexes and ipsilaterally (right) rotates the trunk and neck at the spinal joints. This stretch is particularly effective for the multifidus and rotatores of the TS group. The semispinalis can also be effectively stretched with the stretch shown in Figure 16-18.

QUADRATUS LUMBORUM (QL)—PRONE

❏ **ATTACHMENTS:**

o Inferomedial border of the twelfth rib and the transverse processes of L1-L4 *to the* posteromedial iliac crest

❏ **ACTIONS:**

o Elevates and anteriorly tilts the pelvis at the lumbosacral joint
o Extends and laterally flexes the trunk at the spinal joints
o Depresses the twelfth rib at the costovertebral joint

Starting position (Figure 16-26):

o Client prone
o Therapist standing to the side of the client
o Palpating hand placed just lateral to the lateral border of the erector spinae in the lumbar region
o Support hand sometimes placed directly on the palpation hand for support (not shown)

Palpation steps:

1. First locate the lateral border of the erector spinae musculature (to do so, ask the client to raise the head and upper trunk from the table); then place palpating finger just lateral to the lateral border of the erector spinae.
2. Direct palpating pressure medially, deep to the erector spinae musculature, and feel for the quadratus lumborum (QL).
3. To engage the QL to be certain that you are on it: ask the client to elevate the pelvis on that side at the lumbosacral joint (Note: This involves moving the pelvis along the plane of the table toward the head; in other words, the pelvis should not lift up in the air, away from the table.) and feel for its contraction (Figure 16-27).
4. Once located, palpate medially and superiorly toward the twelfth rib, medially and inferiorly toward the iliac crest, and directly medially toward the transverse processes of the lumbar spine (Figure 16-28).
5. Once the QL has been located, have the client relax it and palpate to assess its baseline tone.

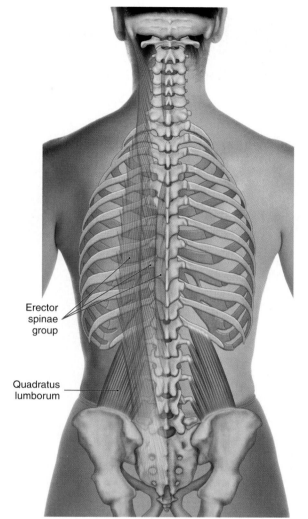

Figure 16-25 Posterior view of the right quadratus lumborum (QL). The left QL and ghosted left erector spinae group have been drawn in as well.

16

Figure 16-26 Starting position for prone palpation of the right quadratus lumborum.

QUADRATUS LUMBORUM (QL)—PRONE—cont'd

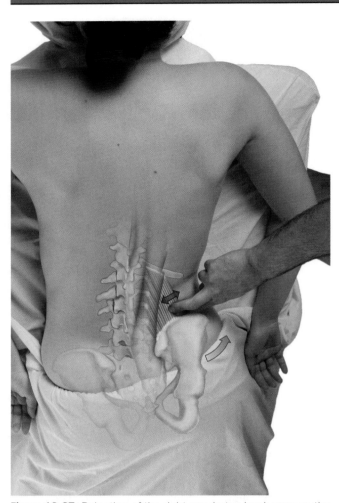

Figure 16-27 Palpation of the right quadratus lumborum as the client elevates the right side of the pelvis. The outline of the right erector spinae group has been ghosted in.

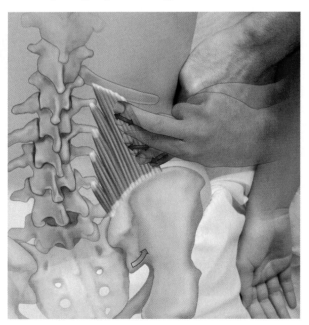

Figure 16-28 Once the quadratus lumborum has been located, palpate in all three directions toward the rib, transverse process, and iliac attachments.

Palpation Notes:

1. The QL cannot be palpated through the erector spinae musculature because the erector spinae is so thick. To successfully palpate the QL, you must be lateral to the erector spinae and then press in firmly with a medial direction to your pressure.

2. The client in Figure 16-28 has a lot of the QL accessible lateral to the erector spinae musculature. However, the amount of exposure of the QL lateral to the erector spinae varies. In some individuals, the erector spinae is wider and/or the QL is narrower, causing very little of the QL to be accessible lateral to the erector spinae musculature.

3. Whenever pressing deeply to palpate a muscle, always press in firmly but slowly! Ask the client to take in a deep breath, and then slowly press in as the client exhales. This procedure may be repeated two to three times, each time pressing in slightly deeper to access the QL.

4. The rib and iliac crest attachments of the QL are usually the easiest to palpate; the transverse processes attachment is usually the most challenging to palpate.

Alternate Palpation Position—Side Lying

Figure 16-29 The quadratus lumborum (QL) can be easily palpated with the client side lying. As with the prone palpation, be sure that your palpating fingers are first located lateral to the erector spinae musculature. In this position, press down toward the table to access the belly and attachments of the QL.

QUADRATUS LUMBORUM (QL)—PRONE—cont'd

TRIGGER POINTS

1. Trigger points (TrPs) in the quadratus lumborum (QL) often result from or are perpetuated by acute or chronic overuse of the muscle (e.g., repeated lifting of heavy objects or bending the trunk into flexion), a sudden overload while stretching the muscle (e.g., when bending the spine into flexion, especially combined with contralateral lateral flexion and/or rotation to either side), joint dysfunction of the thoracolumbar spine, an asymmetrically short lower extremity, or carrying a wallet in a back pocket.

2. TrPs in the QL tend to produce a low back ache that is usually felt deeply, occasional sharp stabs of pain (the pain may be felt at rest, but is usually most severe when sitting or standing), difficulty sleeping (due to referred tenderness to the greater trochanter), difficulty turning over in bed or getting up out of bed or a chair, strong pain when coughing or sneezing, decreased spinal flexion and contralateral lateral flexion, an ipsilaterally elevated pelvis, and a scoliosis with convexity to the opposite side. Pain may also refer to the groin, and even into the scrotum and testicle of a male.

3. The referral patterns of QL TrPs must be distinguished from the referral patterns of TrPs in the erector spinae and transversospinalis groups of the trunk, iliopsoas, gluteus maximus, medius, and minimus, piriformis and other deep lateral rotators of the hip joint, and tensor fasciae latae.

4. TrPs in the QL are often incorrectly assessed as sacroiliac joint dysfunction, lumbar disc syndrome, sciatica, or trochanteric bursitis.

5. Associated TrPs often occur in the contralateral QL, and the ipsilateral erector spinae group or transversospinalis group of the trunk, gluteus minimus, medius, and maximus, iliopsoas, piriformis and other deep lateral rotators of the hip joint, and the external abdominal oblique.

Figure 16-30 A, Posterior view of common quadratus lumborum (QL) TrPs and their corresponding referral zones. **B,** Anterolateral view showing the remainder of the referral zones.

16

QUADRATUS LUMBORUM (QL)—PRONE—cont'd

STRETCHING THE QUADRATUS LUMBORUM

Palpation Key:
Lateral to the erector spinae and press in medially.

Figure 16-31 A stretch of the right quadratus lumborum. The client places the left foot in front of the right and then left laterally flexes the trunk with the arm raised overhead and brought to the left side. See also page 405, Figure 17-18, for another stretch of the quadratus lumborum.

16

INTERSPINALES—SEATED

❑ **ATTACHMENTS:**

o From a spinous process *to the* spinous process immediately superior (in the lumbar and cervical regions)

❑ **ACTIONS:**

o Extends the neck and trunk at the spinal joints

Starting position (Figure 16-33):

o Client seated
o Therapist seated behind the client
o Palpating finger placed between two spinous processes in the lumbar region (Figures 16-33 and 16-34 show two interspinales muscles being palpated, hence two palpating fingers are seen contacting the client)
o Stabilizing hand placed on the upper trunk of the client

Palpation steps:

1. With palpating finger between two adjacent spinous processes of the lumbar spine, ask the client to slightly flex forward and feel for the interspinous muscle between the spinous processes.
2. From this position of flexion, ask the client to extend back to anatomic position and feel for the contraction of the interspinalis muscle. If desired, resistance can be given to the client's trunk extension with your support hand (see Figure 16-34).
3. This procedure can be repeated for other interspinales muscles between other spinous processes.
4. Once the interspinales muscles have been located, have the client relax them and palpate to assess their baseline tone.

Figure 16-32 Posterior view of the right and left interspinales.

Figure 16-33 Starting position for seated palpation of the interspinales.

Figure 16-34 Palpation of the interspinales as the client extends the trunk back to anatomic position from a position of slight flexion.

16

INTERSPINALES—SEATED—cont'd

Palpation Notes:

1. Note that the interspinales are generally located in the lumbar and cervical regions only. More specifically, they are usually located between C2 and T2, T11 and T12, and L1 and L5. However, variations exist and they are often found in other locations, most often in the upper or lower thoracic spine.

2. Flexing the lumbar spine opens up the spaces between spinous processes, making access to the interspinales muscles easier. However, if the client flexes too far, more superficial soft tissues in this region will become stretched and taut, restricting access to the interspinales muscles.

3. Because of the lordotic curve of the lumbar and cervical spinal regions, the interspinales can be difficult to palpate and discern. Generally, lumbar interspinales are easier to palpate than cervical interspinales.

Alternate Palpation Position—Prone

The interspinales can also be palpated with the client prone. It is helpful to place a roll under the client's abdomen to help open up the spaces between the spinous processes in the lumbar region.

TRIGGER POINTS

Note: The patterns of trigger points (TrPs) and TrP referral zones for the interspinales have not been discerned and mapped out.

STRETCHING THE INTERSPINALES

Figure 16-35 A stretch of the bilateral interspinales.

Palpation Key:
Palpate between spinous processes.

DETOUR

Intertransversarii and Levatores Costarum: Muscles called *intertransversarii* are located between adjacent transverse processes of the lumbar and cervical regions of the spine. They laterally flex the trunk and neck at the spinal joints. These muscles are very small and very deep, making palpation and discernment of them relative to adjacent soft tissues nearly impossible.

Muscles called the *levatores costarum* are located in the thoracic region of the spine between the transverse processes of C7-T11 and ribs one to twelve. Their action is to elevate the ribs. Levatores costarum are also quite small and deep, making their palpation and discernment extremely challenging. If their palpation is attempted, have the client prone and place palpating fingers between the mass of the erector spinae musculature and the angles of the ribs while asking the client to slowly and deeply breathe in and out; try to feel for their contraction as the client inhales.

Note: The patterns of trigger points (TrPs) and TrP referral zones for the intertransversarii and levatores costarum have not been discerned and mapped out.

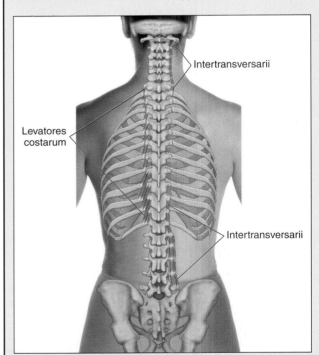

Figure 16-36 Posterior view showing the intertransversarii on the right and the levatores costarum on the left.

16

EXTERNAL AND INTERNAL INTERCOSTALS—SIDE LYING

❏ **ATTACHMENTS:**

o From a rib *to the* rib immediately superior (within an intercostal space)

❏ **ACTIONS:**

o The intercostal muscles can elevate and depress the ribs at the sternocostal and costospinal joints for breathing (the upper intercostals are generally more active with elevation for inhalation; the lower intercostals are generally more active with depression for exhalation).

o Both external and internal intercostals laterally flex the trunk at the spinal joints.

o The external intercostals contralaterally rotate the trunk at the spinal joints.

o The internal intercostals ipsilaterally rotate the trunk at the spinal joints.

Starting position (Figure 16-38):

o Client side lying

o Therapist standing behind the client

o Palpating finger(s) placed in an intercostal space (between two ribs) in the lateral trunk (two levels of intercostals are seen being palpated in Figures 16-38 and 16-39)

Palpation steps:

1. To locate an intercostal space, feel for the hard texture of the ribs in the lateral trunk and then drop your palpating fingers into the intercostal space between them (see Figure 16-39).

2. Once located, palpate in the intercostal space as far anteriorly and posteriorly as possible.

3. Once the intercostals have been located, make sure that the client is breathing lightly so that they are relaxed, and palpate to assess their baseline tone.

A   B   C

16

Figure 16-37 Views of the right intercostals. **A,** Anterior view of the right external intercostals. **B** and **C,** Anterior and posterior views of the right internal intercostals, respectively.

EXTERNAL AND INTERNAL INTERCOSTALS—SIDE LYING—cont'd

Figure 16-38 Starting position for side lying palpation of the right external and internal intercostal muscles.

Figure 16-39 Palpation of right intercostal muscles between the ribs in the lateral trunk.

Palpation Notes:
1. If you ask the client to take in a deep breath, the ribs move apart slightly, increasing the size of the intercostal space and allowing better access to the intercostal muscles.
2. Discerning an external intercostal muscle from its underlying internal intercostal muscle (or vice versa) is extremely difficult.
3. All muscles of the trunk (except for the subcostales and the transversus thoracis) are located superficial to the intercostals, making their palpation more challenging. In some cases, these more superficial muscles are thin enough and loose enough to allow palpation of the deeper intercostals. But in others, these more superficial muscles are either too thick or too tight to allow discernment of the underlying intercostal muscles.
4. Only the internal intercostals are located in the spaces between the costal cartilages. Fibers of the external intercostals extend farther posteriorly to the spine.

Alternate Palpation Position—Prone or Supine
Given that the intercostal muscles are located posteriorly, anteriorly, and laterally in the trunk, they can also be palpated with the client prone or supine.

TRIGGER POINTS

1. Trigger points (TrPs) in the intercostals often result from or are perpetuated by acute or chronic overuse of the muscle (e.g., excessive exercise requiring prolonged forceful breathing, chronic coughing, retching, or trunk rotation), trauma (physical trauma or from thoracic surgery), rib fracture or joint dysfunction, herpes zoster, and heart and lung conditions within the thoracic cavity.
2. TrPs in the intercostals tend to produce local pain that spreads anteriorly from the site of the TrP or to adjacent intercostal spaces if more severe, decreased range of motion of the trunk in contralateral lateral flexion and/or rotation in either direction, restricted and often painful range of motion of the arm (due to fascial pulls on the ribcage), pain and therefore difficulty when breathing in deeply, coughing, and sneezing, or difficulty lying on and thereby causing pressure on the TrPs.
3. The referral patterns of intercostal TrPs must be distinguished from the referral patterns of TrPs in the pectoralis major and minor, serratus anterior, serratus posterior inferior, subclavius, erector spinae and transversospinalis muscles of the trunk, rectus abdominis, external abdominal oblique, levator scapulae, scalenes, rhomboids, and latissimus dorsi.
4. TrPs in the intercostals are often incorrectly assessed as rib joint dysfunction, costochondritis, myocardial infarction (or other intrathoracic conditions), or herpes zoster.
5. Associated TrPs often occur in the other accessory muscles of respiration and the pectoralis major.
6. Notes: 1) Generally, there is no distinction of pain referral patterns for the external versus the internal intercostals. 2) Intercostal TrPs tend to be located anterolaterally or posterolaterally (or between the costal cartilages far anteriorly).

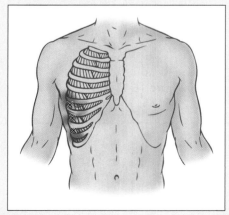

Figure 16-40 Anterior view showing common intercostal muscle TrPs and their corresponding referral zones.

EXTERNAL AND INTERNAL INTERCOSTALS—SIDE LYING—cont'd

STRETCHING THE INTERCOSTALS

Figure 16-41 A stretch of the right intercostal muscles. It is important to isolate the bending to the thoracic region as much as possible.

Palpation Key:

First locate in an intercostal space that is not deep to other musculature.

DETOUR 16-2

Subcostales and Transversus Thoracis: The subcostales and transversus thoracis are deep to the ribcage and extremely challenging if not impossible to palpate and discern from adjacent musculature.

The subcostales (seen on the right side in Figure 16-42, A) attach from ribs ten to twelve to ribs eight to ten; their action is to depress ribs eight to ten. To palpate the subcostales, palpate just lateral to the lateral border of the erector spinae in the posterior intercostal spaces between ribs eight to twelve.

The transversus thoracis (seen on the right side in Figure 16-42, B) attaches from the internal surfaces of the sternum, xiphoid process, and adjacent costal cartilages to the internal surfaces of costal cartilages two to six; its action is to depress ribs two to six. To palpate the transversus thoracis, either palpate just lateral to the xiphoid process of the sternum or in the anteromedial intercostal spaces between ribs two to six, just lateral to the sternum.

Note: The patterns of trigger points (TrPs) and TrP referral zones for the subcostales and transversus thoracis have not been discerned and mapped out.

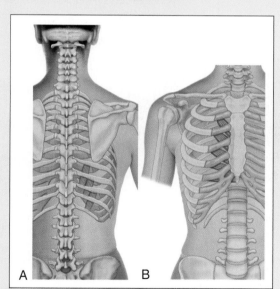

A   B

Figures 16-42 The subcostales and transversus thoracis are deep to the ribcage and extremely challenging to palpate and discern from adjacent musculature.

16

EXTERNAL AND INTERNAL INTERCOSTALS—SIDE LYING—cont'd

DETOUR

Other Muscles of the Anterior Chest:

Figure 16-43 Palpation of the right pectoralis major. **A**, Palpation of the sternocostal head as the client adducts the arm against resistance. **B**, Palpation of the clavicular head as the client flexes and adducts the arm against resistance. See page 172 for more information on pectoralis major palpation.

Figure 16-44 Palpation of the right pectoralis minor. The client is supine with his hand under his low back (not well visualized in this figure). Feel for the contraction of the pectoralis minor as the client presses the hand and forearm down against the table. See page 175 for more information on pectoralis minor palpation.

Figure 16-45 Palpation of the right subclavius. Ask the client to depress the clavicle at the sternoclavicular joint (i.e., to depress the shoulder girdle [scapula and clavicle]), and feel for the contraction of the subclavius. See page 177 for more information on subclavius palpation.

16

RECTUS ABDOMINIS—SUPINE

❏ **ATTACHMENTS:**

o Crest and symphysis of the pubic bone *to the* xiphoid process of the sternum and the costal cartilages of ribs five to seven

❏ **ACTIONS:**

o Flexes and laterally flexes the trunk at the spinal joints
o Posteriorly tilts the pelvis at the lumbosacral joint

Starting position (Figure 16-47):

o Client supine with a small roll under the knees
o Therapist standing to the side of the client
o Palpating hand placed just off center of the midline of the abdomen

Palpation steps:

1. Ask the client to slightly flex the trunk at the spinal joints (slightly curl the trunk upward) and feel for the contraction of the rectus abdominis (Figure 16-48).
2. With the rectus abdominis contracted, strum laterally (perpendicularly) across its fibers to locate its medial and lateral borders.
3. Continue palpating to the superior attachment and then to the inferior attachment by strumming perpendicularly across the fibers.
4. Once the rectus abdominis has been located, have the client relax it and palpate to assess its baseline tone.

Figure 16-46 Anterior view of the right rectus abdominis.

Figure 16-47 Starting position for supine palpation of the right rectus abdominis.

Figure 16-48 Palpation of the right rectus abdominis as the client flexes the trunk against gravity. Palpation should be done perpendicular to the fibers as shown.

16

RECTUS ABDOMINIS—SUPINE—cont'd

Palpation Notes:

1. The rectus abdominis is superficial, and in a well-developed individual it can be visualized. Because of the tendinous inscriptions of the muscle, four separate boxes can usually be seen. For this reason, the rectus abdominis is often called the *six-pack muscle*; perhaps *four-pack muscle* (or *eight-pack* for the two sides of it bilaterally) would be more appropriate.

2. Inexperienced therapists are often apprehensive about palpating all the way to the inferior attachment on the pubic bone, because they are afraid of accidentally passing the pubic bone and contacting the client's genitals. To prevent this, it is helpful to press gently into the abdomen with the rectus abdominis relaxed, feeling for the softness of the abdominal wall. This way, when the pubic bone (and hence the inferior attachment of the rectus abdominis) is reached, the hard feel of the pubic bone will be easily distinguished from the softness of the abdominal wall. Carrying out this palpation with the ulnar side of the hand pressing into the client at a 45-degree angle oriented inferiorly is very effective for locating the pubic bone.

3. In the midline of the anterior abdominal wall, the rectus abdominis is the only muscle present. The other three anterior abdominal wall muscles are located lateral to the rectus abdominis.

TRIGGER POINTS

1. Trigger points (TrPs) in the rectus abdominis often result from or are perpetuated by acute or chronic overuse of the muscle (e.g., excessive exercise doing crunches/curl-ups, straining at stool if constipated, chronic coughing, prolonged forceful abdominal breathing), direct trauma (physical trauma or from surgical incisions), visceral disease (e.g., gastrointestinal disease), or emotional stress (resulting in guarding, which tightens the abdominal wall).

2. TrPs in the rectus abdominis may produce pain felt over the lower aspect of the heart (if upper left–sided TrPs), diffuse abdominal discomfort, and visceral symptoms, such as heartburn, indigestion, abdominal cramping, nausea, and even diarrhea or vomiting. They may also entrap an anterior branch of a spinal nerve, resulting in lower abdominal and pelvic pain.

3. The referral patterns of rectus abdominis TrPs must be distinguished from the referral patterns of TrPs in the erector spinae, transversospinalis, external and internal abdominal obliques, transversus abdominis, intercostals, pectoralis major, and serratus posterior inferior.

4. TrPs in the rectus abdominis are often incorrectly assessed as a multitude of visceral diseases (e.g., peptic ulcer, hiatal hernia, appendicitis, intestinal disease, urinary tract disease, cholecystitis, and gynecologic diseases such as dysmenorrhea) or sacroiliac and/or lumbar joint dysfunction.

5. Associated TrPs often occur in the other muscles of the anterior abdominal wall (contralateral rectus abdominis and ipsilateral and contralateral transversus abdominis and external and internal abdominal obliques) and hip joint adductor muscles.

6. Note: The rectus abdominis pattern of pain that refers to the back of the trunk often crosses the midline of the body, so it is felt on both ipsilateral and contralateral sides of the back.

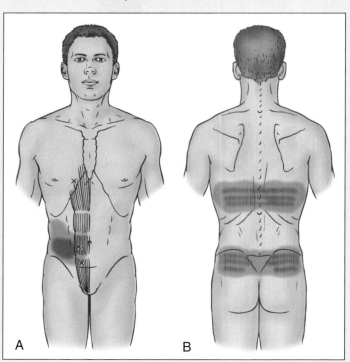

Figure 16-49 A, Anterior view showing common rectus abdominis TrPs and their corresponding referral zone. **B**, Posterior view showing the remainder of the referral zone. Note that posteriorly the referral zones may cross the midline to the contralateral side of the body.

16

RECTUS ABDOMINIS—SUPINE—cont'd

STRETCHING THE RECTUS ABDOMINIS

Figure 16-50 A stretch of the bilateral rectus abdominis muscles. The client lies prone and uses his forearms to help push his trunk into extension. The stretch of one side muscle can be enhanced by adding some lateral flexion to the opposite side.

Palpation Key:
Curl up and palpate the midline.

16

External Abdominal Oblique:

❏ **ATTACHMENTS:**

o Abdominal aponeurosis, pubic bone, inguinal ligament, and the anterior iliac crest *to the* lower eight ribs (Figure 16-51, A)

❏ **ACTIONS:**

o Flexes, laterally flexes, and contralaterally rotates the trunk at the spinal joints
o Posteriorly tilts, elevates, and ipsilaterally rotates the pelvis at the lumbosacral joint
o Compresses the abdominal contents

Internal Abdominal Oblique:

❏ **ATTACHMENTS:**

o Inguinal ligament, iliac crest, and thoracolumbar fascia *to the* lower three ribs and abdominal aponeurosis (Figure 16-51, B)

❏ **ACTIONS:**

o Flexes, laterally flexes, and ipsilaterally rotates the trunk at the spinal joints
o Posteriorly tilts, elevates, and contralaterally rotates the pelvis at the lumbosacral joint
o Compresses the abdominal contents

Starting position (Figure 16-52):
o Client supine with a small roll under the knees
o Therapist standing to the side of the client
o Palpating hand placed on the anterolateral abdominal wall

Palpation steps:
1. With palpating hand on the anterolateral abdominal wall between the iliac crest and the lower ribs (be sure that you are lateral to the rectus abdominis), ask the client to rotate the trunk to the opposite side of the body (contralateral rotation) and feel for the contraction of the external abdominal oblique (Figure 16-53, A).
2. Try to feel for the diagonal orientation of the external abdominal oblique fibers by strumming perpendicular to them.

3. Continue palpating the external abdominal oblique toward its superior and inferior attachments.
4. Repeat the same procedure for the internal abdominal oblique, asking the client to instead flex and ipsilaterally rotate the trunk at the spinal joints (Figure 16-53, B).
5. Once the external abdominal and internal abdominal obliques have been located, have the client relax them and palpate to assess their baseline tone.

A   B

Figure 16-51 The right abdominal obliques. **A**, Lateral view of the right external abdominal oblique. **B**, Lateral view of the right internal abdominal oblique.

Figure 16-52 Starting position for supine palpation of the right external and internal abdominal obliques.

EXTERNAL AND INTERNAL ABDOMINAL OBLIQUES—SUPINE—cont'd

A   B

Figure 16-53 Palpation of he right external and internal abdominal obliques. **A**, Palpation of the right external abdominal oblique as the client flexes and contralaterally (left) rotates the trunk against gravity. **B**, Palpation of the right internal abdominal oblique as the client flexes and ipsilaterally (right) rotates the trunk against gravity.

Palpation Notes:
1. When asking the client to contralaterally rotate (to isolate the external abdominal oblique) and ipsilaterally rotate (to isolate the internal abdominal oblique), try to have the client do as little flexion as possible, or both abdominal obliques on that side will contract.
2. The fiber direction of the external abdominal oblique is similar to the orientation of a coat pocket.
3. Feeling the fiber direction of each of the abdominal obliques and distinguishing between the external and internal abdominal obliques on one side can be challenging.
4. Technically, the inguinal ligament is not an attachment of the external abdominal oblique; rather it is part of its aponeurosis.

Alternate Palpation Position—Side Lying or Prone
Given that the abdominal obliques are also located in the lateral trunk and even attach as far posterior as the thoracolumbar fascia (which attaches into the spine), they can be palpated with the client side lying or even prone.

Palpation Key:
Flex and contralaterally rotate for the external abdominal oblique; flex and ipsilaterally rotate for the internal abdominal oblique.

16

EXTERNAL AND INTERNAL ABDOMINAL OBLIQUES—SUPINE—cont'd

TRIGGER POINTS

1. Trigger points (TrPs) in the abdominal obliques often result from or are perpetuated by acute or chronic overuse of the muscle (e.g., excessive exercise doing crunches/curl-ups, straining at stool if constipated, chronic coughing, prolonged forceful abdominal breathing, prolonged posture of rotation of the trunk), direct trauma (physical trauma or from surgical incisions), visceral disease (e.g., gastrointestinal disease), or emotional stress (resulting in guarding causing tightening of the abdominal wall).
2. TrPs in the abdominal obliques tend to produce pain in the chest (especially the more superior TrPs), abdomen, pelvis, and groin (especially the more inferior TrPs); and visceral symptoms, such as heartburn, indigestion, abdominal cramping, nausea, and even diarrhea or vomiting.
3. The referral patterns of abdominal obliques TrPs must be distinguished from the referral patterns of TrPs in the rectus abdominis, transversus abdominis, intercostals, and pectoralis major.
4. TrPs in the abdominal obliques are often incorrectly assessed as a multitude of visceral diseases (e.g., peptic ulcer, hiatal hernia, appendicitis, intestinal disease, urinary tract disease, cholecystitis, and gynecologic diseases such as dysmenorrhea).
5. Associated TrPs often occur in the other muscles of the anterior abdominal wall (contralateral abdominal obliques, and ipsilateral and contralateral transversus abdominis and rectus abdominis) and hip joint adductor muscles.
6. Notes: 1) For the most part, the external and internal abdominal obliques are next to each other, superficial and deep, and their referral pain patterns have not been discerned from each other. Therefore they are discussed together (the only exception to this is the presence of TrPs in the upper region of the external abdominal oblique where it does not overlie the internal abdominal oblique). 2) The abdominal obliques' pattern of referral pain often crosses the midline of the body and is felt on both the ipsilateral and contralateral sides of the body.

Figure 16-54 Anterior view showing common right-sided external and internal abdominal oblique TrPs and their corresponding referral zones. The upper TrP pictured here is an external abdominal oblique TrP. The lower ones can be in the external or internal abdominal oblique muscles. Note that the referral zones can cross the midline to the contralateral side of the body.

STRETCHING THE ABDOMINAL OBLIQUES

Figure 16-55 Stretches of the right abdominal obliques. **A**, A stretch of the right internal abdominal oblique; the client extends, left laterally flexes, and contralaterally (left) rotates the trunk. **B**, A stretch of the right external abdominal oblique; the client extends, left laterally flexes, and ipsilaterally (right) rotates the trunk.

EXTERNAL AND INTERNAL ABDOMINAL OBLIQUES—SUPINE—cont'd

DETOUR

Transversus Abdominis: The transversus abdominis (TA) attaches from the inguinal ligament, iliac crest, thoracolumbar fascia, and costal cartilages of ribs seven to twelve *to the* abdominal aponeurosis. It acts like a corset, compressing the abdominal contents within the abdominal cavity. Palpate the client's anterolateral abdominal wall, and ask the client to compress the abdominal contents by forcefully breathing out; feel for the contraction of the transversus abdominis. The transversus abdominis is deep to the external and internal abdominal obliques and extremely difficult to discern from these muscles, because they also contract when compressing the abdominal contents.

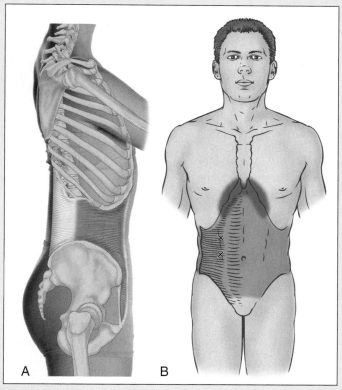

Figure 16-56 Views of the transversus abdominis (TA). **A,** Lateral view of the right TA. **B,** Anterior view showing common right-sided TA TrPs and their corresponding referral zone. Note that the referral zone can cross the midline to the contralateral side of the body.

16

DIAPHRAGM—SUPINE

❏ **ATTACHMENTS:**

o   Internal surfaces of the lower six ribs, the xiphoid process of the sternum, and the anterior surfaces of L1-L3 *to the* central tendon of the diaphragm (located in the center of the muscle)

❏ **ACTIONS:**

o   Increases the volume of the thoracic cavity, allowing the lungs to expand for inspiration

Starting position (Figure 16-58):

o   Client supine with a roll under the knees to flex the thighs at the hip joint
o   Therapist seated to the side of the client
o   Palpating fingers curled under the inferior margin of the anterior ribcage

Palpation steps:

1. With your palpating fingers curled around the inferior margin of the anterior ribcage, ask the client to take in a deep breath and then slowly exhale. As the client exhales, curl your fingertips under (inferior and then deep to) the ribcage and feel for the diaphragm on the internal surface of the ribcage (Figure 16-59).
2. Repeat this procedure anteriorly and posteriorly as far as possible on both sides of the ribcage.
3. Assessment of the diaphragm should only be made when it is totally relaxed, which occurs at the end of the exhalation.

Figure 16-57 Anterior view of the diaphragm.

Figure 16-58 Starting position for supine palpation of the diaphragm.

Palpation Key:
Curl your fingers around the ribcage.

16

DIAPHRAGM—SUPINE—cont'd

Figure 16-59 Palpation of the diaphragm. **A**, Palpation of the right side of the diaphragm as the client slowly exhales. **B**, Close-up showing palpation of the diaphragm by curling the fingers around the ribcage so that the finger pads are oriented against the muscle.

Palpation Notes:
1. By placing a roll under the client's knees, the thighs are passively flexed at the hip joints, causing the pelvis to passively posteriorly tilt, slackening the anterior abdominal wall and allowing better access to the diaphragm.
2. As with any muscle palpation that is fairly deep, it is important to use gentle but firm pressure and to sink *slowly* into the tissue.

3. Successful palpation of the diaphragm requires a relaxed and slackened abdominal wall. For this reason, the diaphragm is easiest to palpate anteriorly because the anterior abdominal wall is easiest to relax and slacken. As the lateral abdominal wall is reached, the diaphragm becomes increasingly harder to palpate. It is extremely difficult if not impossible to palpate the diaphragm through the posterior abdominal wall.

Alternate Palpation Positions—Side Lying or Seated

Figure 16-60 The diaphragm can also be palpated with the client side lying or seated. If the client is side lying, have the client's trunk flexed and the thighs passively flexed at the hip joints. This allows for relaxation and slackening of the anterior abdominal wall, allowing better access to the diaphragm. Similarly, if the client is seated, have the client's trunk slightly flexed to slacken the anterior abdominal wall, allowing better access to the diaphragm.

DIAPHRAGM—SUPINE—cont'd

TRIGGER POINTS

1. Trigger points (TrPs) in the diaphragm often result from or are perpetuated by acute or chronic overuse of the muscle (e.g., vigorous exercise leading to excessive forceful breathing, chronic hiccups) or chronic coughing.

2. TrPs in the diaphragm tend to produce pain upon exertion (especially at deep exhalation) at the anterolateral ribcage, often described as a "stitch in the side" or shortness of breath.

3. The referral patterns of diaphragm TrPs must be distinguished from the referral patterns of TrPs in the external abdominal oblique, subclavius, and pectoralis minor.

4. TrPs in the diaphragm are often incorrectly assessed as peptic ulcer, gallbladder disease, gastroesophageal reflux, or hiatal hernia.

5. Associated TrPs often occur in the intercostal muscles, rectus abdominis, and external and internal abdominal obliques.

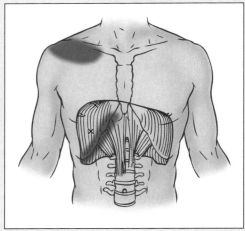

Figure 16-61 Anterior view showing common diaphragm TrPs and their corresponding referral zones.

STRETCHING THE DIAPHRAGM

Figure 16-62 A stretch of the diaphragm. The client breathes out forcefully, expelling as much air from the lungs a possible, while slightly flexing the trunk.

16

ILIOPSOAS—SEATED   `16-4` `16-5`

❑ ATTACHMENTS:

o Anterolaterally (bodies, discs, and transverse processes) on vertebrae T12-L5 (psoas major) and the internal surface of the ilium (iliacus) *to the* lesser trochanter of the femur

❑ ACTIONS:

o The psoas major flexes, laterally flexes, and contralaterally rotates the trunk at the spinal joints.
o Both the psoas major and the iliacus flex and laterally rotate the thigh at the hip joint, and anteriorly tilt the pelvis at the hip joint.

Starting Position (Figure 16-64):

o Client seated with the trunk slightly flexed
o Therapist seated to the side and slightly to the front of the client
o Palpating hand placed anterolaterally on the client's abdominal wall, approximately halfway between the umbilicus and the ASIS (anterior superior iliac spine); ensure placement is lateral to the lateral border of the rectus abdominis
o Fingers of support hand placed over fingers of palpating hand to increase strength and stability of palpating fingers (not shown in Figure 16-64)

Palpation Steps:

1. Ask the client to take in a deep but relaxed breath; as the client exhales, slowly (but firmly) sink in toward the belly of the psoas major by pressing diagonally in toward the spine. You may need to repeat this procedure two to three times before arriving at the psoas major belly at the spine.
2. To confirm that you are on the psoas major, ask the client to gently flex the thigh at the hip joint by lifting the foot slightly off the floor and feel for the contraction of the psoas major (Figure 16-65).
3. Strum perpendicularly across the fibers to feel for the width of the muscle.
4. Continue palpating the psoas major toward its superior vertebral attachment and inferiorly as far as possible within the abdominopelvic cavity.
5. To palpate the iliacus, curl your fingers around the iliac crest with your finger pads oriented toward the internal

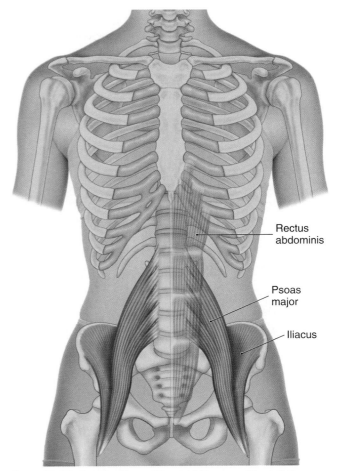

Figure 16-63 Anterior view of the right iliopsoas. The left iliopsoas and ghosted left rectus abdominis have been drawn in as well.

surface of the ilium, and feel for the iliacus (Figure 16-66). To engage the iliacus, ask the client to flex the thigh at the hip joint by lifting the foot slightly off the floor.
6. Once the iliopsoas major has been located, have the client relax it and palpate to assess its baseline tone.

16

Figure 16-64 Starting position for seated palpation of the right iliopsoas.

ILIOPSOAS—SEATED—cont'd

Figure 16-65 Palpation of the right psoas major as the client gently flexes the thigh at the hip joint by lifting her foot up slightly from the floor.

Palpation Notes:

1. The iliopsoas is composed of the psoas major muscle and the iliacus muscle.
2. The client's trunk begins in slight flexion to slacken and thereby relax the muscles of the anterior abdominal wall, allowing easier entry and discernment of the psoas major and iliacus.
3. Before beginning the palpation procedure, have the client demonstrate how he/she will lift the foot off the floor (flexing the thigh at the hip joint), so that no time will be wasted once you are palpating into the abdomen and ready for this step.
4. Only the fibers of the iliacus closest to the iliac crest are palpable; the rest are too deep to be accessed.
5. **Be careful when palpating deep into the abdominal cavity for the belly of the psoas major; major blood vessels (aorta and iliac arteries) are located nearby. If you feel a pulse under your fingers, move your palpating fingers off the artery.**
6. Palpating the distal belly and tendon of the iliopsoas is most easily done with the client supine (see Figure 16-67).
7. **Be careful when palpating the iliopsoas in the proximal anterior thigh because the femoral nerve, artery, and vein are located over the iliopsoas and pectineus in this region (see Figure 16-2). If you feel a pulse under your fingers, either gently move the artery out of the way or slightly move your palpating fingers off the artery. Similarly, if you are pressing on the femoral nerve and the client feels shooting pain into the thigh, move your palpating fingers off the nerve.**

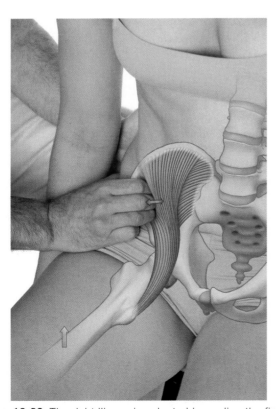

Figure 16-66 The right iliacus is palpated by curling the fingers around the iliac crest so that the finger pads are oriented against the muscle.

Alternate Palpation Position—Supine or Side Lying

Figure 16-67 The psoas major can also be palpated with the client supine or side lying. The disadvantage of supine palpation position is that when the client flexes the thigh at the hip joint, the muscles of the abdominal wall may contract to stabilize the pelvis. This can interfere with feeling the psoas major, located deep to these muscles. This may also occur to some degree with the side lying palpation position.

16

ILIOPSOAS—SEATED—cont'd

DETOUR

Iliopsoas Distal Belly and Tendon: With the client supine, first locate the sartorius (by asking the client to laterally rotate and flex the thigh at the hip joint); then drop off the sartorius medially onto the iliopsoas distal belly/tendon. To confirm your location, ask the client to flex the trunk by doing a small curl-up of the trunk and feel for the tensing of the psoas major belly and tendon (the psoas major is the more medial portion of the iliopsoas). No other muscle in the anterior thigh contracts with trunk flexion (Figure 16-68, A). Now passively hold the client's thigh into flexion and follow the belly/tendon distally to the lesser trochanter by asking the client to alternately contract and relax the psoas major by gently initiating a curling up of the trunk and then relaxing (Figure 16-68, B). The texture of the distal belly/tendon will harden only when the muscle contracts, whereas the lesser trochanter will be palpably hard regardless of whether the muscle is contracted. Note: Be aware of the presence of the femoral nerve, artery, and vein in this region (see Palpation Note #6).

Figure 16-68 Palpation of the distal belly and tendon of the psoas major in the proximal thigh as the client flexes (curls) the trunk at the spinal joints against gravity. **A,** Palpation of the distal belly immediately distal to the inguinal ligament; the sartorius has been ghosted in. **B,** Palpation of the distal tendon and its femoral attachment at the lesser trochanter.

TRIGGER POINTS

1. Trigger points (TrPs) in the iliopsoas often result from or are perpetuated by acute or chronic overuse of the muscle (e.g., excessive exercise doing curl-ups/crunches, excessive running, or excessive kicking when playing soccer), prolonged shortening of the muscle (e.g., sitting with the hip joints flexed, sleeping in fetal position, having an excessive lumbar lordosis), an asymmetrically short lower extremity, or carrying a wallet in a back pocket.

2. TrPs in the iliopsoas tend to produce decreased extension of the thigh at the hip joint or pain in a characteristic vertical pattern along the lumbar spine that is worst when standing and relieved when lying down (pain is also often relieved when the hip joint is passively flexed). TrPs in the psoas major may entrap the femoral nerve or genitofemoral nerve as they exit the abdominal cavity into the pelvis (causing possible altered sensation into the thigh).

3. The referral patterns of iliopsoas TrPs must be distinguished from the referral patterns of TrPs in the quadratus lumborum, erector spinae or transversospinalis of the trunk, piriformis, gluteus medius and maximus, sartorius, pectineus, adductors longus and brevis, and rectus abdominis.

4. TrPs in the iliopsoas are often incorrectly assessed as lower thoracic, lumbar, or sacroiliac joint dysfunction, or appendicitis.

5. Associated TrPs often occur in the erector spinae and transversospinalis muscles of the trunk, quadratus lumborum, rectus abdominis, gluteals, hamstrings, tensor fasciae latae, rectus femoris, pectineus, and contralateral iliopsoas.

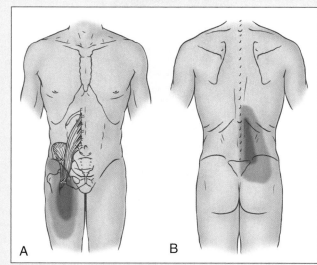

Figure 16-69 A, Anterior view showing common iliopsoas TrPs and their corresponding referral zone. **B,** Posterior view showing the remainder of the referral zone.

16

ILIOPSOAS—SEATED—cont'd

STRETCHING THE ILIOPSOAS

Figure 16-70 A stretch of the right iliopsoas. The client lunges forward with the pelvis and trunk, creating an extension force across the right hip joint. Note: It is important to keep the trunk straight or slightly extended, or the psoas major will not be stretched.

DETOUR

Psoas Minor: The psoas minor is a small muscle that attaches from the anterolateral bodies of T12 and L1 to the pubic bone. It flexes the trunk at the spinal joints and posteriorly tilts the pelvis at the lumbosacral joint.

Given that the psoas major also does these actions and that the psoas minor sits directly on the belly of the psoas major, it can be very difficult to discern the psoas minor from the psoas major by engaging the psoas minor with trunk flexion. Furthermore, trunk flexion will likely engage the more superficial abdominal obliques, blocking palpation of the psoas minor. If psoas minor palpation is attempted, first locate the psoas major (see page 385) and then feel for a small band of muscle that sits anteriorly on it. To then discern these two muscles from each other, feel for a band of musculature on the psoas major that does not contract with flexion of the thigh at the hip joint.

The psoas minor can be stretched with the same stretch used for the rectus abdominis (see Figure 16-50). TrPs and TrP referral zones for the psoas minor have not been clearly mapped out and separated from TrPs in the belly of the psoas major. Note: The psoas minor is often absent.

Palpation Key:

Psoas major: Press in diagonally toward the spine, slowly but firmly. Iliacus: Curl your fingers around the iliac crest.

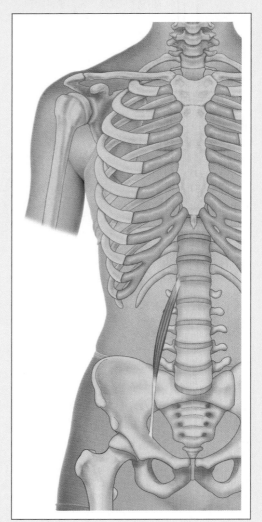

Figure 16-71 Anterior view of the right psoas minor.

Whirlwind Tour   **Muscles of the Trunk**

Client Prone:

1. **Latissimus dorsi:** The client is prone with the arm relaxed on the table at the side of the body; you are sitting or standing to the side of the client. Feel for the contraction of the latissimus dorsi at the posterior aspect of the axillary fold as the client extends the arm against resistance. Once felt, continue palpating the latissimus dorsi toward the spinal and pelvic attachment as the client alternately contracts and relaxes the muscle. Then palpate to the humeral attachment in the axilla by strumming perpendicular to the muscle as the client alternately contracts and relaxes the muscle. Note: It can be challenging to discern the latissimus dorsi from the teres major. At the humeral attachment, the latissimus dorsi attachment is located anterior to the teres major attachment, and therefore much easier to palpate directly and feel.

2. **Erector spinae group:** The client is prone; you are standing to the side of the client. Feel for the contraction of the erector spinae group just lateral to the lumbar spine as the client extends the trunk, neck, and head at the spinal joints by lifting the trunk slightly up into the air. Once felt, palpate transversely across the erector spinae to determine its width. Now palpate it to its inferior attachment, and then palpate it as far superior as possible by strumming perpendicular to its fibers as the client alternately contracts and relaxes the muscle. Note: It is usually difficult to palpate and discern the erector spinae musculature in the neck.

3. **Transversospinalis group:** The client is prone; you are standing to the side of the client. Feel for the contraction of the transversospinalis musculature within the laminar groove of the lumbar spine as the client slightly extends and contralaterally rotates the trunk at the spinal joints. (Note: It is primarily the multifidus that is present at this level.) Once located, try to strum perpendicular to the direction of fibers and feel for the multifidus deep to the erector spinae. Repeat this procedure superiorly up the spine. To palpate the semispinalis group (primarily the semispinalis capitis) in the cervical region, have the client prone with the hand in the small of the back. Place your palpating fingers over the laminar groove of the cervical spine and ask the client to slightly extend the neck at the spinal joints, feeling for the contraction of the semispinalis deep to the upper trapezius. Once located, follow the semispinalis up to the attachment on the head by strumming perpendicular to the direction of fibers as the client alternately contracts and relaxes the muscle.

4. **Quadratus lumborum (QL):** The client is prone; you are standing to the side of the client. Locate the lateral border of the erector spinae group in the lumbar region. Once located, palpate immediately lateral to that. Sink into the tissue slowly but firmly with a direction to your pressure that is anterior and medial toward the QL. To engage the QL to be certain that you are on it, ask the client to elevate the pelvis at the lumbosacral joint. (Note: Elevation of the pelvis involves moving the pelvis along the plane of the table toward the head.) Once felt, palpate the QL supero-

medially to the twelfth rib, inferomedially to the iliac crest, and medially toward the transverse processes as the client alternately contracts and relaxes the muscle.

Client Seated:

5. **Interspinales:** The client is seated with the trunk slightly flexed at the spinal joints; you are standing or seated behind the client. Place your palpating finger in the interspinous space between two adjacent vertebrae in the lumbar spine, and feel for the interspinous muscle located there. Then ask the client to extend back to anatomic position and feel for the contraction of the interspinalis muscle. If desired, resistance can be given. Repeat this procedure for other interspinalis muscles. Note: The vertebrae must be flexed to allow access to the interspinalis muscle. However, if the vertebrae are flexed too much, all soft tissues between the vertebrae become taut and it is not possible to palpate into the interspinous space.

Client Side Lying:

6. **External and internal intercostals:** The client is side lying; you are standing behind the client. Intercostal muscles are located between ribs in the anterior, posterior, and lateral trunk. However, it is usually easiest to palpate them laterally, so look to locate them there first. Place your palpating fingers in an intercostal space in the lateral trunk and feel for the intercostal musculature. Once felt, continue palpating the intercostal musculature at that level as far anteriorly and posteriorly as possible. Repeat this procedure for the other levels of intercostal muscles.

Client Supine with a Small Roll Under the Knees:

7. **Rectus abdominis:** The client is supine with a small roll under the knees; you are standing to the side of the client. Place your palpating fingers on the anterior abdomen, just lateral to the midline, and feel for the contraction of the rectus abdominis as the client slightly flexes the trunk at the spinal joints. Once felt, strum across the rectus abdominis to determine its width. Then continue palpating to its superior and inferior attachments by strumming perpendicularly to its fibers as the client alternately contracts and relaxes the muscle. Note: It is easiest to locate the inferior attachment on the pubic bone when the rectus femoris is relaxed.

8 **Anterolateral abdominal wall muscles (external abdominal oblique [EAO], internal abdominal oblique [IAO], and transversus abdominis [TA]):** The client is supine with a small roll under the knees; you are standing to the side of the client. Place your palpating hand on the anterolateral abdominal wall (lateral to the rectus

16

abdominis) and feel for the contraction of the EAO as the client slightly flexes and contralaterally rotates the trunk at the spinal joints. Once a muscle contraction is felt, try to feel for the orientation of the EAO's fibers by strumming perpendicular to them; then continue palpating the EAO superiorly and inferiorly toward its attachments. Repeat the same procedure for the deeper IAO by asking the client to instead slightly flex and ipsilaterally rotate the trunk at the spinal joints and feeling for their fiber direction running perpendicular in orientation to the fibers of the EAO. If successful, strum perpendicular to the IAO's fibers and palpate from attachment to attachment. To palpate the TA deep to the abdominal obliques, ask the client to compress the abdominal contents (but keep in mind that this can also engage the external and internal abdominal obliques). Note: It can be very difficult to discern the muscles of the anterolateral abdominal wall from each other because both abdominal obliques contract with flexion of the trunk at the spinal joints, and all of them contract with compression of the abdominal contents.

9. **Diaphragm:** The client is supine with a small roll under the knees; you are seated or standing to the side of the client. First curl your palpating fingers under the inferior margin of the client's anterior ribcage with your finger pads oriented toward the muscle. Then ask the client to take in a deep breath and slowly exhale. As the client exhales, reach in and feel for the diaphragm. Repeat this procedure as far anteriorly and posteriorly as possible on both sides of the ribcage.

Client Seated:

10. **Iliopsoas (psoas major and iliacus):** The client is seated with the trunk slightly flexed; you are seated diagonally in front of the client. Place your palpating fingers on the client's anterolateral abdominal wall, halfway between the umbilicus and ASIS (make sure you are lateral to the lateral border of the rectus abdominis). Ask the client to take in a slow deep breath, and firmly but slowly sink in toward the spine as the client slowly exhales (repeat this step once or twice if necessary until you reach the psoas major). Once you believe that you have reached the psoas major, confirm by asking the client to flex the thigh at the hip joint by gently lifting the foot from the floor a small amount. Once felt, strum perpendicularly across the fibers to feel its width. Then continue palpating to its superior attachment and as far inferiorly as possible by strumming across the muscle as the client alternately contracts and relaxes it. To palpate the iliacus, curl your palpating fingers around the iliac crest toward the iliacus on the internal ilium and feel for its contraction as the client once again gently lifts the foot from the floor a small amount. Once felt, palpate as much of the iliacus as possible.

11. **Psoas minor:** To feel the psoas minor, first locate the belly of the psoas major and then feel for a band of muscle that sits anteriorly on the psoas major's belly. The psoas minor will not contract with flexion of the thigh at the hip joint (i.e., lifting the foot from the floor).

Chapter 17

Tour #8—Palpation of the Pelvic Muscles

Overview

This chapter is a palpation tour of the muscles of the pelvis. The tour begins with the gluteal muscles and then covers the piriformis, quadratus femoris, and other "deep lateral rotators" of the thigh at the hip joint. Palpation for each of the muscles is shown in the prone position, except for the gluteus medius, which is described in side lying position. Alternate palpation positions are also described. The major muscles of the region are each given a separate layout; there are also a few detours to other muscles of the region. Trigger point (TrP) information and stretching is given for each of the major muscles covered in this chapter (as well as the gluteus minimus). The chapter closes with an advanced *Whirlwind Tour* that explains the sequential palpation of all of the muscles of the chapter.

Chapter Outline

Chapter Objectives

After completing this chapter, the student should be able to perform the following for each of the muscles covered in this chapter:

1. State the attachments.
2. State the actions.
3. Describe the starting position for palpation.
4. Describe and explain the purpose of each of the palpation steps.
5. Palpate each muscle.
6. State the "Palpation Key."
7. Describe alternate palpation positions.

8. State the locations of the most common TrP(s).
9. Describe the TrP referral zones.
10. State the most common factors that create and/or perpetuate TrPs.
11. State the symptoms most commonly caused by TrPs.
12. Describe and perform a stretch.

Video demonstrations of the muscle palpations in this chapter are presented in Chapter 17 on DVD 1.

Figure 17-1 Posterior views of the muscles of the pelvis. **A**, Superficial view on the left and an intermediate view on the right.

- Psoas major
- Iliac crest
- Gluteus medius (cut)
- Gluteus minimus
- Gluteus minimus
- Piriformis
- Superior gemellus
- Obturator internus
- Obturator externus
- Inferior gemellus
- Obturator externus
- Intertrochanteric crest
- Iliopsoas distal tendon
- Quadratus femoris (cut)

B

Figure 17-1, cont'd B, Deeper views.

17

Figure 17-2 Right lateral views of the muscles of the pelvis. **A**, Superficial view.

YOU ARE HERE

17

A

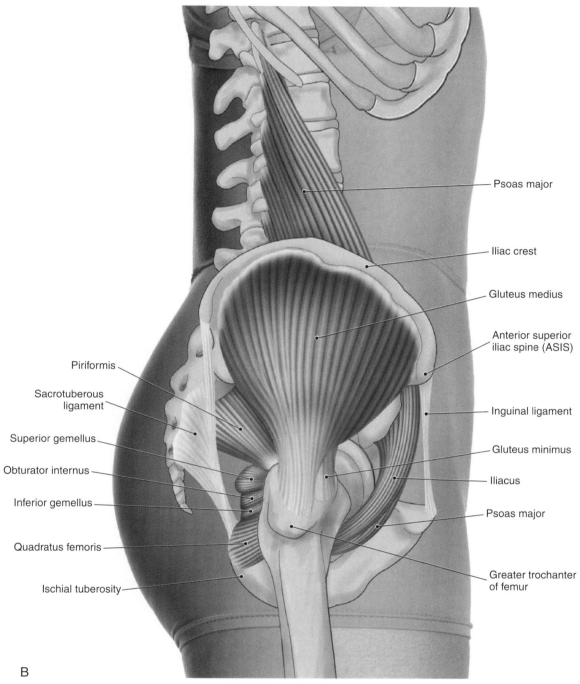

Psoas major

Iliac crest

Gluteus medius

Anterior superior
iliac spine (ASIS)

Inguinal ligament

Gluteus minimus

Iliacus

Psoas major

Greater trochanter
of femur

Piriformis

Sacrotuberous
ligament

Superior gemellus

Obturator internus

Inferior gemellus

Quadratus femoris

Ischial tuberosity

B

Figure 17-2, cont'd B, Intermediate view.

YOU ARE HERE

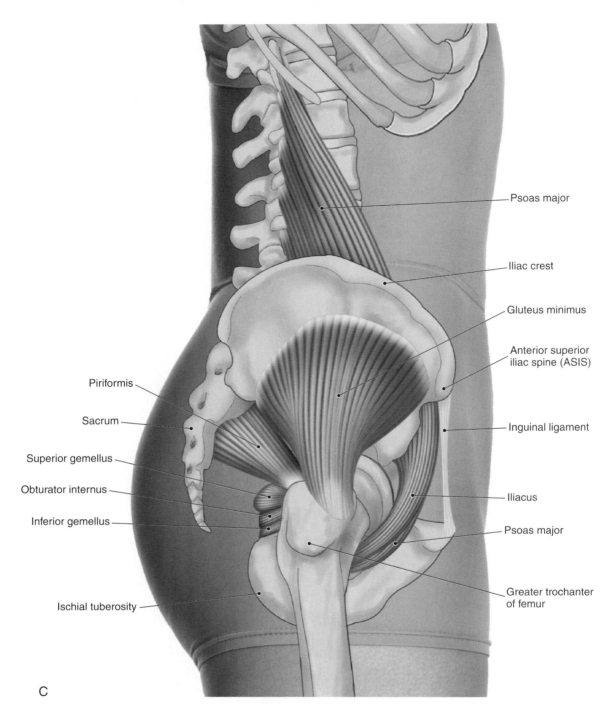

Figure 17-2, cont'd C, Deep view.

C

17

A

B

Figure 17-3 Medial views of the muscles of the right side of the pelvis. **A,** Superficial view. **B,** Deeper view.

17

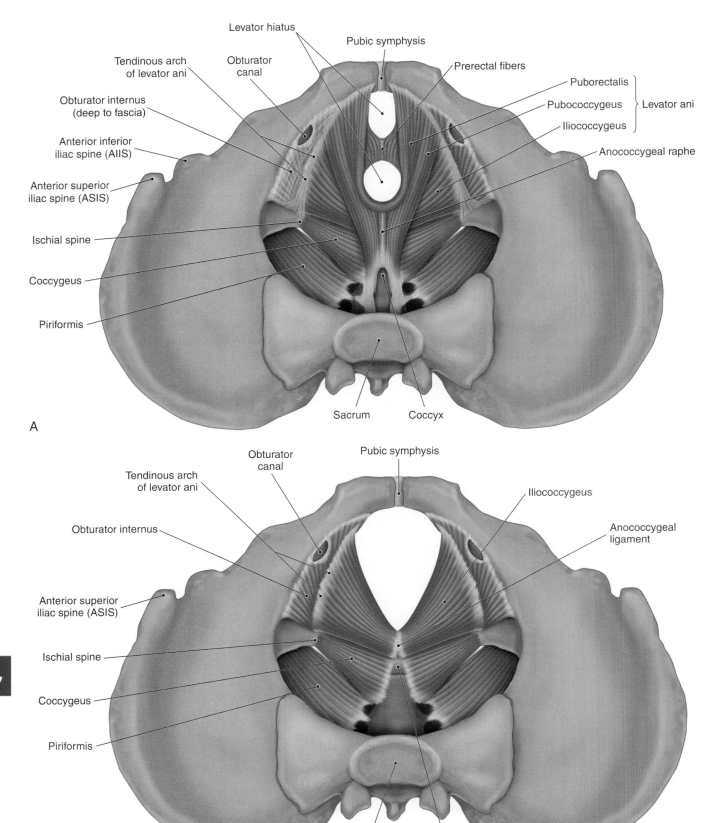

Figure 17-4 Superior views of the muscles of the pelvic floor; female pelvis. **A**, Superficial view. **B**, Deeper view.

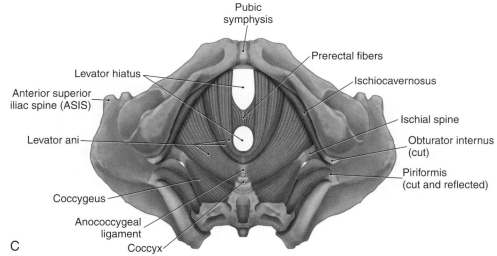

Figure 17-5 Inferior views of the muscles of the pelvic floor; female pelvis. **A**, Superficial view. **B**, Intermediate view. **C**, Deep view.

GLUTEUS MAXIMUS—PRONE

❏ **ATTACHMENTS:**

o Posterior iliac crest, posterolateral sacrum, and the coccyx *to the* gluteal tuberosity of the femur and the iliotibial band

❏ **ACTIONS:**

o Extends and laterally rotates the thigh at the hip joint
o The upper fibers abduct and the lower fibers adduct the thigh at the hip joint
o Posteriorly tilts the pelvis at the hip joint

Starting position (Figure 17-7):

o Client prone
o Therapist standing to the side of the client
o Palpating hand placed lateral to the sacrum
o Support hand placed on the distal posterior thigh if resistance is needed

Palpation steps:

1. Ask the client to extend and laterally rotate the thigh at the hip joint, and feel for the contraction of the gluteus maximus (Figure 17-8).
2. With the muscle contracted, strum perpendicular to the fibers to discern the borders of the muscle.
3. Continue palpating the gluteus maximus laterally and inferiorly (distally) to its distal attachments by strumming perpendicular to its fibers.
4. If desired, you may add resistance to the client's thigh extension to better engage the gluteus maximus.
5. Once the gluteus maximus has been located, have the client relax it and palpate to assess its baseline tone.

Figure 17-6 Posterior view of the right gluteus maximus. The tensor fasciae latae and iliotibial band have been ghosted in.

17

Figure 17-7 Starting position for prone palpation of the right gluteus maximus.

Figure 17-8 Palpation of the right gluteus maximus as the client extends and laterally rotates the thigh at the hip joint against resistance.

GLUTEUS MAXIMUS—PRONE—cont'd

Palpation Notes:
1. The gluteus maximus is superficial and easy to palpate.
2. The gluteus maximus is known as the principle muscle of the posterior buttock. However, it does not cover the entire buttock. The gluteus medius is superficial superolaterally. When following the gluteus maximus from the sacrum toward its distal attachment, be sure to follow it laterally and inferiorly (distally).

Alternate Palpation Position—Side Lying

Figure 17-9 The gluteus maximus can also be palpated with the client side lying. Palpate the gluteus maximus on the side of the body away from the table while asking the client to actively extend and laterally rotate the thigh at the hip joint. However, because extension of the thigh is not against gravity when the client is side lying, the therapist must use the support hand to add resistance to extension to engage the gluteus maximus.

TRIGGER POINTS

1. Trigger points (TrPs) in the gluteus maximus often result from or are perpetuated by acute or chronic overuse (often with a strong eccentric contraction, such as walking uphill, especially if leaning over; or by concentric contraction, such as swimming the crawl stroke), prolonged lengthened position (e.g., sleeping with the hip joint flexed), prolonged sitting (especially if sitting on a thick wallet), direct trauma, irritation from injections, and Morton's foot.
2. TrPs in the gluteus maximus may produce restlessness and pain with prolonged sitting, difficulty sleeping, pain walking uphill (especially if leaning over), pain when bending over, and restricted hip joint flexion.
3. The referral patterns of gluteus maximus TrPs must be distinguished from the referral patterns of TrPs in the gluteus medius, gluteus minimus, piriformis, tensor fasciae latae, vastus lateralis, semitendinosus, semimembranosus, quadratus lumborum, and pelvic floor muscles.
4. TrPs in the gluteus maximus are often incorrectly assessed as sacroiliac joint dysfunction, lumbar facet joint syndrome, trochanteric bursitis, coccygodynia, or disc compression upon a nerve.
5. Associated TrPs often occur in the gluteus medius, gluteus minimus, hamstrings, erector spinae group, rectus femoris, and iliopsoas.

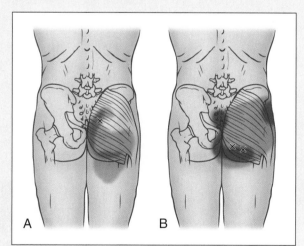

Figure 17-10 Posterior views of common gluteus maximus TrPs and their corresponding referral zones.

17

GLUTEUS MAXIMUS—PRONE—cont'd

STRETCHING THE GLUTEUS MAXIMUM

Figure 17-11 A stretch of the right gluteus maximus. With the knee joint flexed, the client uses the hands to pull the right thigh up and across the body toward the opposite shoulder. To better stretch the lower fibers of the gluteus maximus, the thigh should be brought straight up toward the same side shoulder. Note: If the client experiences a pinching sensation in the groin with this stretch, it is helpful to either first stretch the hip flexors (especially the sartorius and ilio-psoas) before doing this stretch, or to first laterally rotate and abduct the thigh at the hip joint to untwist and slacken the hip joint capsule before doing the stretch.

Palpation Key:
Extend and laterally
rotate the thigh.

GLUTEUS MEDIUS—SIDE LYING

❏ ATTACHMENTS:
o External surface of the ilium (from just inferior to the iliac crest) *to the* lateral surface of the greater trochanter of the femur

❏ ACTIONS:
o Posterior fibers:
  o Abduct, extend, and laterally rotate the thigh at the hip joint
  o Posteriorly tilt and depress the same side of the pelvis at the hip joint
o Middle fibers:
  o Abduct the thigh at the hip joint
  o Depress the same side of the pelvis at the hip joint
o Anterior fibers:
  o Abduct, flex, and medially rotate the thigh at the hip joint
  o Anteriorly tilt and depress the same side of the pelvis at the hip joint

Starting position (Figure 17-13):
o Client side lying
o Therapist standing behind the client
o Palpating hand placed just distal to the middle of the iliac crest, between the iliac crest and the greater trochanter of the femur
o Support hand placed on the lateral surface of the distal thigh

Palpation steps:
1. Palpating just distal to the middle of the iliac crest, ask the client to abduct the thigh at the hip joint and feel for the contraction of the middle fibers of the gluteus medius (Figure 17-14). If desired, resistance can be added to the client's thigh abduction with the support hand.
2. Strum perpendicular to the fibers, palpating the middle fibers of the gluteus medius distally toward the greater trochanter.

Figure 17-12 Lateral view of the right gluteus medius. The piriformis has been ghosted in.

3. To palpate the anterior fibers, place palpating hand immediately distal and posterior to the ASIS, ask the client to flex and medially rotate the thigh at the hip joint, and feel for the contraction of the anterior fibers of the gluteus medius (Figure 17-15, A) (see Palpation Note #1). It may be necessary to add resistance.
4. To palpate the posterior fibers, place palpating hand over the posterosuperior portion of the gluteus medius, ask the client to extend and laterally rotate the thigh at the hip joint, and feel for the contraction of the posterior fibers of the gluteus medius (Figure 17-15, B) (see Palpation Note #1). It may be necessary to add resistance.
5. Once the gluteus medius has been located, have the client relax it and palpate to assess its baseline tone.

Figure 17-13 Starting position for side lying palpation of the right gluteus medius. Note: The therapist usually stands behind the client, but is shown standing in front of the client here so that the reader's view is not obstructed.

GLUTEUS MEDIUS—SIDE LYING—cont'd

Figure 17-14 Palpation of the middle fibers of the right gluteus medius immediately distal to the center of the iliac crest as the client attempts to abduct the thigh at the hip joint against resistance.

Palpation Notes:
1. The middle fibers of the gluteus medius are superficial and easy to palpate. The anterior fibers are next to and deep to the tensor fasciae latae (TFL) and are difficult to distinguish from the TFL. The posterior fibers are next to the piriformis and deep to the gluteus maximus and difficult to distinguish from these two muscles.
2. During walking, when one lower limb is off the ground and the body weight is being supported by the other lower limb, contraction of the gluteus medius on the weight-bearing side can be easily felt. Its role is to create a depression force on that side of the pelvis, which creates an elevation force on the other side of the pelvis, preventing the other side from falling (depressing) to the unsupported side of the body.

Figure 17-15 Side lying palpation of the anterior and posterior fibers of the right gluteus medius. **A,** Palpation of the anterior fibers of the gluteus medius as the client abducts and medially rotates the thigh. **B,** Palpation of the posterior fibers of the gluteus medius as the client abducts and laterally rotates the thigh.

Alternate Palpation Position—Standing

Figure 17-16 The middle fibers of the gluteus medius can be easily palpated with the client standing. Palpate just distal to the middle of the iliac crests, and ask the client to slowly walk in place or simply shift her body weight from one foot to the other. You will feel the contraction of the gluteus medius on the weight-bearing side.

GLUTEUS MEDIUS—SIDE LYING—cont'd

TRIGGER POINTS

1. Trigger points (TrPs) in the gluteus medius often result from or are perpetuated by acute or chronic overuse (e.g., excessive walking or running, walking on soft sand, prolonged standing on one lower extremity), prolonged immobility, sacroiliac joint dysfunction, sitting on a thick wallet, direct trauma, injections, and Morton's foot.
2. TrPs in the gluteus medius may produce pain when sleeping on the involved side or walking, restricted hip joint adduction, hip joint pain, antalgic gait, sciatica-like pain referral, and a posturally depressed pelvis (with resultant scoliosis).
3. The referral patterns of gluteus medius TrPs must be distinguished from the referral patterns of TrPs in the gluteus maximus, gluteus minimus, and piriformis.
4. TrPs in the gluteus medius are often incorrectly assessed as low back pain, sacroiliac joint dysfunction, lumbar facet joint syndrome, or trochanteric bursitis.
5. Associated TrPs often occur in the gluteus maximus, gluteus minimus, piriformis, tensor fasciae latae, and quadratus lumborum.

Figure 17-17 Posterolateral views of common gluteus medius TrPs and their corresponding referral zones.

Figure 17-18 A stretch of the right gluteus medius and minimus. The client adducts the right thigh behind the body while using the wall for support. Note: It is important to not place too much weight on the ankle joint of the foot in back. See also page 368, Figure 16-31, for another stretch of the gluteus medius.

Palpation Key:
Palpate just distal to the middle of the iliac crest and have the client abduct the thigh.

17

GLUTEUS MEDIUS—SIDE LYING—cont'd

DETOUR 17-1

Gluteus Minimus: The gluteus minimus attaches from the external ilium to the greater trochanter of the femur and is deep to the gluteus medius. It also has the same actions as the gluteus medius. Therefore it is extremely difficult to discern from the gluteus medius.

Trigger Points:

1. Trigger points (TrPs) in the gluteus minimus often result from or are perpetuated by the same activities that create TrPs in the gluteus medius.
2. TrPs of the gluteus minimus generally produce the same symptoms as gluteus medius TrPs. However, the referral pain pattern for gluteus minimus TrPs often extends much farther distally (as far as the ankle joint) than the

pattern of either the gluteus medius or maximus. Furthermore, the pain of gluteus minimus TrPs is often persistent and severe.

3. The referral patterns of gluteus minimus TrPs must be distinguished from the referral patterns of TrPs in the gluteus maximus, gluteus medius, piriformis, hamstrings, tensor fasciae latae (TFL), gastrocnemius, soleus, fibularis longus and brevis, popliteus, and tibialis posterior.
4. TrPs in the gluteus minimus are often incorrectly assessed as L5 or S1 nerve compression, or trochanteric bursitis.
5. Associated TrPs often occur in the gluteus medius, piriformis, vastus lateralis, fibularis longus, gluteus maximus, TFL, and quadratus lumborum.

Gluteus minimus

Piriformis

A

B

C

Figure 17-19 Views of the right gluteus minimus. **A**, Lateral view of the right gluteus minimus. The piriformis has been ghosted in. **B** and **C**, Posterolateral views of common gluteus minimus TrPs and their corresponding referral zones.

PIRIFORMIS—PRONE

❏ ATTACHMENTS:

o Anterior surface of the sacrum *to the* greater trochanter of the femur

❏ ACTIONS:

o Laterally rotates the thigh at the hip joint
o If the thigh is first flexed approximately 60 degrees or more, the piriformis becomes an abductor and medial rotator of the thigh at the hip joint.

Starting Position (Figure 17-21):

o Client prone with the leg flexed to 90 degrees at the knee joint
o Therapist standing to the side of the client
o Palpating hand placed just lateral to the sacrum, halfway between the posterior superior iliac spine (PSIS) and the apex of the sacrum.
o Support hand placed on the medial surface of the distal leg, just proximal to the ankle joint

Palpation Steps:

1. Begin by finding the point on the lateral sacrum that is halfway between the PSIS and the apex of the sacrum. Drop just off the sacrum laterally at this point and you will be on the piriformis.
2. Resist the client from laterally rotating the thigh at the hip joint and feel for the contraction of the piriformis (Figure 17-22). Note: Lateral rotation of the client's thigh involves the client's foot moving medially toward the midline (and opposite side) of the body.
3. Continue palpating the piriformis laterally toward the superior border of the greater trochanter of the femur by strumming perpendicular to the fibers as the client alternately contracts (against resistance) and relaxes the piriformis.
4. Once the piriformis has been located, have the client relax it and palpate to assess its baseline tone.

A

B

Figure 17-20 Views of the piriformis. **A**, Posterior view. The piriformis has been drawn on both sides. The gluteus medius and superior gemellus have been ghosted in on the left. **B**, Anterior view of the right piriformis, showing its attachment onto the anterior surface of the sacrum.

Figure 17-21 Starting position for prone palpation of the right piriformis.

Figure 17-22 Palpation of the right piriformis as the client attempts to laterally rotate the thigh at the hip joint against gentle to moderate resistance.

PIRIFORMIS—PRONE—cont'd

Palpation Notes:

1. As soon as the midline of the sacrum is found, it is helpful to find the greater trochanter of the femur and trace the course of the piriformis from the midline of the sacrum to the greater trochanter before beginning the palpation. This way, you do not have to interrupt the palpation protocol to find the greater trochanter.
2. When giving resistance to the client's lateral rotation of the thigh at the hip joint, do not let the client contract too forcefully, or the more superficial gluteus maximus (also a lateral rotator) may be engaged, blocking palpation of the deeper piriformis.
3. It can be challenging to discern the borders between the piriformis and the gluteus medius superiorly and superior gemellus inferiorly, because these muscles are also lateral rotators of the thigh at the hip joint and may be engaged when the client contracts the piriformis.
4. The sciatic nerve usually exits from the anterior pelvis into the buttock between the piriformis and the superior gemellus. Approximately 10% to 20% of the time, all or part of the sciatic nerve emerges through the belly of the piriformis itself. With either representation, be aware of the proximity of the sciatic nerve when palpating the piriformis.
5. The sacral attachment of the piriformis can be palpated on the anterior sacrum. To accomplish this, the therapist must use a gloved hand and access the piriformis through the rectum. However, local licensure laws may not allow this palpation.
6. If the thigh is first flexed at the hip joint approximately 60 degrees or more, the piriformis can abduct the thigh at the hip joint and also changes from being a lateral rotator to a medial rotator of the thigh at the hip joint. This change in action can change how the piriformis is stretched (Figure 17-23).

TRIGGER POINTS

1. Trigger points (TrPs) in the piriformis often result from or are perpetuated by acute or chronic overuse of the muscle, prolonged shortening of the muscle (e.g., driving with foot on the gas pedal, sleeping on one's side with the upper thigh flexed and adducted), sacroiliac joint sprain, hip joint arthritis, Morton's foot, leg length discrepancy, and hyperpronation of the foot at the subtalar joint.
2. TrPs in the piriformis may produce restlessness and discomfort when sitting, lateral rotation of the thigh at the hip joint resulting in turn-out of the foot, restricted medial rotation of the thigh at the hip joint, and sacroiliac joint dysfunction.
3. The referral patterns of piriformis TrPs must be distinguished from the referral patterns of TrPs in the gluteus maximus, medius, and minimus; quadratus lumborum; and pelvic floor muscles.
4. TrPs in the piriformis are often incorrectly assessed as sacroiliac joint dysfunction, piriformis syndrome (compression of the sciatic nerve), herniated disc compression upon spinal nerves L5 or S1, or facet syndrome.
5. Associated TrPs often occur in the gluteus minimus, superior and inferior gemelli, obturator internus, coccygeus, and levator ani.

Figure 17-24 Posterior view of common piriformis TrPs and their corresponding referral zones.

STRETCHING THE PIRIFORMIS

Figure 17-23 A stretch of the right piriformis. With the right leg crossed in front of the left thigh, the client uses the hands to pull the left thigh further into flexion. Note: Because the thigh is flexed so much, the piriformis being a medial rotator is stretched by lateral rotation. See also page 410, Figure 17-28, for another stretch of the piriformis.

Palpation Key:
Find the midpoint of the lateral border of the sacrum. Then draw a line from there to the greater trochanter.

17

QUADRATUS FEMORIS—PRONE

17-3

❏ **ATTACHMENTS:**

o Lateral border of the ischial tuberosity *to the* intertrochanteric crest of the femur

❏ **ACTIONS:**

o Laterally rotates the thigh at the hip joint

Starting Position (Figure 17-26):

o Client prone with the leg flexed to 90 degrees at the knee joint
o Therapist standing to the side of the client
o Palpating hand placed just lateral to the lateral border of the ischial tuberosity
o Support hand placed on the medial surface of the distal leg, just proximal to the ankle joint

Palpation Steps:

1. Begin by finding the lateral border of the ischial tuberosity. This is usually best accomplished by first finding the inferior (distal) border and then palpating around to the lateral side. Once located, place palpating hand just lateral to the lateral border of the ischial tuberosity.
2. With gentle to moderate force, resist the client from laterally rotating the thigh at the hip joint and feel for the contraction of the quadratus femoris (Figure 17-27). Note: Lateral rotation of the client's thigh involves the client's

Figure 17-25 Posterior view of the quadratus femoris drawn on both sides. The inferior gemellus and adductor magnus have been ghosted in on the left side.

foot moving medially toward the midline (and opposite side) of the body.

3. Continue palpating the quadratus femoris laterally toward the intertrochanteric crest by strumming perpendicular to the fibers as the client alternately contracts (against resistance) and relaxes the quadratus femoris.
4. Once the quadratus femoris has been located, have the client relax it and palpate to assess its baseline tone.

Figure 17-26 Starting position for prone palpation of the right quadratus femoris.

Figure 17-27 Palpation of the quadratus femoris as the client attempts to laterally rotate the thigh at the hip joint against gentle to moderate resistance.

17

Palpation Key:
Find the lateral border of the ischial tuberosity.

QUADRATUS FEMORIS—PRONE—cont'd

Palpation Notes:

1. When giving resistance to the client's lateral rotation of the thigh at the hip joint, do not let the client contract too forcefully, or the more superficial gluteus maximus (also a lateral rotator) may be engaged, blocking palpation of the deeper quadratus femoris.
2. Of all six "deep lateral rotators" of the thigh at the hip joint, the piriformis is the most well known; however, the quadratus femoris is the largest.

3. If the thigh is first flexed at the hip joint approximately 60 degrees or more, the quadratus femoris can abduct the thigh at the hip joint.
4. **Proceed with caution when palpating the quadratus femoris because the sciatic nerve courses directly over it.**

STRETCHING THE QUADRATUS FEMORIS

Figure 17-28 A stretch of the right quadratus femoris is shown. The client uses the hands to pull the thigh up and across the body. Note: If the client experiences a pinching sensation in the groin with this stretch, it is helpful to first stretch the hip flexors (especially the sartorius and iliopsoas) before doing this stretch or to first laterally rotate and abduct the thigh at the hip joint to untwist and slacken the hip joint capsule before doing the stretch. See also page 408, Figure 17-23, for another stretch of this region.

TRIGGER POINTS

Note: The patterns of trigger points (TrPs) and TrP referral zones for the quadratus femoris and the other deep lateral rotators (see Detour to Other Deep Lateral Rotators on the next page) have not been differentiated from the patterns for the piriformis.

Furthermore, factors that create or perpetuate TrPs in the quadratus femoris and other deep lateral rotators are likely to be the same as those for the piriformis.

DETOUR

Other Deep Lateral Rotators: Of the six deep lateral rotators of the thigh at the hip joint (piriformis, superior gemellus, obturator internus, inferior gemellus, obturator externus, quadratus femoris), the piriformis is the most superior of the group and the quadratus femoris is the most inferior. The other deep lateral rotators are quite small and difficult to discern from each other, so it is best to palpate them as a group. To palpate these other deep lateral rotators, either find the piriformis and palpate inferior to it, or find the quadratus femoris and palpate superior to it. Follow the same procedure used to palpate the piriformis and quadratus femoris by giving gentle to moderate resistance to the client's lateral rotation of the thigh at the hip joint. Note: Given that the obturator externus is deeper than the rest, it is usually the most difficult of the group to palpate.

Figure 17-29 The deep lateral rotators of the thigh at the hip joint. **A,** Posterior view of the deep lateral rotators. The piriformis and quadratus femoris have been ghosted in on the left side and deleted on the right side. **B,** Palpation of the other deep lateral rotators by first locating the piriformis and then dropping inferiorly off it. This palpation is done as the client attempts to laterally rotate the thigh against gentle to moderate resistance.

17

Muscles of the Pelvis

Client Prone:

1. **Gluteus maximus:** The client is prone; you are standing to the side of the client. Place your palpating hand just lateral to the sacrum and feel for the contraction of the gluteus maximus as the client extends and laterally rotates the thigh at the hip joint (resistance can be added if desired). Once felt, continue to palpate the gluteus maximus toward its distal attachment by strumming perpendicular to its fibers as the client alternately contracts and relaxes the muscle.

Client Side Lying:

2. **Gluteus medius:** The client is side lying; you are standing behind the client. Place palpating hand immediately distal to the middle of the iliac crest and feel for the contraction of the middle fibers of the gluteus medius as the client abducts the thigh at the hip joint (resistance can be added if desired). Once felt, continue palpating the middle fibers distally to the greater trochanter of the femur by strumming perpendicular to the fibers as the client alternately contracts and relaxes the muscle. The anterior fibers and posterior fibers are mostly deep to other muscles and more difficult to palpate and discern. To palpate the anterior fibers, place your palpating hand immediately distal and posterior to the ASIS, ask the client to flex and medially rotate the thigh at the hip joint, and feel for the contraction of the anterior fibers of the gluteus medius deep to the tensor fasciae latae (TFL). If felt, try to palpate the rest of the anterior fibers deep to the TFL. To palpate the posterior fibers, place your palpating hand over the posterosuperior portion of the gluteus maximus, ask the client to extend and laterally rotate the thigh at the hip joint, and feel for the contraction of the posterior fibers of the gluteus medius deep to the gluteus maximus. If felt, try to palpate the rest of the posterior fibers deep to the gluteus maximus. Note: The gluteus minimus is wholly deep to and has the same actions as the gluteus medius. Therefore, although it can be palpated, it is extremely difficult to discern from the gluteus medius.

3. **Piriformis:** The client is prone with the leg flexed to 90 degrees at the knee joint; you are standing to the side of the client. Place your palpating fingers just lateral to the sacrum, halfway between the PSIS and the apex of the sacrum, and feel for the contraction of the piriformis as the client laterally rotates the thigh at the hip joint against gentle to moderate resistance. Note: Lateral rotation of the thigh in this position requires the client's foot to move medially toward the midline (i.e., the opposite side) of the body. Once felt, continue palpating the piriformis toward the greater trochanter attachment by strumming perpendicular to its fibers as the client alternately contracts and relaxes the muscle. Note: It can be difficult to discern the superior border between the piriformis and gluteus medius and the inferior border between the piriformis and superior gemellus.

4. **Quadratus femoris:** The client is prone with the leg flexed to 90 degrees at the knee joint; you are standing to the side of the client. Place your palpating fingers just lateral to the lateral border of the ischial tuberosity and feel for the contraction of the quadratus femoris as the client laterally rotates the thigh at the hip joint against gentle to moderate resistance. Note: Lateral rotation of the thigh in this position requires the client's foot to move medially toward the midline (i.e., the opposite side) of the body. Once felt, continue palpating the quadratus femoris toward its femoral attachment by strumming perpendicular to its fibers as the client alternately contracts and relaxes the muscle.

5. **Detour: Other deep lateral rotators (superior gemellus, obturator internus, inferior gemellus, obturator externus):** The client is prone with the leg flexed to 90 degrees at the knee joint; you are standing to the side of the client. These other deep lateral rotators located between the piriformis and quadratus femoris are small and deep, but they can usually be palpated. However, it is difficult to discern them from each other (the obturator externus is deeper than the others and generally the most difficult to palpate). To palpate these muscles, follow the same palpation procedure as for the piriformis and quadratus femoris by adding gentle to moderate resistance to the client's lateral rotation of the thigh at the hip joint, and palpate between the piriformis and quadratus femoris.

Chapter 18

Tour #9—Palpation of the Thigh Muscles

Overview

This chapter is a palpation tour of the muscles of the thigh. The tour begins with the hamstring muscles in the posterior thigh, then addresses muscles primarily located in the anterior thigh, including the quadriceps femoris group, and then concludes with the muscles of the adductor group in the medial thigh. Except for the hamstring muscles, which are palpated prone, palpation for the rest of the muscles is shown in the supine position, with the client's thighs resting on the table and the legs hanging off the table. Although the client is rarely placed in this position for treatment, it is an extremely effective position for palpation of the muscles of the thigh, because it affords the possibility of easily isolating contraction of each target muscle of the thigh. However, maintaining this position for a prolonged period can be uncomfortable for the client's lower back. One way to remedy this is to ask the client to flex their hip and knee joints on the side not being palpated, placing that foot on the table. This will serve to stabilize the pelvis, removing strain from their lower back. If desired, each of these palpations can be done with the client supine with the entire lower extremity on the table instead. Other alternate palpation positions are also described. The major muscles or muscle groups of the region are each given a separate layout. There are also a few detours to other muscles of the region. Trigger point (TrP) information and stretching is given for each of the muscles covered in this chapter. The chapter closes with an advanced *Whirlwind Tour* that explains the sequential palpation of all the muscles of the chapter.

Chapter Outline

Chapter Objectives

After completing this chapter, the student should be able to perform the following for each of the muscles covered in this chapter:

1. State the attachments.
2. State the actions.
3. Describe the starting position for palpation.
4. Describe and explain the purpose of each of the palpation steps.
5. Palpate each muscle.
6. State the "Palpation Key."
7. Describe alternate palpation positions.
8. State the locations of the most common TrP(s).
9. Describe the TrP referral zones.
10. State the most common factors that create and/or perpetuate TrPs.
11. State the symptoms most commonly caused by TrPs.
12. Describe and perform a stretch.

Video demonstrations of the muscle palpations in this chapter are presented in Chapter 18 on DVD 1.

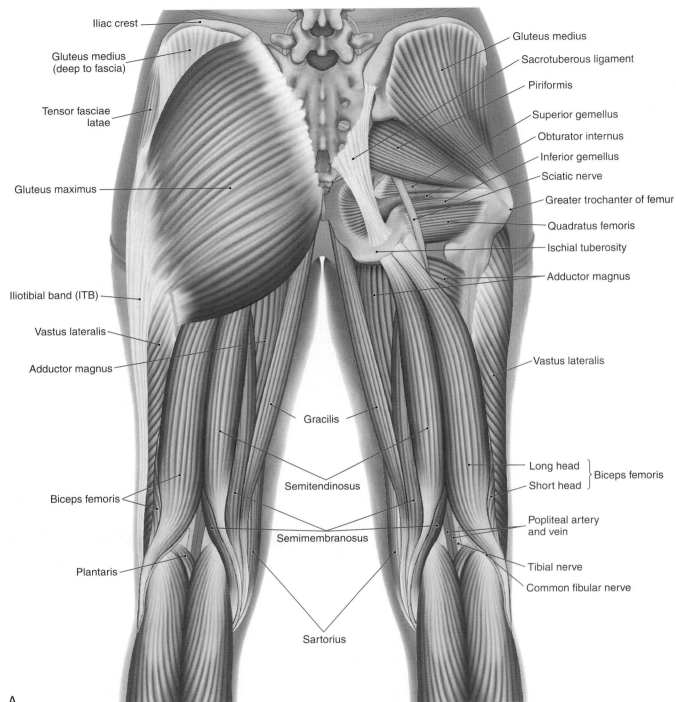

Iliac crest
Gluteus medius (deep to fascia)
Tensor fasciae latae
Gluteus maximus
Iliotibial band (ITB)
Vastus lateralis
Adductor magnus
Biceps femoris
Plantaris

Gluteus medius
Sacrotuberous ligament
Piriformis
Superior gemellus
Obturator internus
Inferior gemellus
Sciatic nerve
Greater trochanter of femur
Quadratus femoris
Ischial tuberosity
Adductor magnus
Vastus lateralis
Long head
Short head } Biceps femoris
Popliteal artery and vein
Tibial nerve
Common fibular nerve

Gracilis
Semitendinosus
Semimembranosus
Sartorius

A

18

Figure 18-1 Posterior views of the muscles of the pelvis and thigh. **A,** Superficial view on the left and an intermediate view on the right.

Figure 18-1, cont'd B, Deeper views.

Posterior superior
iliac spine (PSIS)

Sciatic nerve

Femoral artery

Lesser trochanter

Anterior
head

Posterior
head

Adductor
magnus

Vastus lateralis

Popliteal artery
and vein

Sciatic nerve

Tibial nerve

Common fibular nerve

Sacrotuberous ligament

Ischial tuberosity

Adductor magnus

Vastus lateralis

Gracilis

Biceps femoris
short head

Semimembranosus

Plantaris

Sartorius

Medial
head

Lateral
head

Gastrocnemius

B

18

12th rib
Psoas minor
Psoas major
Inferior vena cava
Abdominal aorta
Iliacus
Piriformis
Inguinal ligament
Gluteus medius
Tensor fasciae latae
Gluteus medius
Gluteus minimus
Piriformis
Sartorius
Iliopsoas distal belly/tendon
Femoral nerve, artery, and vein
Greater trochanter of femur
Pectineus
Adductor longus
Iliotibial band (ITB)
Gracilis
Adductor magnus
Vastus lateralis
Quadriceps femoris { Rectus femoris
Vastus medialis
Patella
Head of fibula
Tibial tuberosity
Tibialis anterior
Gastrocnemius
Extensor digitorum longus
Fibularis longus
Soleus
Pes anserine tendon { Sartorius
Gracilis
Semitendinosus

A

Figure 18-2 Views of the anterior thigh. **A,** Superficial view on the right and an intermediate view on the left.

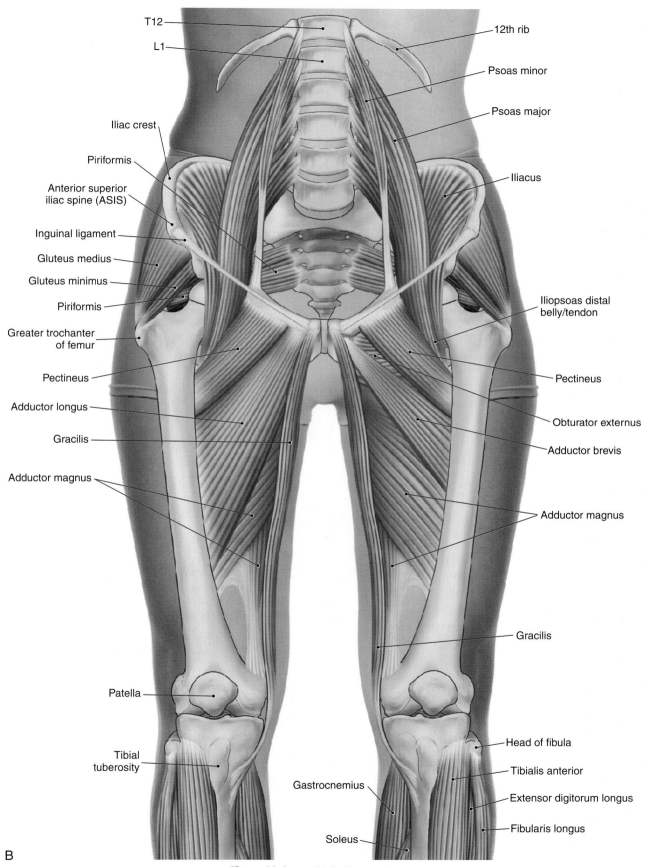

Figure 18-2, cont'd B, Deeper views.

B

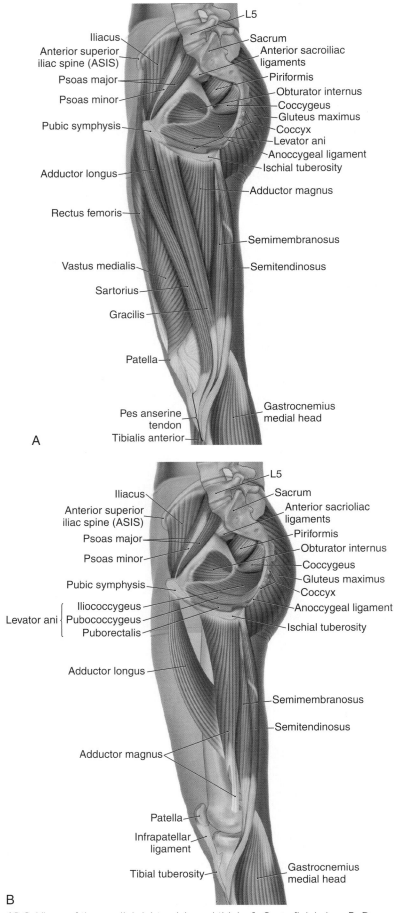

A

L5
Iliacus
Anterior superior iliac spine (ASIS)
Psoas major
Psoas minor
Pubic symphysis
Adductor longus
Rectus femoris
Vastus medialis
Sartorius
Gracilis
Patella
Pes anserine tendon
Tibialis anterior

Sacrum
Anterior sacroiliac ligaments
Piriformis
Obturator internus
Coccygeus
Gluteus maximus
Coccyx
Levator ani
Anoccygeal ligament
Ischial tuberosity
Adductor magnus
Semimembranosus
Semitendinosus
Gastrocnemius medial head

B

L5
Iliacus
Anterior superior iliac spine (ASIS)
Psoas major
Psoas minor
Pubic symphysis
Levator ani { Iliococcygeus Pubococcygeus Puborectalis
Adductor longus
Adductor magnus
Patella
Infrapatellar ligament
Tibial tuberosity

Sacrum
Anterior sacrioliac ligaments
Piriformis
Obturator internus
Coccygeus
Gluteus maximus
Coccyx
Anoccygeal ligament
Ischial tuberosity
Semimembranosus
Semitendinosus
Gastrocnemius medial head

18

Figure 18-3 Views of the medial right pelvis and thigh. **A**, Superficial view. **B**, Deeper view.

Figure 18-4 Views of the right lateral thigh. **A,** Superficial view. **B,** Deep view (with only the quadriceps femoris group and biceps femoris of the hamstring group drawn in).

HAMSTRING GROUP—PRONE

Lateral hamstrings: biceps femoris, long head and short head
Medial hamstrings: semitendinosus and semimembranosus

❏ ATTACHMENTS:

o Biceps femoris: ischial tuberosity (long head) and the linea aspera of the femur (short head) *to the* head of the fibula and the lateral tibial condyle
o Semitendinosus: ischial tuberosity *to the* pes anserine tendon at the proximal anteromedial tibia
o Semimembranosus: ischial tuberosity *to the* posterior surface of the medial tibial condyle

❏ ACTIONS:

o All three hamstrings flex the leg at the knee joint, extend the thigh at the hip joint, and posteriorly tilt the pelvis at the hip joint
o Lateral hamstrings laterally rotate the leg at the knee joint; medial hamstrings medially rotate the leg at the knee joint
o Note: The short head of the biceps femoris does not cross the hip joint and therefore does not have an action at the hip joint.

Starting position (Figure 18-6):

o Client prone with leg partially flexed at the knee joint
o Therapist standing to the side of the client
o Palpating hand placed just distal to the ischial tuberosity
o Support hand placed around the distal leg, just proximal to the ankle joint

Palpation steps:

1. Palpating just distal to the ischial tuberosity, resist the client from further flexion of the leg at the knee joint and feel for the contraction of the hamstrings.
2. Strumming perpendicular to the fibers, follow the biceps femoris toward the head of the fibula. Repeat this procedure from the ischial tuberosity to follow the medial hamstrings toward the medial side of the leg (Figure 18-7).
3. Once each of the hamstrings has been located, have the client relax it and palpate to assess its baseline tone.

A

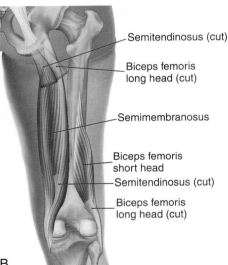

B

Figure 18-5 Posterior views of the right hamstring group. **A,** Superficial view of all three hamstring muscles. **B,** Deeper view. The proximal and distal tendons of the semitendinosus and the long head of the biceps femoris have been cut and ghosted in.

18

Figure 18-6 Starting position for prone palpation of the right hamstrings.

HAMSTRING GROUP—PRONE—cont'd

Figure 18-7 Palpation of the superficial hamstring muscles of the right thigh as the client attempts to flex the leg at the knee joint against resistance. **A,** Palpation of the long head of the biceps femoris on the lateral side. **B,** Palpation of the semitendinosus on the medial side.

Palpation Notes:

1. Distally, the tendons of the medial and lateral hamstrings are quite far apart and easy to distinguish. Proximally they are closer to each other and more difficult to distinguish. Using rotation of the leg at the knee joint is an excellent way to discern between them. The medial hamstrings are medial rotators and the lateral hamstrings are lateral rotators. Keep in mind that the knee joint only allows rotations to occur if it is first flexed; the recommended flexion of the knee joint is 90 degrees.

2. When the client is not contracting the hamstrings to try to flex the leg at the knee joint against the resistance of your support hand, use your support hand to support the client's leg so that the hamstrings are allowed to fully relax. Otherwise, if the client has to hold the leg partially flexed in the air, the hamstrings will not relax between contractions. Full relaxation between contractions creates a greater change in muscle tone, making it easier to palpate and locate the target hamstring muscle.

3. It can be difficult to discern the bellies of the two medial hamstrings from each other. Note that the distal tendon of the semitendinosus is very prominent and easy to find. The semimembranosus can be palpated on either side of the distal semitendinosus, especially the medial side (Figure 18-8).

4. Directly anterior to the belly of the biceps femoris is the vastus lateralis muscle; use flexion versus extension of the leg to discern their border. Directly anterior to the medial hamstrings in the proximal thigh is the adductor magnus; use flexion of the leg to discern this border. The adductor magnus does not cross the knee joint and will stay relaxed with leg flexion, whereas the hamstrings will contract with flexion.

Figure 18-8 The distal semimembranosus can be palpated on either side of the distal tendon of the semitendinosus. Palpation on its lateral side is shown here.

18

HAMSTRING GROUP—PRONE—cont'd

Alternate Palpation Position—Seated

Having the client seated with the foot flat on the floor allows for easy use of rotations of the leg at the knee joint to locate the distal tendons of the biceps femoris, semitendinosus, and gracilis. With lateral rotation, the biceps femoris is easily palpable on the lateral side. With medial rotation, two tendons stand out on the medial side, the semitendinosus and gracilis. The semitendinosus is the larger of the two and more lateral (closer to the midline of the thigh).

Figure 18-9 Palpation of the distal tendons of the biceps femoris, semitendinosus, and gracilis as the client rotates the leg at the knee joint. **A**, Palpation of the biceps femoris as the client laterally rotates the leg. **B**, Palpation of the semitendinosus and gracilis as the client medially rotates the leg. Note: For the purpose of these photos, the client is standing with the foot on a stool.

TRIGGER POINTS

1. Trigger points (TrPs) in the hamstrings often result from or are perpetuated by acute or chronic overuse of the muscle and ischemia caused by compression on the distal posterior thigh from sitting in an ill-fitting chair. They also commonly result from prolonged shortening of the muscle due to sleeping in the fetal position.
2. TrPs in the medial hamstrings tend to produce pain that is superficial and sharper in quality, whereas lateral hamstring TrPs tend to produce pain that is deeper and duller in quality. TrPs in the lateral hamstrings often wake clients at night, resulting in nonrestful sleep.
3. The referral patterns of hamstring TrPs must be distinguished from the referral patterns of TrPs in the piriformis, gluteus medius and minimus, obturator internus, vastus lateralis, popliteus, plantaris, and gastrocnemius.
4. TrPs in the hamstrings are often incorrectly assessed as sciatica or degenerative joint disease of the knee.
5. Associated TrPs often occur in the adductor magnus, vastus lateralis, gastrocnemius, iliopsoas, and quadriceps femoris muscles.

Figure 18-10 Posterior views of common lateral and medial hamstring TrPs, with their corresponding referral zones. **A**, Lateral hamstring (biceps femoris). **B**, Medial hamstrings (semitendinosus and semimembranosus).

18

HAMSTRING GROUP—PRONE—cont'd

STRETCHING THE HAMSTRING GROUP

Figure 18-11 A stretch of the right hamstring group. The client sits with the right knee joint fully extended and rocks the pelvis forward into anterior tilt at the hip joint. Note: The spine does not need to bend in this stretch.

Palpation Key:
Resist flexion of the leg at the knee joint.

DETOUR

Adductor Magnus: Once the medial hamstrings have been located in the proximal thigh, drop just medial (anterior) to their medial border and you will be on the adductor magnus. The adductor magnus is located between the medial hamstrings and the gracilis. To confirm your location, ask the client to flex the leg at the knee joint. This will engage the hamstrings and the gracilis, but not the adductor magnus between them. Resisted adduction of the thigh at the hip joint will engage the adductor magnus (and the gracilis) (Figure 18-12).

Figure 18-12 The adductor magnus can be palpated between the medial hamstrings and the gracilis. The medial hamstrings and the gracilis contract when the client flexes the leg at the knee joint, but the adductor magnus does not.

18

TENSOR FASCIAE LATAE (TFL)—SUPINE

❑ **ATTACHMENTS:**

o Anterior superior iliac spine (ASIS) and the anterior iliac crest *to the* iliotibial band, ⅓ of the way down the thigh

❑ **ACTIONS:**

o Medially rotates, flexes, and abducts the thigh at the hip joint
o Anteriorly tilts and ipsilaterally depresses the pelvis at the hip joint

Starting position (Figure 18-14):

o Client supine with thighs on the table and legs hanging off the table
o Therapist standing to the side of the client
o Palpating fingers placed just distal and lateral to the ASIS
o If resistance is necessary, support hand placed on the distal anterolateral thigh

Palpation steps:

1. Ask the client to medially rotate and flex the thigh at the hip joint and feel for the contraction of the tensor fasciae latae (TFL) immediately distal and slightly lateral to the ASIS (Figure 18-15).
2. Continue palpating the TFL distally to its iliotibial band attachment by strumming perpendicular to the fibers.
3. Having the client contract to lift the medially rotated thigh up into flexion against gravity is usually sufficient resistance to bring out the TFL. However, if needed, additional resistance can be given with the support hand placed on the distal anterior thigh.
4. Once the TFL has been located, have the client relax it and palpate to assess its baseline tone.

Figure 18-13 Lateral view of the right tensor fasciae latae (TFL). The gluteus maximus has been ghosted in. *ITB*, Iliotibial band.

Figure 18-14 Starting position for supine palpation of the right TFL.

Figure 18-15 The right TFL is palpated by asking the client to medially rotate and flex the thigh at the hip joint.

18

TENSOR FASCIAE LATAE (TFL)—SUPINE—cont'd

Palpation Notes:

1. The TFL is superficial and easy to palpate.
2. It is interesting to compare the palpation procedures for the TFL and sartorius. Both muscles attach to the ASIS and are flexors of the thigh at the hip joint. However, the TFL is also a medial rotator of the thigh, and the sartorius is also a lateral rotator of the thigh. Therefore, to palpate the TFL, palpate immediately distal and lateral to the ASIS and ask the client to medially rotate and flex the thigh at the hip joint. To palpate the sartorius, palpate immediately distal and medial to the ASIS and ask the client to laterally rotate and flex the thigh at the hip joint.
3. Between the proximal attachments of the TFL and sartorius is the rectus femoris of the quadriceps femoris group.
4. The reason that the supine client is lying with the legs off the table is that it allows for immediate and easy palpation and discernment of the rectus femoris by asking the client to straighten out (extend) the leg at the knee joint without contracting any flexors of the thigh at the hip joint. Locating the rectus femoris allows for better distinction between the TFL and the rectus femoris. This position also allows for easy palpation of other anterior and medial thigh muscles.

Alternate Palpation Position—Side Lying

Figure 18-16 Because the TFL is located in the anterolateral thigh, it can also be easily palpated with the client in side lying position. Ask the client to medially rotate and flex (slight abduction may also be added) the thigh at the hip joint and feel for the contraction of the TFL.

TRIGGER POINTS

1. Trigger points (TrPs) in the tensor fasciae latae (TFL) often result from or are perpetuated by acute or chronic overuse of the muscle, and prolonged shortening of the muscle due to sitting and sleeping in the fetal position.
2. The referral patterns of TFL TrPs must be distinguished from the referral patterns of TrPs in the anterior fibers of the gluteus medius and minimus, vastus lateralis, and quadratus lumborum.
3. TrPs in the TFL are often incorrectly assessed as trochanteric bursitis, sacroiliac joint syndrome, or meralgia paresthetica.
4. Associated TrPs often occur in the anterior gluteus minimus, rectus femoris, iliopsoas, and sartorius.

Figure 18-17 Lateral view of a common tensor fasciae latae (TFL) TrP with its corresponding referral zone.

18

TENSOR FASCIAE LATAE (TFL)—SUPINE—cont'd

STRETCHING THE TENSOR FASCIAE LATAE (TFL)

Palpation Key:
Medially rotate
and flex the thigh.

Figure 18-18 A stretch of the right TFL. The client adducts the right thigh behind the body while using the wall for support. Note: It is important to not place too much weight on the ankle joint of the foot in back. See Figure 16-31, page 368, for another stretch of the TFL.

18

SARTORIUS—SUPINE

❏ ATTACHMENTS:

o Anterior superior iliac spine (ASIS) *to the* pes anserine tendon at the proximal anteromedial tibia

❏ ACTIONS:

o Laterally rotates, flexes, and abducts the thigh at the hip joint
o Anteriorly tilts and ipsilaterally depresses the pelvis at the hip joint
o Flexes and medially rotates the leg at the knee joint

Starting position (Figure 18-20):

o Client supine with thighs on the table and legs hanging off the table
o Therapist standing to the side of the client
o Palpating fingers placed just distal and medial to the ASIS
o If resistance is necessary, support hand placed on the distal anteromedial thigh

Palpation steps:

1. Ask the client to laterally rotate and flex the thigh at the hip joint and feel for the contraction of the sartorius immediately distal and slightly medial to the ASIS (Figure 18-21).
2. If necessary, use the support hand to add resistance when the client flexes the laterally rotated thigh.
3. Continue palpating the sartorius toward its distal attachment by strumming perpendicular to the fibers.
4. Once the sartorius has been located, have the client relax it and palpate to assess its baseline tone.

Figure 18-19 Anterior view of the right sartorius. The tensor fasciae latae (TFL) and iliotibial tract (ITB) have been ghosted in.

Figure 18-20 Starting position for supine palpation of the right sartorius.

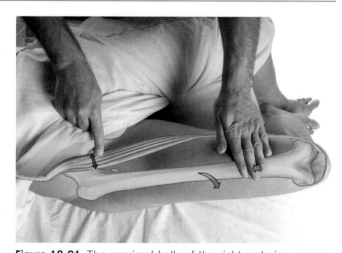

Figure 18-21 The proximal belly of the right sartorius engages and is easily palpable when the client laterally rotates and flexes the thigh at the hip joint. Note: The therapist usually palpates from the same side of the table, but is shown here standing on the opposite side of the table for the purpose of this photo.

18

SARTORIUS—SUPINE—cont'd

Palpation Notes:

1. Even though it is superficial, the distal ½ of the sartorius is often difficult to palpate and discern from the adjacent musculature. One method to locate it is to first locate the vastus medialis in the distal thigh (it is usually fairly prominent and often forms a bulge in well-developed individuals). To engage the vastus medialis, have the client extend the leg at the knee joint. Once the vastus medialis has been found, move just medial (posterior) off it onto the sartorius. Then ask the client to flex the leg at the knee joint to engage the sartorius. In this position, this can be accomplished by asking the client to press the leg against the table (Figure 18-22).

2. In addition to asking the client to laterally rotate and flex the thigh at the hip joint, it can be helpful to ask the client to also abduct the thigh at the hip joint and flex the leg at the knee joint. These four actions are all the actions of the sartorius upon the thigh and leg.

3. The sartorius and tensor fasciae latae (TFL) are palpated in a similar manner. To palpate the sartorius, palpate immediately distal and slightly medial to the ASIS and ask the client to laterally rotate and flex the thigh at the hip joint. To palpate the TFL, palpate immediately distal and slightly lateral to the ASIS and ask the client to medially rotate and flex the thigh at the hip joint. Note: Between the proximal attachments of the TFL and sartorius is the rectus femoris of the quadriceps femoris group.

4. Proximally, the medial border of the sartorius forms the lateral border of the femoral triangle. Located within the femoral triangle are the iliopsoas and pectineus muscles, and the femoral nerve, artery, and vein.

Figure 18-22 Palpation of the distal belly of the right sartorius by first locating the vastus medialis. **A**, Palpation of the engaged vastus medialis as the client extends the leg at the knee joint. **B**, Once the vastus medialis is located, the therapist palpates the distal belly of the sartorius immediately medial (posterior) to the vastus medialis as the client engages the sartorius by flexing the leg at the knee joint against the resistance of the table.

Alternate Palpation Position—Supine with Entire Lower Extremity on the Table

Figure 18-23 The sartorius can be palpated with the client supine with the thighs and legs on the table. The right sartorius is engaged and palpated here by asking the client to laterally rotate and flex the thigh at the hip joint.

18

SARTORIUS—SUPINE—cont'd

TRIGGER POINTS

1. Trigger points (TrPs) in the sartorius often result from or are perpetuated by acute or chronic overuse of the muscle, or a prolonged shortening of the muscle due to sitting in the cross-legged lotus position or sleeping in the fetal position.
2. TrPs in the sartorius tend to produce superficial sharp pain or tingling compared with the usual deep dull pain typical of myofascial TrPs.
3. The referral patterns of sartorius TrPs must be distinguished from the referral patterns of TrPs in the vastus medialis, vastus intermedius, pectineus, iliopsoas, and the three "adductors" of the thigh.
4. TrPs in the sartorius are often incorrectly assessed as meralgia paresthetica or medial knee joint dysfunction.
5. Associated TrPs often occur in the quadriceps femoris and the three "adductor" muscles of the thigh.

Figure 18-24 Anteromedial view of common sartorius TrPs with their corresponding referral zone.

STRETCHING THE SARTORIUS

Figure 18-25 A stretch of the right sartorius. The client medially rotates, extends, and adducts the right thigh while leaning forward with the pelvis (posterior tilting it) and trunk to increase the stretch across the hip joint. Note: It is important to not let the pelvis fall into anterior tilt and to make sure that excessive weight is not placed on the ankle joint of the foot in back.

18

SARTORIUS—SUPINE—cont'd

DETOUR

Iliopsoas Distal Belly and Tendon: Slide medially off the proximal tendon of the sartorius and you will be on the distal belly and tendon of the iliopsoas; confirm by asking the client to gently flex the trunk at the spinal joints (by doing a small abdominal curl-up) and feel for the tensing of the psoas major portion of the iliopsoas distal belly and tendon (the psoas major portion is the more medial portion of the iliopsoas). Be aware of the presence of the femoral nerve, artery, and vein overlying the iliopsoas distal belly and tendon. For more details, see page 387).

Palpation Key:
Laterally rotate and flex the thigh.

Figure 18-26 Palpation of the distal belly and tendon of the right psoas major portion of the iliopsoas medial to the sartorius as the client flexes the spine by doing a curl-up.

18

The quadriceps femoris group is composed of the rectus femoris, vastus medialis, vastus lateralis, and vastus intermedius.

❑ ATTACHMENTS:

o Rectus femoris: anterior inferior iliac spine (AIIS) *to the* tibial tuberosity
o Vastus medialis, lateralis, and intermedius: linea aspera of the femur *to the* tibial tuberosity

❑ ACTIONS:

o All four quadriceps femoris muscles extend the leg at the knee joint.
o The rectus femoris also flexes the thigh and anteriorly tilts the pelvis at the hip joint.

Starting position (Figure 18-28):

o Client supine with thighs on the table and legs hanging off the table
o Therapist standing to the side of the client
o Palpating fingers placed on the proximal anterior thigh
o If resistance is necessary, support hand placed on the distal leg, just proximal to the ankle joint

Palpation steps:

1. Proximally, the rectus femoris is located between the tensor fasciae latae (TFL) and sartorius. Either locate the proximal tendon of the TFL (see page 424) and drop off it medially, or locate the proximal tendon of the sartorius (see page 427) and drop off it laterally, and you will be on the rectus femoris.

2. Ask the client to extend the leg at the knee joint and feel for the contraction of the rectus femoris (Figure 18-29, A). If necessary, use the support hand to add resistance when the client extends the leg.

3. Continue palpating the rectus femoris distally to the tibial tuberosity by strumming perpendicular to its fibers.

4. For the vastus medialis, palpate in the anteromedial thigh, just proximal to the patella while the client extends the leg at the knee joint, and feel for its contraction. Then strum perpendicular to the fibers and palpate as much of the vastus medialis as possible (Figure 18-29, B).

5. For the vastus lateralis, palpate in the anterolateral thigh, just proximal to the patella while the client extends the leg at the knee joint, and feel for its contraction. Then strum perpendicular to the fibers and palpate the vastus lateralis in the anterolateral thigh, in the lateral thigh deep to the iliotibial band (ITB) and in the posterolateral thigh immediately posterior to the ITB (Figure 18-29, C).

6. Once the quadriceps femoris muscles have been located, have the client relax them and palpate to assess their baseline tone.

A   B

Figure 18-27 Views of the quadriceps femoris group. **A,** Superficial and deep anterior views. The right side is a superficial view. The rectus femoris has been removed on the left side to expose the vastus intermedius. **B,** Right lateral view.

18

QUADRICEPS FEMORIS GROUP—SUPINE—cont'd

Figure 18-28 Starting position for supine palpation of the right quadriceps femoris group.

Figure 18-29 Palpation of the quadriceps femoris muscles as the client extends the leg at the knee joint. **A,** Anterolateral view showing palpation of the rectus femoris. **B,** Anteromedial view showing palpation of the vastus medialis. **C,** Anterolateral view showing palpation of the vastus lateralis.

18

QUADRICEPS FEMORIS GROUP—SUPINE

Palpation Notes:

1. Proximally, the rectus femoris is located between the TFL and the sartorius. Either of these two muscles can be used as a landmark to find the rectus femoris.

2. The rectus femoris can be palpated and followed all the way to the AIIS. Follow the rectus femoris proximally as far as possible with the client in the starting position (see Figure 18-28). Then passively flex the client's thigh at the hip joint as you continue palpating farther proximally toward the AIIS. Ask the client to alternately contract and relax the rectus femoris by extending the leg at the knee joint and feel for the tensing of the proximal tendon. When you have reached the AIIS itself, make sure that the rectus femoris is relaxed and passively slackened so that the hard texture of the AIIS will be discernable from the adjacent soft tissue texture of the proximal tendon of the rectus femoris (Figure 18-30).

3. In well-developed clients, it is usually possible to discern the borders between the rectus femoris and the vastus lateralis on the lateral side, and rectus femoris and vastus medialis on the medial side. While the quadriceps femoris group is contracted, strum perpendicularly across the rectus femoris, feeling for the side-to-side width of the muscle. Then feel for a palpable indent/groove running vertically between the rectus femoris and the vastus muscles on either side.

4. The vastus medialis is superficial and easy to palpate in the distal thigh. However, proximally it is deeper and can be difficult to palpate and discern from adjacent musculature.

5. The vastus lateralis is superficial in the anterolateral thigh and deep only to the ITB in the lateral thigh. In these locations, it is easy to palpate. It is also superficial and fairly easy to palpate immediately posterior to the ITB in the posterolateral thigh. However, the linea aspera attachment is quite deep and can be difficult to palpate and discern.

6. Because the vastus lateralis muscle is deep to the iliotibial band, tension in this muscle is often blamed on the iliotibial band.

7. The vastus intermedius is extremely difficult to palpate and discern because it is deep to the rectus femoris and vastus lateralis and has the same action as these other muscles.

8. The patella is a sesamoid bone that developed evolutionarily within the distal tendon of the quadriceps femoris tendon. Its major function is to increase the leverage force and therefore the strength of the quadriceps femoris muscles.

Figure 18-30 Palpation of the proximal tendon of the rectus femoris at the AIIS (see Palpation Note #2).

Alternate Palpation Position—Side Lying

Figure 18-31 Because the vastus lateralis is located so far laterally, it is easily palpable with the client in side lying position. Palpate anterior, deep to, and posterior to the iliotibial band and feel for the contraction of the vastus lateralis as the client extends the leg at the knee joint. Note: In this position, because extension of the leg is not against gravity, it is usually necessary to add resistance to leg extension with the support hand to increase the strength of the vastus lateralis contraction, thereby making it more easily palpable.

18

QUADRICEPS FEMORIS GROUP—SUPINE—cont'd

TRIGGER POINTS

1. Trigger points (TrPs) in the quadriceps femoris often result from or are perpetuated by acute or chronic overuse of the musculature (e.g., running, cycling), direct trauma, or a lack of stretching of the quadriceps femoris due to a lack of full knee flexion (this may occur in sedentary individuals as well as those recovering from surgery or fracture of the hip or knee joints). Other factors include placing a heavy weight on the lap when sitting (e.g., laptop computer, child) or receiving repeated intramuscular injections.

2. TrPs in the quadriceps femoris often produce knee joint pain (this is common in children and adults); at times weakness of the knee joint occurs, sometimes resulting in a buckling of the knee joint when walking. Clients with vastus lateralis TrPs are often unable to sleep on the affected side.

3. The referral patterns of quadriceps femoris TrPs must be distinguished from the referral patterns of gluteus minimus, gluteus medius, sartorius, tensor fasciae latae, the three "adductors" of the thigh, gracilis, and possibly pectineus and iliopsoas.

4. TrPs in the quadriceps femoris are often incorrectly assessed as knee joint dysfunction, trochanteric bursitis, or meralgia paresthetica.

5. Associated TrPs often occur in the other quadriceps femoris muscles, hamstrings, iliopsoas, sartorius, the three "adductors" of the thigh, and gluteus minimus.

Figure 18-32 Views of the quadriceps femoris muscles' common TrPs with their referral zones. **A**, Anterior view of the rectus femoris. **B**, Anterior view of the vastus medialis. **C**, Lateral view of the vastus lateralis. **D**, Anterior view of the vastus intermedius.

18

QUADRICEPS FEMORIS GROUP—SUPINE—cont'd

STRETCHING THE QUADRICEPS FEMORIS

Palpation Key:
Extension of
the leg.

Figure 18-33 A stretch of the right quadriceps femoris group. The client stands and uses his hand to pull the knee joint into full flexion. If the hip joint is extended while doing this stretch, it targets the stretch more to the rectus femoris, but if the hip joint is flexed, it targets the stretch more to the vastus muscles. Note: It is important when doing this stretch to make sure that the knee joint is not rotated.

18

PECTINEUS—SUPINE

❑ ATTACHMENTS:

o Superior pubic ramus *to the* pectineal line on the proximal posterior shaft of the femur

❑ ACTIONS:

o Adducts and flexes the thigh at the hip joint
o Anteriorly tilts the pelvis at the hip joint

Starting position (Figure 18-35, A):

o Client supine with thighs on the table and legs hanging off the table
o Therapist standing to the side of the client
o Place palpating fingers on the proximal anteromedial thigh and locate the proximal tendon of the adductor longus. To locate it, simply palpate along the pubic bone from lateral to medial until you encounter a prominent tendon (it is the most prominent tendon in the region) (Figure 18-35, B)
o Support hand placed on the distal anteromedial thigh, just proximal to the knee joint

Palpation steps:

1. After locating the proximal tendon of the adductor longus, drop off it anteriorly (laterally) and you will be on the pectineus (Figure 18-35, C).
2. To engage the pectineus, palpate against the pubic bone while asking the client to adduct the thigh at the hip joint. Using your support hand to add resistance is usually helpful (Figure 18-36).

Figure 18-34 Anterior view of the right pectineus. The adductor longus has been cut and ghosted in.

3. Once located, strum perpendicular to the fibers and continue palpating the pectineus distally as far as possible.
4. Once the pectineus has been located, have the client relax it and palpate to assess its baseline tone.

Figure 18-35 Locating the pectineus by first finding the adductor longus tendon. **A**, Starting position for supine palpation of the pectineus. **B**, The therapist first locates and palpates the proximal tendon of the adductor longus, which is the most prominent tendon in the region. **C**, The therapist drops anteriorly (laterally) immediately off the adductor longus tendon onto the pectineus.

18

PECTINEUS—SUPINE—cont'd

Figure 18-36 This figure shows engagement and palpation of the pectineus as the client adducts the thigh against resistance.

Palpation Notes:

1. When locating the pectineus, the adductor longus tendon is an excellent landmark to use because it is the most prominent tendon in this region of the thigh. When locating it, it is necessary to palpate directly next to the pubic bone. If you are too far distal in the thigh, you will not be able to feel it.

2. Another way to find the pectineus is to first locate the distal tendon of the iliopsoas (see page 387) and then drop off it medially (posteriorly) and you will be on the pectineus. The border between the iliopsoas and pectineus can be distinguished by asking the client to perform a curl-up of the trunk. This will tense the psoas major tendon but not the pectineus. If you are still on the iliopsoas, keep moving medially along the pubic bone; once you reach tissue that does not engage and tense with this trunk motion, you are on the pectineus.

3. Even though much of the pectineus is superficial, it is recessed compared with the adjacent muscles. When palpating for the pectineus, it often feels as though the palpating fingers drop into a depression or pocket. For this reason, it is sometimes slightly difficult to locate at first and may require either deeper pressure or greater resistance to adduction of the thigh at the hip joint.

4. Keep in mind that asking the client to actively adduct the thigh at the hip joint will cause the other adductors in the region to contract as well.

5. If asking the client to adduct the thigh at the hip joint does not engage the pectineus, you can try asking the client to flex the thigh instead (resistance can be added with your support hand). However, keep in mind that all muscles in the anterior thigh will contract with thigh flexion.

6. **Be careful when palpating the proximal anterior thigh, because the femoral nerve, artery, and vein are located over the iliopsoas and pectineus in this region. If you feel a pulse under your fingers, either gently move the artery out of the way or slightly move your palpating fingers off the artery. Similarly, if you are pressing on the femoral nerve and the client feels shooting pain, move your palpating fingers off the nerve.**

TRIGGER POINTS

1. Trigger points (TrPs) in the pectineus often result from or are perpetuated by acute or chronic overuse of the muscle (during such activities as horseback riding, gymnastics, or sexual intercourse), or prolonged shortening of the muscle due to sitting cross-legged or sleeping in the fetal position. They may also occur secondary to degenerative joint disease of the hip.

2. TrPs in the pectineus tend to produce deep dull pain in the groin.

3. The referral patterns of pectineus TrPs must be distinguished from the referral patterns of TrPs in the iliopsoas, sartorius, gracilis, and the three "adductors" of the thigh.

4. TrPs in the pectineus are often incorrectly assessed as degenerative joint disease of the hip or obturator nerve entrapment.

5. Associated TrPs often occur in the iliopsoas, gracilis, and the three "adductors" of the thigh.

Figure 18-37 Anteromedial view showing a common pectineus TrP with its corresponding referral zone.

18

PECTINEUS—SUPINE—cont'd

STRETCHING THE PECTINEUS

Palpation Key:
Drop anteriorly off the adductor longus tendon.

Figure 18-38 A stretch of the right pectineus. The client extends, abducts, and laterally rotates the right thigh while leaning forward with the pelvis (posteriorly tilting it) and trunk to increase the stretch across the hip joint. Note: It is important to not let the pelvis fall into anterior tilt and to make sure that excessive weight is not placed on the ankle joint of the foot in back. See Figure 18-43, page 441, and Figure 18-57, page 449, for two other stretches of the pectineus.

18

ADDUCTOR LONGUS—SUPINE

❑ ATTACHMENTS:
o Body of the pubic bone *to the* linea aspera of the femur

❑ ACTIONS:
o Adducts and flexes the thigh at the hip joint
o Anteriorly tilts the pelvis at the hip joint

Starting position (Figure 18-40):
o Client supine with thighs on the table and legs hanging off the table
o Therapist standing to the side of the client
o Palpating fingers placed on the prominent tendon of the adductor longus in the proximal anterior thigh
o Support hand placed on the distal anteromedial thigh, just proximal to the knee joint

Palpation steps:
1. The proximal tendon of the adductor longus is the most prominent tendon in the medial thigh and usually easily palpable. To locate it, simply palpate along the pubic bone from lateral to medial until you encounter a prominent tendon.
2. Once located, to confirm that you are on it, ask the client to adduct the thigh at the hip joint against resistance and feel for it to tense (Figure 18-41).
3. Strum perpendicular to the tendon to palpate its width.
4. Continue to palpate it distally as far as possible toward its linea aspera attachment.
5. Once the adductor longus has been located, have the client relax it and palpate to assess its baseline tone.

Figure 18-39 Anterior view of the right adductor longus. The pectineus has been cut and ghosted in.

Figure 18-40 Palpation of the right adductor longus. **A,** Starting position for supine palpation of the adductor longus. **B,** Location of the proximal tendon of the adductor longus, which is the most prominent tendon of the region.

18

ADDUCTOR LONGUS—SUPINE—cont'd

Figure 18-41 Engagement and palpation of the right adductor longus as the client adducts the thigh at the hip joint against resistance.

Palpation Notes:
1. The proximal tendon of the adductor longus is very prominent and easily palpable, even when the muscle is relaxed. It is also an excellent landmark to use to find the pectineus (located anterior to the adductor longus) and the gracilis (located posterior to the adductor longus). If you encounter difficulty locating the adductor longus' proximal tendon, then you are probably not palpating proximally enough. It is necessary to palpate directly along the pubic bone.
2. Proximally, the medial border of the adductor longus forms the medial border of the femoral triangle. Located within the femoral triangle are the iliopsoas and pectineus muscles, and the femoral nerve, artery, and vein.

TRIGGER POINTS

1. Trigger points (TrPs) in the adductor longus often result from or are perpetuated by acute or chronic overuse of the muscle (during such activities as horseback riding), or prolonged shortening of the muscle due to sleeping on one's side with the thigh in adduction, or sitting for prolonged periods, especially with the legs crossed.
2. TrPs in the adductor longus may be the leading cause of groin pain, and often restrict abduction of the thigh at the hip joint.
3. The referral patterns of adductor longus TrPs must be distinguished from the referral patterns of TrPs in the other two "adductor" muscles, pectineus, sartorius, and the vastus medialis.
4. TrPs in the adductor longus are often incorrectly assessed as an adductor tendinitis/periostitis, degenerative joint disease of the hip, inguinal hernia, prostatitis, or nerve entrapment of the obturator or genitofemoral nerves.
5. Associated TrPs often occur in the other two "adductor" muscles, the gracilis, pectineus, and the vastus medialis.

Figure 18-42 Anterior view showing a common adductor longus TrP with its corresponding referral zone.

ADDUCTOR LONGUS—SUPINE—cont'd

STRETCHING THE ADDUCTOR LONGUS

Palpation Key:
Most prominent tendon in the groin region.

Figure 18-43 A stretch of the bilateral adductors longus and brevis. The client sits and lets gravity pull the thighs into abduction and extension; the client can then use his hands to increase the stretch. See Figure 18-38, page 438, and Figure 18-57, page 449, for two other stretches of the adductors longus and brevis.

18

ADDUCTOR LONGUS—SUPINE—cont'd

DETOUR

Adductor Brevis: The adductor brevis attaches from the pubic bone to the linea aspera of the femur and is usually located entirely deep to other adductors of the hip joint, principally the adductor longus. It also has the same actions (adduction and flexion of the thigh at the hip joint) as the nearby adductors. For this reason, it is extremely difficult to palpate and discern the adductor brevis. However, a small part of it is sometimes accessible between the adductor longus and the gracilis. To palpate the adductor brevis, find the border between the adductor longus and gracilis and try to press between these two muscles, palpating deeper for the adductor brevis (Figure 18-44, B). Alternatively, you can try palpating the adductor brevis through the adductor longus. Keep in mind that if you ask the client to adduct the thigh, all adductors in the region will likely engage, obscuring discernment of the palpation of the adductor brevis.

Trigger Points:
1. Factors that create and/or perpetuate TrPs in the adductor brevis and symptoms caused by TrPs in the adductor brevis are the same as for the adductor longus.
2. TrP referral patterns for the adductor brevis have not been distinguished from the referral patterns for the adductor longus.
3. Note: Due to its depth, palpating and discerning TrPs in the adductor brevis can be difficult.

Adductor brevis

Adductor longus (cut)

Adductor brevis

Adductor longus (cut)

A

B

Figure 18-44 The adductor brevis. **A**, Anterior view. The adductor longus has been cut and ghosted in on the left. **B**, Palpation of the right adductor brevis proximally between the adductor longus (ghosted in) and gracilis as the client adducts the thigh against resistance.

Palpation Key:
Palpate between the adductor longus and gracilis.

18

GRACILIS—SUPINE

❑ **ATTACHMENTS:**

o Body and inferior ramus of the pubic bone *to the* pes anserine tendon at the proximal anteromedial tibia

❑ **ACTIONS:**

o Flexes and medially rotates the leg at the knee joint
o Adducts and flexes the thigh at the hip joint
o Anteriorly tilts the pelvis at the hip joint

Starting position (Figure 18-46, A):

o Client supine with thighs on the table and legs hanging off the table
o Therapist standing to the side of the client
o Palpating fingers placed on the proximal medial thigh, on the proximal tendon of the adductor longus

Palpation steps:

1. First locate the proximal tendon of the adductor longus; it is the most prominent tendon in the region. To locate it, simply palpate along the pubic bone from lateral to medial until you encounter a prominent tendon (Figure 18-46, B and C). Then drop just off it posteriorly (medially) and you will be on the gracilis (Figure 18-47, A).
2. Ask the client to engage the gracilis by flexing the leg at the knee joint; this can be easily accomplished by asking the client to press the leg against the table. This will engage the gracilis, but not the adductor longus and adductor magnus on either side of it, making it easy to discern the gracilis in the proximal thigh (Figure 18-47, B).

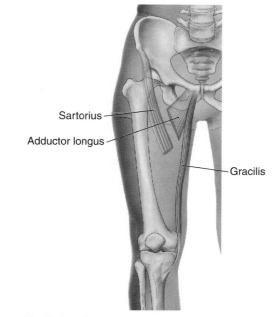

Figure 18-45 Anterior view of the right gracilis. The adductor longus and sartorius have been cut and ghosted in.

3. Once located, strum perpendicular to the fibers and continue palpating the gracilis distally as far as possible.
4. Once the gracilis has been located, have the client relax it and palpate to assess its baseline tone.

Figure 18-46 Locating the right proximal gracilis by first locating the adductor longus tendon. **A**, Starting position for supine palpation of the right gracilis. **B** and **C**, The therapist first locates and palpates the proximal tendon of the adductor longus, which is the most prominent tendon in the region.

18

GRACILIS—SUPINE—cont'd

Figure 18-47 Palpation of the right proximal gracilis. **A,** The therapist locates the proximal tendon of the gracilis by dropping medially off the adductor longus tendon. **B,** Engagement and palpation of the gracilis as the client flexes the leg against the resistance of the table.

Palpation Notes:

1. In the proximal thigh, the gracilis is bordered by the adductor longus anteriorly and the adductor magnus posteriorly. Because neither of these other two muscles crosses the knee joint, having the client flex the leg at the knee joint against the table engages the gracilis but not these adjacent muscles. This allows for effective palpation and discernment of the gracilis proximally.

2. To distinguish the gracilis from the sartorius in the distal thigh, use abduction and adduction of the thigh at the hip joint. The sartorius will engage with abduction; the gracilis will engage with adduction.

3. The distal tendon of the gracilis can also be easily located. Palpate the distal posteromedial thigh while the client medially rotates the leg at the knee joint (the knee joint must be flexed to be able to rotate), and feel for two tendons to noticeably tense (Figure 18-48). The gracilis is the smaller and more medial one of the two (the semitendinosus is the other one and is larger and more lateral; in other words, closer to the midline of the thigh). Once located, strum perpendicular and palpate the gracilis proximally toward the pubic bone.

Figure 18-48 Seated palpation of the distal tendon of the right gracilis as the client medially rotates the leg at the knee joint. The semitendinosus has been ghosted in. Note: For the purpose of this photo, the client is standing with the foot on a stool.

GRACILIS—SUPINE—cont'd

Alternate Palpation Position—Seated, Prone, or Side Lying
The gracilis can be palpated with the client in a number of positions. Seated palpation is effective (see Palpation Note #3 and Figure 18-48). The gracilis can also be palpated with the client prone; from this perspective it is located beyond (anterior to) the adductor magnus. The gracilis can also be palpated with the client side lying. In this position, palpate the gracilis of the lower extremity that is against the table. Note: To access this gracilis, it is necessary to have the client's thigh of the lower extremity that is away from the table flexed at the hip and knee joints. Use resisted flexion of the leg at the knee joint to engage the gracilis and feel for its contraction (Figure 18-49).

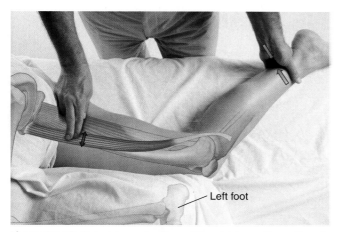

— Left foot

Figure 18-49 Side lying palpation of the right gracilis as the client flexes the leg at the knee joint against resistance. The adductor magnus has been ghosted in. Note: To access the right gracilis, the client's left lower extremity is flexed at the hip and knee joints.

TRIGGER POINTS

1. Trigger points (TrPs) in the gracilis often result from or are perpetuated by acute or chronic overuse of the muscle (during such activities as horseback riding), or prolonged shortening of the muscle due to sleeping on one's side with the thigh in adduction, or sitting for prolonged periods, especially with the legs crossed.
2. TrPs in the gracilis may produce either a hot stinging pain or a dull ache, and may result in a decrease in range of the motion of abduction of the thigh at the hip joint. Clients with TrPs in the gracilis often have difficulty finding a position of comfort.
3. The referral patterns of gracilis TrPs must be distinguished from the referral patterns of TrPs in the three "adductors" of the thigh, pectineus, sartorius, and vastus medialis.
4. TrPs in the gracilis are often incorrectly assessed as an adductor tendinitis/periostitis, inguinal hernia, pes anserine bursitis, prostatitis, or nerve entrapment of the obturator or genitofemoral nerves.
5. Associated TrPs often occur in the distal sartorius.

Figure 18-50 Medial view showing common gracilis TrPs with their corresponding referral zone.

18

GRACILIS—SUPINE—cont'd

STRETCHING THE GRACILIS

Palpation Key:
Drop posteriorly off the adductor longus tendon.

Figure 18-51 A stretch of the right gracilis. The client extends, abducts, and laterally rotates the right thigh at the hip joint while keeping the knee joint extended and leaning forward with the pelvis (posteriorly tilting it) and trunk to increase the stretch across the hip joint. Note: It is important to not let the pelvis fall into anterior tilt and to make sure that excessive weight is not placed on the ankle joint of the foot in back. See Figure 18-57, page 449, for another stretch of the gracilis.

18

ADDUCTOR MAGNUS—SUPINE

❑ **ATTACHMENTS:**

o Ischial tuberosity and the ischiopubic ramus *to the* linea aspera and adductor tubercle of the femur

❑ **ACTIONS:**

o Adducts and extends the thigh at the hip joint
o Posteriorly tilts the pelvis at the hip joint

Starting position (Figure 18-53):

o Client supine with the thighs on the table and the legs hanging off the table
o Therapist standing to the side of the client
o Palpating fingers placed on the proximal medial thigh (between the gracilis and medial hamstrings)
o Support hand placed on the distal medial thigh

Palpation steps:

1. The adductor magnus is actually quite easily palpable in the proximal medial thigh between the gracilis and the medial hamstring muscles (semitendinosus and semi-membranosus), where it is located in a depression between these muscles.
2. Locate the adductor magnus by first locating the gracilis and medial hamstrings, which contract with flexion of the leg at the knee joint, performed by asking the client to press the leg against the table. Once you feel these muscles palpably harden with leg flexion, feel for the adductor magnus between them (it will stay relaxed and soft during this joint action) (Figure 18-54, A).
3. To engage the adductor magnus and confirm that you are on it, ask the client to either adduct the thigh against resistance supplied by your support hand, or to extend the

Figure 18-52 Posterior view of the right adductor magnus.

thigh at the hip joint against the resistance of the table (as shown in Figure 18-54, B).
4. Continue palpating the adductor magnus distally as far as possible by strumming perpendicular to the fibers as the client alternately contracts and relaxes it.
5. Once the adductor magnus has been located, have the client relax it and palpate to assess its baseline tone.

Figure 18-53 Starting position for supine palpation of the right adductor magnus.

18

ADDUCTOR MAGNUS—SUPINE—cont'd

Figure 18-54 Palpation of the right adductor magnus in the medial thigh between the gracilis and medial hamstrings. **A,** The gracilis and medial hamstrings engage when the client flexes the leg at the knee joint by pressing the leg against the table. **B,** Engagement and palpation of the adductor magnus between these muscles as the client extends the thigh at the hip joint by pressing the thigh down against the table.

Palpation Notes:

1. The easiest way to confirm that you are on the adductor magnus is to ask the client to flex the leg at the knee joint. The gracilis and medial hamstring musculature (semitendinosus and semimembranosus) located on either side of the adductor magnus will contract with this joint action and become palpably hard, whereas the adductor magnus will not contract and will remain relaxed and soft. If you are between these two other muscles, you are on the adductor magnus.

2. The adductor magnus itself can be engaged by asking the client to adduct or extend the thigh at the hip joint against resistance. Note that the gracilis will also contract with adduction, but not with extension. Also, the medial hamstrings will also contract with extension, but not with adduction. Therefore these actions can also be used to distinguish the borders of the adductor magnus with these two adjacent muscles.

3. The adductor magnus sits in a slightly recessed depression in the medial thigh between the gracilis and the medial hamstrings. Therefore it is usually necessary to gently but firmly press in to feel this muscle.

4. Other than the portion of the adductor magnus that is superficial in the proximal medial thigh, most of the rest of the muscle is deep and difficult to discern from adjacent musculature. From the anterior perspective, the adductor magnus can be looked at as a floor for the other more anterior adductor muscles of the thigh. From the posterior perspective, the adductor magnus can be looked at as a floor for the more posterior hamstring muscles of the thigh.

5. The attachment on the adductor tubercle at the medial side of the knee joint is often palpable.

Alternate Palpation Position—Prone or Side Lying

The adductor magnus can also be accessed with the client prone or side lying. In prone position, the adductor magnus is located directly anterior to the medial hamstring muscles (see Figure 18-1, A). In side lying position, the client's lower extremity that is away from the table must be flexed at the hip and knee joints so that the adductor magnus of the thigh that is against the table can be accessed.

Figure 18-55 Side lying palpation of the right adductor magnus.

ADDUCTOR MAGNUS—SUPINE—cont'd

TRIGGER POINTS

1. Trigger points (TrPs) in the adductor magnus often result from or are perpetuated by acute or chronic overuse of the muscle (during such activities as skiing or horseback riding), or prolonged shortening of the muscle due to sleeping on one's side with the thigh in adduction, or sitting for prolonged periods, especially with the legs crossed.

2. Clients with adductor magnus TrPs often experience difficulty positioning their lower extremity at night. The more proximal TrP (Figure 18-56, B) of the adductor magnus can create pain that is felt within the pelvis; in some clients, this pain occurs during sexual intercourse.

3. The referral patterns of adductor magnus TrPs must be distinguished from the referral patterns of TrPs in the other two "adductors," pectineus, sartorius, vastus medialis, and perhaps the iliopsoas.

4. TrPs in the adductor magnus are often incorrectly assessed as an adductor tendinitis/periostitis, inguinal hernia, prostatitis, visceral or gynecologic disease, or nerve entrapment of the obturator or genitofemoral nerves.

5. Associated TrPs often occur in the other two "adductor" muscles, the pectineus, and the vastus medialis.

6. Note: Because much of the adductor magnus is deep, palpating TrPs in this muscle can be difficult.

Figure 18-56 Views of the right adductor magnus with common TrPs and their corresponding referral zones. **A**, Anterior view. **B**, Medial view of a sagittal section through the pelvis showing another common adductor magnus TrP with its internal visceral referral zone.

STRETCHING THE ADDUCTOR MAGNUS

Figure 18-57 A stretch of the bilateral adductor magnus muscles. The client lies against a wall and lets gravity pull his thighs into abduction. See Figure 18-43, page 441, for another stretch of the adductor magnus. Figure 18-51, page 446, shows a good stretch of the most proximal fibers of the anterior head (the adductor minimus portion) of the adductor magnus.

Palpation Key:
Between the gracilis and medial hamstrings.

18

Whirlwind Tour   **Muscles of the Thigh**

For all palpations of the muscles of the thigh, the therapist is standing to the side of the client.

Client Supine:

For all palpations of the muscles of the thigh except the prone palpation of the hamstrings at the end, the client is supine with the thighs on the table and the legs hanging off the table.

1. **Tensor fasciae latae (TFL):** Have the client first medially rotate the thigh at the hip joint and then flex the thigh into the air. Palpating just distal and lateral to the anterior superior iliac spine (ASIS), feel for the contraction of the TFL. Strum perpendicular and palpate to the distal attachment.

2. **Sartorius:** Have the client first laterally rotate the thigh at the hip joint and then flex the thigh into the air. Palpating just distal and medial to the ASIS, feel for the contraction of the sartorius. Strum perpendicular and palpate toward the distal attachment as far as possible. Distally, the sartorius is directly posterior to the vastus medialis; use extension of the leg at the knee joint to locate the vastus medialis. Confirm that you are on the distal sartorius by asking the client to flex the leg at the knee joint against the resistance of the table.

3. **Quadriceps femoris group:** Proximally, the rectus femoris is between the sartorius and the TFL. Find either one of these muscles and then drop onto the rectus femoris. Ask the client to extend the leg at the knee joint and feel for the contraction of the rectus femoris. Strum perpendicular and palpate to the distal attachment. Palpate in the distal anteromedial thigh for the vastus medialis and in the anterolateral, lateral, and posterolateral thigh for the vastus lateralis, always using leg extension to engage these muscles.

4. **Iliopsoas distal belly and tendon:** Find the proximal attachment of the sartorius and drop immediately medial onto the distal belly and tendon of the iliopsoas. Ask the client to do a gentle curl-up of the trunk and feel for the tensing of the belly and tendon of the psoas major. Be aware of the presence of the femoral nerve, artery, and vein in this region.

5. **Adductor longus:** Palpate along the pubic bone within the anteromedial thigh, feeling for the prominent tendon of the adductor longus. Once located, ask the client to adduct the thigh against gentle to moderate resistance and feel for the contraction of the adductor longus. Strum perpendicular and continue palpating distally as far as possible. Be aware that all adductors in this region will contract with resisted adduction of the thigh.

6. **Pectineus:** First locate the proximal tendon of the adductor longus and then drop immediately off it laterally (anteriorly) onto the pectineus. Ask the client to either adduct and/or flex the thigh at the hip joint and feel for its contraction. Pressing deeper and/or adding greater resistance may be necessary. Strum perpendicular and continue palpating the pectineus distally as far as possible. Be aware of the presence of the femoral nerve, artery, and vein in this region.

7. **Gracilis:** First find the proximal tendon of the adductor longus and then drop off it immediately medially (posteriorly) onto the gracilis. Ask the client to flex the leg at the knee joint by pressing the leg against the table and feel for the contraction of the gracilis. Strum perpendicular to the fibers and follow distally to the pes anserine. Note: The distal tendon can also be located by palpating the distal posteromedial thigh and asking the client to medially rotate the leg at the knee joint, feeling for the gracilis and semitendinosus tendons to noticeably tense. The gracilis is the smaller and more medially located of the two tendons. Strum perpendicular and palpate it proximally to the pubic bone.

8. **Adductor magnus:** Palpate immediately posterior from the gracilis onto the adductor magnus. You know you are on the adductor magnus when you do not feel a contraction when the client presses the leg against the table (flexion of the leg at the knee joint). Confirm you are on the adductor magnus by resisting the client from adducting the thigh at the hip joint (be aware that all adductors in this region may engage with this action) or by extending the thigh at the hip joint by pressing the thigh against the table (be aware that the hamstrings will likely engage with this action). Palpate distally as far as possible by strumming perpendicular to the fibers. Note: The adductor magnus is located between the gracilis and medial hamstring muscles; these muscles can be felt to contract when the client presses the leg against the table (flexion of the leg at the knee joint). The adductor magnus does not cross the knee joint and will stay relaxed when the leg flexes at the knee joint.

9. **Hamstrings (supine):** From the adductor magnus, palpate immediately posterior onto the medial hamstrings (semitendinosus and semimembranosus). Confirm that you are on the hamstrings by feeling their contraction when the client presses the leg against the table (flexion of the leg at the knee joint).

Client Prone with the Leg Partially Flexed at the Knee Joint:

10. **Entire hamstring group:** Resist the client from further flexing the leg at the knee joint and feel for the common proximal attachment of the hamstring group just distal to the ischial tuberosity. Strum perpendicular to the fibers and continue palpating the biceps femoris distally toward the head of the fibula. Then strum perpendicularly and continue palpating the medial hamstrings distally toward the medial side of the leg. The medial and lateral hamstrings are side by side in the proximal thigh, but they diverge in the distal thigh. Note: The semitendinosus is generally superficial to the semimembranosus, and its distal tendon is very prominent. Palpate on either side of the distal semitendinosus for the semimembranosus.

18

Chapter 19

Tour #10—Palpation of the Leg Muscles

Overview

This chapter is a palpation tour of the muscles of the leg. The tour begins with the muscles of the anterior compartment, then covers the muscles of the lateral compartment, and concludes with the muscles of the superficial and deep posterior compartments. Palpation of the muscles of the anterior compartment is shown supine; palpation of the muscles of the lateral compartment is shown side lying; and palpation of the muscles of the posterior compartments is shown prone. Alternate palpation positions for most of the muscles are also described. The major muscles or muscle groups of the region are each given a separate layout. There are also a few detours to other muscles of the region. Trigger point (TrP) information and stretching is given for each of the muscles covered in this chapter. The chapter closes with an advanced *Whirlwind Tour* that explains the sequential palpation of all of the muscles of the chapter.

Chapter Outline

Chapter Objectives

After completing this chapter, the student should be able to perform the following for each of the muscles covered in this chapter:

1. State the attachments.
2. State the actions.
3. Describe the starting position for palpation.
4. Describe and explain the purpose of each of the palpation steps.
5. Palpate each muscle.
6. State the "Palpation Key."
7. Describe alternate palpation positions.
8. State the locations of the most common TrP(s).
9. Describe the TrP referral zones.
10. State the most common factors that create and/or perpetuate TrPs.
11. State the symptoms most commonly caused by TrPs.
12. Describe and perform a stretch.

Video demonstrations of the muscle palpations in this chapter are presented in Chapter 19 on DVD 1.

A

B

Figure 19-1 Anterior views of the right leg. **A**, Superficial view.
B, Deeper view (the tibialis anterior has been removed).

Quadriceps femoris
Iliotibial band (ITB)
Sartorius
Patella
Head of fibula
Pes anserine tendons
Fibularis longus
Gastrocnemius medial head
Tibialis anterior
Extensor digitorum longus
Soleus
Fibularis brevis
Flexor digitorum longus
Fibularis tertius
Superior and inferior extensor retinacula
Extensor hallucis longus
Lateral malleolus of fibula

Iliotibial band (ITB)
Patella
Quadriceps femoris
Head of fibula
Sartorius
Fibularis longus
Pes anserine tendons
Gastrocnemius medial head
Extensor digitorum longus
Soleus
Fibularis brevis
Extensor hallucis longus
Fibularis tertius
Flexor digitorum longus
Medial malleolus of tibia
Lateral malleolus of fibula

19

Semitendinosus

Gracilis

Sartorius

Semimembranosus

Vastus lateralis

Biceps femoris

Femoral artery and vein, tibial nerve

Plantaris

Common fibular nerve

Gastrocnemius lateral head

Gastrocnemius medial head

Soleus

Fibularis longus

Plantaris tendon

Fibularis brevis

Flexor digitorum longus

Flexor hallucis longus

Medial malleolus of tibia

Calcaneus

Lateral malleolus of fibula

Tibialis posterior

Fibularis brevis tendon

Tibialis anterior

Flexor digitorum longus tendon

Flexor hallucis longus

Fibularis longus tendon

A

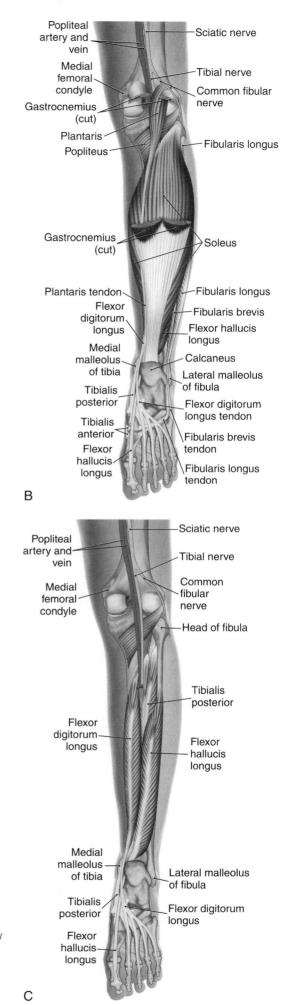

Popliteal artery and vein

Medial femoral condyle

Gastrocnemius (cut)

Plantaris

Popliteus

Sciatic nerve

Tibial nerve

Common fibular nerve

Fibularis longus

Gastrocnemius (cut)

Soleus

Plantaris tendon

Flexor digitorum longus

Medial malleolus of tibia

Tibialis posterior

Tibialis anterior

Flexor hallucis longus

Fibularis longus

Fibularis brevis

Flexor hallucis longus

Calcaneus

Lateral malleolus of fibula

Flexor digitorum longus tendon

Fibularis brevis tendon

Fibularis longus tendon

B

Popliteal artery and vein

Medial femoral condyle

Flexor digitorum longus

Medial malleolus of tibia

Tibialis posterior

Flexor hallucis longus

Sciatic nerve

Tibial nerve

Common fibular nerve

Head of fibula

Tibialis posterior

Flexor hallucis longus

Lateral malleolus of fibula

Flexor digitorum longus

C

Figure 19-2 Posterior views of the right leg. **A**, Superficial view. **B**, Intermediate view (the gastrocnemius has been cut). **C**, Deep view (the gastrocnemius, soleus, and plantaris have been removed).

19

YOU ARE HERE

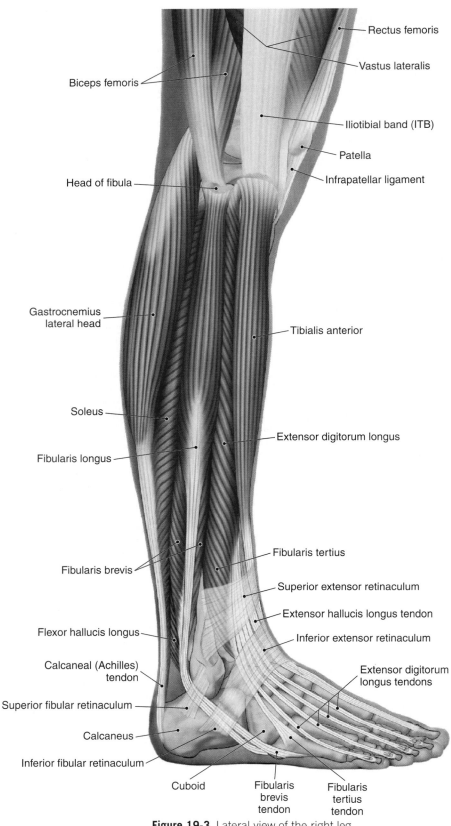

Figure 19-3 Lateral view of the right leg.

19

Rectus femoris

Vastus medialis

Patella

Retinacular fibers

Pes anserine tendons

Tibialis anterior

Tibia

Superior extensor retinaculum

Extensor digitorum longus tendons

Extensor hallucis longus tendon

1st metatarsal

A

Sartorius

Gracilis

Semitendinosus

Semimembranosus

Gastrocnemius medial head

Soleus

Tibialis posterior

Flexor digitorum longus

Flexor hallucis longus

Medial malleolus of tibia

Calcaneal (Achilles) tendon

Flexor retinaculum

Inferior extensor retinaculum

Tibialis posterior

Flexor hallucis longus

Flexor digitorum longus

Medial malleolus of tibia

B

19

Figure 19-4 Medial views of the right leg. **A**, Superficial view. **B**, Deep view.

❑ ATTACHMENTS:

o Lateral tibial condyle and the proximal ⅔ of the anterior border of the tibia *to the* first cuneiform and the base of the first metatarsal (Figure 19-5)

❑ ACTIONS:

o Dorsiflexes the foot at the ankle joint; inverts the foot at the tarsal joints

Starting position (Figure 19-6):

o Client supine
o Therapist standing to the side of the client
o Palpating hand not yet placed on the client
o Support hand placed on the medial side of the distal foot

Palpation steps:

1. Resist the client from dorsiflexing and inverting the foot and look for the distal tendon of the tibialis anterior on the medial side of the ankle joint and foot; it is usually visible (Figure 19-7).
2. Palpate the distal tendon by strumming perpendicular across it. Continue palpating the tibialis anterior proximally to the lateral tibial condyle by strumming perpendicular to the fibers. Its belly is located directly lateral to the border of the tibia in the anterior leg (Figure 19-8).
3. Once the tibialis anterior has been located, have the client relax it and palpate to assess its baseline tone.

Figure 19-5 Anterior view of the right tibialis anterior.

Figure 19-6 Starting position for supine palpation of the right tibialis anterior.

Figure 19-7 With resisted dorsiflexion and inversion of the foot, the distal tendon of the tibialis anterior is usually easily visible.

TIBIALIS ANTERIOR—SUPINE—cont'd

Figure 19-8 Palpation of the belly of the right tibialis anterior.

Palpation Notes:

1. As with all superficial muscles, it is always best to look before placing your palpating hand over the muscle. Otherwise your hand may block your view, making it difficult to see and locate the muscle and its tendon.
2. The distal tendon of the tibialis anterior is usually very prominent and visible. The belly is also usually prominent and visible directly lateral to the shaft of the tibia in the anterior leg. If the tendon and belly are not visible, they can usually be easily palpated by strumming perpendicularly.
3. The distal attachment of the tibialis anterior can be discerned with careful palpation. Follow the tibialis anterior toward the first cuneiform and base of the first metatarsal while having the client alternately contract and relax it against gentle resistance (see Figure 19-7).
4. To clearly discern the border between the tibialis anterior and the adjacent extensor digitorum longus (EDL), do not ask the client to dorsiflex the foot because it will engage both muscles. Instead use inversion and eversion. Inversion will engage the tibialis anterior but not the EDL; eversion will engage the EDL but not the tibialis anterior.
5. The belly and tendon of the extensor hallucis longus (EHL) are located directly next to the tibialis anterior, and this muscle also contracts with dorsiflexion and inversion of the foot. If the presence of this muscle makes it difficult to discern the tibialis anterior, ask the client to flex the big toe while you gently resist foot dorsiflexion and inversion. Flexion of the big toe will reciprocally inhibit the EHL (remember that strong resistance to foot dorsiflexion/inversion will likely override reciprocal inhibition of the EHL).

Alternate Palpation Position—Seated
The tibialis anterior can also be easily palpated with the client seated.

TRIGGER POINTS

1. Trigger points (TrPs) in the tibialis anterior often result from or are perpetuated by acute or chronic overuse of the muscle, trauma, postures that result in chronic shortening of the muscle, and tight antagonistic ankle joint plantarflexor muscles.
2. TrPs in the tibialis anterior may produce weakness of dorsiflexion of the foot (which may result in foot drop or foot slap).
3. The referral patterns of tibialis anterior TrPs must be distinguished from the referral patterns of TrPs in the extensor hallucis longus, extensor digitorum longus, fibularis tertius, extensor digitorum brevis, extensor hallucis brevis, and first dorsal interosseus pedis.
4. TrPs in the tibialis anterior are often incorrectly assessed as anterior compartment syndrome, anterior shin splints, L5 nerve compression, or first metatarsophalangeal joint dysfunction.
5. Associated TrPs often occur in the fibularis longus, extensor hallucis longus, and extensor digitorum longus.

Figure 19-9 Anteromedial view showing a common tibialis anterior TrP and its corresponding referral zone.

19

YOU ARE HERE

TIBIALIS ANTERIOR—SUPINE—cont'd

STRETCHING THE TIBIALIS ANTERIOR

Palpation Key:
First look for the distal tendon.

Figure 19-10 A stretch of the bilateral tibialis anterior muscles. The client plantarflexes and everts the feet. The stool is used for support and to prevent the client from placing excessive weight upon the toes and feet.

19

EXTENSOR DIGITORUM LONGUS (EDL)—SUPINE

❑ **ATTACHMENTS:**

o Proximal ²/₃ of the anterior fibula and the lateral tibial condyle *to the* dorsal surface of the middle and distal phalanges of toes two to five (Figure 19-11)

❑ **ACTIONS:**

o Extends toes two to five at the metatarsophalangeal (MTP) and interphalangeal (IP) joints
o Dorsiflexes the foot at the ankle joint; everts the foot at the tarsal joints

Starting position (Figure 19-12):

o Client supine
o Therapist standing to the side of the client
o Palpating hand not yet placed on the client
o Fingers of the support hand placed on the dorsal surfaces of toes two to five

Palpation steps:

1. Resist the client from extending toes two to five at the metatarsophalangeal and interphalangeal joints and look for the tendons of the extensor digitorum longus (EDL) to become visible on the dorsum of the foot.
2. Palpate the distal tendons by strumming perpendicularly across them (Figure 19-13, A).
3. Continue palpating the EDL proximally by strumming perpendicular to the fibers (Figure 19-13, B). Most of its belly is located between the tibialis anterior and the fibularis longus (see Figure 19-1, A).
4. Once the EDL has been located, have the client relax it and palpate to assess its baseline tone.

Figure 19-11 Anterior view of the right extensor digitorum longus. The fibularis tertius has been ghosted in.

Extensor digitorum longus

Fibularis tertius

Figure 19-12 Starting position for supine palpation of the right extensor digitorum longus.

19

EXTENSOR DIGITORUM LONGUS (EDL)—SUPINE—cont'd

Figure 19-13 Palpation of the right extensor digitorum longus as the client extends toes two to five against resistance. **A**, Palpation of the distal tendons on the dorsum of the foot. **B**, Palpation of the belly in the anterolateral leg.

Palpation Notes:

1. Many people have difficulty isolating motion of their toes. The client may be unable to extend toes two to five without also extending the big toe. If this occurs, do not restrain the big toe from extending. This may stop the big toe from moving, but will not stop the extensor hallucis longus (EHL) muscle from isometrically contracting. It is the contraction of the belly of the EHL that we do not want.

2. As with all superficial muscles, it is always best to look before placing your palpating hand over the muscle. Otherwise your hand may block your view, making it difficult to see and locate the muscle and its tendon. The distal tendons of the EDL are usually very prominent and visible and can be palpated by strumming perpendicularly.

4. To clearly discern the border between the EDL and the adjacent tibialis anterior, do not ask the client to dorsiflex the foot because it will engage both muscles. Instead use inversion and eversion. Eversion will engage the EDL but not the tibialis anterior; inversion will engage the tibialis anterior but not the EDL.

5. To clearly discern the border between the EDL and the adjacent fibularis longus, do not ask the client to evert the foot because it will engage both muscles. Instead use dorsiflexion and plantarflexion. Dorsiflexion will engage the EDL but not the fibularis longus; plantarflexion will engage the fibularis longus but not the EDL.

Alternate Palpation Position—Seated
The extensor digitorum longus can also be easily palpated with the client seated.

19

EXTENSOR DIGITORUM LONGUS (EDL)—SUPINE—cont'd

TRIGGER POINTS

1. Trigger points (TrPs) in the extensor digitorum longus (EDL) often result from or are perpetuated by acute or chronic overuse of the muscle (especially because of a weak fibularis longus), postures that result in chronic shortening of the muscle (e.g., driving with a sharply angled gas pedal), chronic lengthening of the muscle (e.g., wearing high-heeled shoes or sleeping with foot in dorsiflexion), tight antagonistic ankle joint plantarflexor muscles, trauma, tripping (with ankle joint forced into plantarflexion), anterior compartment syndrome, and L4-L5 nerve compression.
2. TrPs in the EDL may produce ankle joint dorsiflexion weakness (which may result in foot drop or foot slap), entrapment of the deep fibular nerve (which may further dorsiflexion weakness), growing pains, and night cramps in the belly of the muscle.
3. The referral patterns of EDL TrPs must be distinguished from the referral patterns of TrPs in the fibularis longus, fibularis brevis, fibularis tertius, extensor digitorum brevis, dorsal interossei pedis, and extensor hallucis brevis.
4. TrPs in the EDL are often incorrectly assessed as tarsal joint dysfunction, metatarsophalangeal joint dysfunction, or L4 nerve compression.
5. Associated TrPs often occur in the fibularis longus, fibularis brevis, fibularis tertius, tibialis anterior, and extensor hallucis longus.

Figure 19-14 Anterolateral view showing a common extensor digitorum longus TrP and its corresponding referral zone.

Figure 19-15 A stretch of the right extensor digitorum longus. The client plantarflexes and inverts the foot while holding on for support and to prevent placing excessive weight upon the foot in back.

Palpation Key:
First look for the distal tendons going to toes two to five.

19

YOU ARE HERE

EXTENSOR DIGITORUM LONGUS (EDL)—SUPINE—cont'd

DETOUR

Fibularis Tertius: The fibularis tertius is actually the most distal and lateral aspect of the extensor digitorum longus (EDL) and attaches from the distal anterior fibula to the fifth metatarsal. First find the distal tendon of the EDL that goes to the little toe on the dorsum of the foot; then palpate directly lateral to it, feeling for a tendon that goes to the fifth metatarsal. It may not be visible, so you may need to strum perpendicular to its fiber direction to feel for it; it may even be necessary to gently use a fingernail to feel it. If it is not readily palpable, then resist the client from everting and dorsiflexing the foot (actions of the fibularis tertius) and palpate again for its tendon (Figure 19-16, B). Once you have located the distal tendon of the fibularis tertius, resist the client once again from performing the actions of this muscle and palpate the fibularis tertius proximally into the leg (Figure 19-16, C). Given its actions of dorsiflexion and eversion of the foot, the fibularis tertius would be stretched by plantarflexing and inverting the foot.

Note: The fibularis tertius is often missing, unilaterally or bilaterally.

Trigger Points:

1. Factors that create and/or perpetuate trigger points (TrPs) in the fibularis tertius and symptoms caused by TrPs in the fibularis tertius are the same as for the extensor digitorum longus (EDL).
2. TrPs in the fibularis tertius may cause pain with active dorsiflexion of the foot at the ankle joint or pain at the end range of motion of plantarflexion of the foot.
3. TrPs in the fibularis tertius are often associated with TrPs in the fibularis longus, fibularis brevis, and EDL.

Palpation Key:
Palpate lateral to the extensor digitorum longus tendon to the little toe.

Extensor digitorum longus

Fibularis tertius

A   B   C   D

Figure 19-16 Views of the right fibularis tertius. **A,** Anterior view of the right fibularis tertius. The extensor digitorum longus (EDL) has been ghosted in. **B** and **C,** Anterolateral views showing palpation of the distal tendon and belly of the fibularis tertius respectively as the client everts and dorsiflexes the foot against resistance. The EDL has been ghosted in. **D,** Lateral view showing common fibularis tertius TrPs and their corresponding referral zone.

19

EXTENSOR HALLUCIS LONGUS (EHL)—SUPINE

❑ **ATTACHMENTS:**

o Middle $^1/_3$ of the anterior fibula *to the* dorsal surface of the distal phalanx of the big toe (Figure 19-17)

❑ **ACTIONS:**

o Extends the big toe at the metatarsophalangeal (MTP) and interphalangeal (IP) joints
o Dorsiflexes the foot at the ankle joint; inverts the foot at the tarsal joints

Starting position (Figure 19-18):
o Client supine
o Therapist standing to the side of the client
o Palpating hand not yet placed on the client
o Fingers of the support hand placed on the dorsal surface of the distal phalanx of the big toe

Palpation steps:
1. Resist the client from extending the big toe at the metatarsophalangeal and interphalangeal joints and look for the tendon of the extensor hallucis longus (EHL) to become visible.
2. Palpate the distal tendon by strumming perpendicular across it (Figure 19-19, A).
3. Continue palpating the EHL proximally by strumming perpendicular to the fibers. Once the EHL goes deep to the tibialis anterior and extensor digitorum longus; do not strum perpendicular to it. Instead feel for its contraction deep to these other muscles when the big toe extends (Figure 19-19, B).
4. Once the EHL has been located, have the client relax it and palpate to assess its baseline tone.

Figure 19-17 Anterior view of the right extensor hallucis longus.

Figure 19-18 Starting position for supine palpation of the right extensor hallucis longus.

19

EXTENSOR HALLUCIS LONGUS (EHL)—SUPINE—cont'd

Figure 19-19 Palpation of the right extensor hallucis longus as the client extends the big toe against resistance. **A**, Palpation of the distal tendon on the dorsum of the foot. **B**, Palpation of the belly in the anterolateral leg.

Palpation Notes:

1. Many people have difficulty isolating motion of their toes. The client may be unable to extend the big toe without extending the other toes. If this occurs, do not restrain the other toes from extending. This may stop them from moving, but will not stop the extensor digitorum longus (EDL) muscle from isometrically contracting; it is the contraction of the belly of the EDL that we do not want.

2. Most of the belly of the EHL is located between and deep to the tibialis anterior and extensor digitorum longus (EDL). As you palpate the EHL proximally, deep to these other muscles, it can be helpful to close your eyes to eliminate visual sensations from distracting you, and press very lightly with your palpating fingers, feeling for the subtle contraction deeper within the tissue of the EHL when the client extends the big toe, either with or without resistance (see Figure 19-19, B).

3. Do not allow the client to dorsiflex the foot at the ankle joint when palpating the EHL, because all muscles of the anterior leg will contract with dorsiflexion. Also, do not allow the client to invert the foot at the tarsal joints because that will engage the tibialis anterior; similarly do not allow the client to evert the foot, because that will engage the EDL. Any other muscles that contract when palpating the EHL will make it more difficult to palpate and discern it.

Alternate Palpation Position—Seated
The extensor hallucis longus can also be easily palpated with the client seated.

TRIGGER POINTS

1. Trigger points (TrPs) in the extensor hallucis longus (EHL) often result from or are perpetuated by acute or chronic overuse of the muscle, postures that result in chronic shortening of the muscle (e.g., driving with a sharply angled gas pedal), chronic lengthening of the muscle (e.g., wearing high-heeled shoes, sleeping with foot in dorsiflexion), tight antagonistic ankle joint plantarflexor muscles, trauma, tripping (with ankle joint forced into plantarflexion), anterior compartment syndrome, and L4 nerve compression.

2. TrPs in the EHL may produce ankle joint dorsiflexion weakness (which may result in foot drop or foot slap), growing pains, and night cramps in the belly of the muscle.

3. The referral patterns of EHL TrPs must be distinguished from the referral patterns of TrPs in the tibialis anterior and extensor hallucis brevis.

4. TrPs in the EHL are often incorrectly assessed as metatarsophalangeal joint dysfunction or L4-L5 nerve compression.

5. Associated TrPs often occur in the tibialis anterior, extensor hallucis brevis, extensor digitorum longus, and fibularis tertius.

Figure 19-20 Anterolateral view showing a common extensor hallucis longus TrP and its corresponding referral zone.

Chapter 19 Tour #10—Palpation of the Leg Muscles

EXTENSOR HALLUCIS LONGUS (EHL)—SUPINE—cont'd

STRETCHING THE EXTENSOR HALLUCIS LONGUS

Figure 19-21 A stretch of the right extensor hallucis longus.

Palpation Key:
First look for the distal tendon to the big toe.

19

❑ **ATTACHMENTS:**

o Fibularis longus: proximal $^1/_2$ of the lateral fibula *to the* first cuneiform and the base of the first metatarsal
o Fibularis brevis: distal $^1/_2$ of the lateral fibula *to the* lateral side of the base of the fifth metatarsal (Figure 19-22)

❑ **ACTIONS:**

o Fibularis longus and brevis: evert the foot at the tarsal joints; plantarflex the foot at the ankle joint

Starting position (Figure 19-23):

o Client side lying
o Therapist standing to the side of the client
o Palpating hand placed on the lateral side of the fibula, just distal to the head of the fibula
o Support hand placed on the lateral side of the foot

Palpation steps:

1. Resist the client from everting the foot at the tarsal joints and feel for the contraction of the fibularis longus (Figure 19-24).
2. Continue palpating the fibularis longus distally by strumming perpendicular to the fibers. Note that the fibularis longus becomes tendon approximately halfway down the leg.
3. The distal tendon of the fibularis longus can usually be fairly easily palpated immediately posterior to the lateral malleolus of the fibula (Figure 19-25).
4. To palpate the fibularis brevis, palpate on either side of the fibularis longus in the distal half of the leg (Figure 19-26, A).
5. The distal tendon of the fibularis brevis is often visible and palpable in the proximal foot distal to the lateral malleolus of the fibula (Figure 19-26, B).
6. Once the fibularis longus and brevis have been located, have the client relax them and palpate to assess their baseline tone.

A   B

Figure 19-22 Lateral views of the right fibularis longus and brevis. **A**, Fibularis longus. **B**, Fibularis brevis.

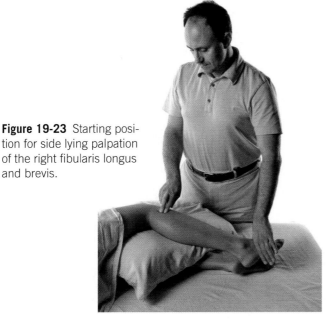

Figure 19-23 Starting position for side lying palpation of the right fibularis longus and brevis.

Figure 19-24 Palpation of the belly of the fibularis longus as the client everts the foot against resistance.

19

FIBULARIS LONGUS AND FIBULARIS BREVIS—SIDE LYING—cont'd

Figure 19-25 When resistance is applied to eversion of the foot, the distal tendon of the fibularis longus is often visible just proximal to the lateral malleolus of the fibula.

A   Fibularis longus tendon

B

Figure 19-26 Palpation of the right fibularis brevis as the client everts the foot against resistance. **A** shows palpation of its belly immediately posterior to the fibularis longus tendon. **B** shows palpation of its distal tendon distal to the lateral malleolus.

Palpation Notes:
1. The distal tendon of the fibularis longus is also often visible and palpable distal to the lateral malleolus of the fibula before it dives around the cuboid to enter the plantar surface of the foot to make its way to the medial side of the foot. Once the distal tendon of the fibularis longus enters the plantar side of the foot, it is located very deep and is not discernable except perhaps at the distal attachment on the first metatarsal and first cuneiform.
2. Having the client do eversion of the foot at the tarsal joints does not help discern the border between the extensor digitorum longus (EDL) and the fibularis longus and brevis. To discern this border, use dorsiflexion and plantarflexion of the foot at the ankle joint. The EDL engages with dorsiflexion, and the fibularis longus and brevis engage with plantarflexion. (Note: Eversion of the foot will discern the border between the fibularis longus and brevis muscles and the soleus because the soleus is an invertor of the foot.)

Alternate Palpation Position—Supine, Prone, or Seated
The fibularis longus and fibularis brevis can also be easily palpated with the client supine, prone, or seated.

19

FIBULARIS LONGUS AND FIBULARIS BREVIS—SIDE LYING—cont'd

TRIGGER POINTS

1. Trigger points (TrPs) in the fibularis longus and brevis often result from or are perpetuated by acute or chronic overuse of the muscle, prolonged shortening of the muscle (e.g., sleeping with the feet plantarflexed), prolonged immobilization (often due to wearing a cast), an ankle joint inversion sprain, chronic tension of the tibialis anterior and/or tibialis posterior, wearing high-heeled shoes, flat feet, running on uneven (slanted side to side) surfaces, habitually sitting with one leg crossed over the other, TrPs in the gluteus minimus, Morton's foot, or even socks with tight elastic bands that constrict circulation.

2. TrPs in the fibularis longus or brevis may produce weak ankles; pain with active eversion of the foot or with end range of motion of active or passive inversion of the foot; and entrapment of the common fibular nerve, deep fibular nerve (either of which may cause foot drop or foot slap), or the superficial fibular nerve.

3. The referral patterns of fibularis longus and brevis TrPs must be distinguished from the referral patterns of TrPs in the tibialis anterior, extensor digitorum longus, extensor hallucis longus, extensor digitorum brevis, extensor hallucis brevis, and gluteus minimus.

4. TrPs in the fibularis longus and brevis are often incorrectly assessed as lateral compartment syndrome or lumbar disc syndrome.

5. Associated TrPs often occur in the other fibularis muscles, extensor digitorum longus, tibialis posterior, and gluteus minimus.

6. Note: The referral patterns of the fibularis longus and fibularis brevis muscles have not been distinguished from each other.

Figure 19-27 Lateral view showing common fibularis longus and brevis TrPs and their corresponding referral zones.

Figure 19-28 A stretch of the right fibularis longus and brevis muscles. The client uses a towel to pull the foot into inversion and dorsiflexion.

Palpation Key:
Palpate the lateral fibula and evert the foot.

19

GASTROCNEMIUS—PRONE
19-3

❑ **ATTACHMENTS:**

o Posterior surfaces of the medial and lateral condyles of the femur *to the* posterior surface of the calcaneus (*via the* calcaneal tendon) (Figure 19-29)

❑ **ACTIONS:**

o Plantarflexes the foot at the ankle joint; inverts the foot at the tarsal joints
o Flexes the leg at the knee joint

Starting position (Figure 19-30):

o Client prone with the knee joint fully or nearly fully extended
o Therapist standing to the side of the client
o Palpating hand placed on the proximal posterior leg
o Support hand placed on the plantar surface of the foot

Palpation steps:

1. Ask the client to plantarflex the foot against your resistance and feel for the contraction of the gastrocnemius (Figure 19-31, A).
2. Palpate the medial and lateral bellies of the gastrocnemius in the proximal posterior leg.
3. Approximately halfway down the leg, the gastrocnemius becomes tendon. Palpate the tendon all the way to its attachment on the posterior surface of the calcaneus via the calcaneal (Achilles) tendon (Figure 19-31, B).
4. Once the gastrocnemius has been located, have the client relax it and palpate to assess its baseline tone.

Figure 19-29 Posterior view of the right gastrocnemius.

Figure 19-30 Starting position for prone palpation of the right gastrocnemius.

19

GASTROCNEMIUS—PRONE—cont'd

Figure 19-31 Palpation of the right gastrocnemius as the client plantarflexes the foot against resistance. **A**, Palpation of the medial belly. **B**, Palpation of the calcaneal (Achilles) tendon with two fingers on either side of the tendon just proximal to the calcaneus.

Palpation Notes:

1. The calcaneal tendon, also known as the Achilles tendon, is the common distal attachment of the gastrocnemius and soleus muscles.

2. The proximal attachments of the gastrocnemius on the posterior surfaces of the femoral condyles can be palpated. One at a time, follow a belly of the gastrocnemius proximally as the client alternately contracts and relaxes the muscle with resisted plantarflexion of the foot (with the knee joint extended). Be sure to stay medial to the biceps femoris distal tendon for the lateral head of the gastrocnemius and lateral to the semitendinosus and semimembranosus tendons for the medial head of the gastrocnemius (Figure 19-32). Once you are in the popliteal region, passively flex the client's knee joint to approximately 90 degrees to slacken the hamstrings, and palpate for the femoral condyle attachments of the two heads of the gastrocnemius. Note: Be careful when palpating in the popliteal region because of the presence of the tibial and common fibular nerves and the popliteal artery and vein in the popliteal fossa (see Figure 19-2).

3. Discerning the proximal attachment of the lateral head of the gastrocnemius from the plantaris is difficult because these muscles are directly next to each other and have the same joint actions (see Figure 19-35, C).

Figure 19-32 Palpation of the proximal attachments of the gastrocnemius. **A**, Medial head. The semitendinosus and semimembranosus have been ghosted in. **B**, Lateral head. The plantaris is drawn in. The biceps femoris long and short heads are cut and ghosted in.

GASTROCNEMIUS—PRONE—cont'd

Alternate Palpation Position—Standing

The gastrocnemius can also be easily palpated with the client standing. Asking the client to go up on the toes will engage the gastrocnemius, and its contours will usually become visible.

TRIGGER POINTS

1. Trigger points (TrPs) in the gastrocnemius often result from or are perpetuated by acute or chronic overuse of the muscle (e.g., walking/running uphill), prolonged shortening of the muscle (e.g., wearing high heels, sleeping with the feet in plantarflexion, driving with the foot plantarflexed on the gas pedal), riding a bicycle with a seat that is too low, chilling of the muscle, immobilization (e.g., wearing a cast), socks with tight elastic bands that constrict circulation, and S1 nerve compression.
2. TrPs in the gastrocnemius may produce calf cramps (including nocturnal cramps), intermittent claudication, and an inability to extend the knee joint when the ankle joint is dorsiflexed.
3. The referral patterns of gastrocnemius TrPs must be distinguished from the referral patterns of TrPs in the soleus, plantaris, popliteus, tibialis posterior, flexor digitorum longus, hamstrings, and gluteus minimus.
4. TrPs in the gastrocnemius are often incorrectly assessed as posterior compartment syndrome, deep vein thrombosis, an S1 nerve compression, or growing pains.
5. Associated TrPs often occur in the soleus, hamstring muscles, tibialis anterior, extensor digitorum longus, extensor hallucis longus, and gluteus minimus.

Figure 19-33 Posterior views showing common gastrocnemius TrPs and their corresponding referral zones. **A**, Medial head. **B**, Lateral head.

STRETCHING THE GASTROCNEMIUS

Figure 19-34 A stretch of the right gastrocnemius. With the knee joint extended, the client leans forward with the leg causing ankle joint dorsiflexion. It is important that the heel stays on the ground. Note: If the knee joint is flexed, this becomes a soleus stretch.

Palpation Key:
Resist foot plantarflexion with the knee joint extended.

19

GASTROCNEMIUS—PRONE—cont'd

DETOUR

Plantaris: The plantaris is a small muscle attaching from the lateral condyle of the femur to the calcaneus (Figure 19-35, A). Its belly is located directly medial to the proximal attachment of the lateral head of the gastrocnemius (see Figure 19-32, B). To palpate the plantaris, begin with gentle palpation in the center of the popliteal fossa and gradually move laterally until you feel the presence of muscle tissue that contracts with plantarflexion of the foot at the ankle joint (Figure 19-35, B). You are now on the plantaris. To discern the plantaris from the lateral head of the gastrocnemius is difficult because these two muscles have identical actions. Stretching the gastrocnemius would also stretch the plantaris.

Note: Trigger points (TrPs) in the plantaris may cause pain at the end range of motion of dorsiflexion of the foot. TrPs in the plantaris are often associated with TrPs in the gastrocnemius (Figure 19-35, C).

Palpation Key:
Palpate medial to the attachment of the lateral head of the gastrocnemius.

Figure 19-35 Views of the right plantaris. **A,** Posterior view of the plantaris. The popliteus has been ghosted in. **B,** Palpation of the plantaris. **C,** Posterior view showing a common plantaris TrP and its corresponding referral zone.

Plantaris
Popliteus

A   B   C

SOLEUS—PRONE

❑ ATTACHMENTS:

o Head and proximal half of the posterior fibula and the soleal line of the posterior tibia *to the* posterior surface of the calcaneus (via the calcaneal tendon) (Figure 19-36)

❑ ACTIONS:

o Plantarflexes the foot at the ankle joint; inverts the foot at the tarsal joints

Starting position (Figure 19-37):
o Client prone with the knee joint flexed to approximately 90 degrees
o Therapist standing to the side of the client
o Palpating hand placed on the proximal posterior leg
o Support hand placed on the plantar surface of the foot

Palpation steps:
1. Ask the client to plantarflex the foot against gentle resistance and feel for the contraction of the soleus deep to the gastrocnemius (Figure 19-38, A).
2. Palpate the soleus to its proximal attachment and palpate it distally to its distal attachment on the posterior calcaneus, via the calcaneal (Achilles) tendon.
3. Although from the posterior perspective, the soleus is deep to the gastrocnemius, from the lateral perspective, the soleus is superficial and can be palpated (Figure 19-38, B). Note: A portion of the soleus is also superficial on the medial side of the proximal leg (see Figure 19-4, A).
4. Once the soleus has been located, have the client relax it and palpate to assess its baseline tone.

Figure 19-36 Posterior view of the right soleus.

Figure 19-37 Starting position for prone palpation of the right soleus.

SOLEUS—PRONE—cont'd

Figure 19-38 Palpation of the right soleus as the client plantarflexes the foot against gentle resistance with the knee joint flexed. **A**, Palpation of the posterior aspect through the gastrocnemius. **B**, Palpation of the lateral aspect where the soleus is superficial.

Palpation Notes:

1. The calcaneal tendon, also known as the Achilles tendon, is the common distal attachment of the soleus and gastrocnemius muscles.

2. The reason that the soleus is palpated with the client's leg flexed at the knee joint is that this position slackens and thereby inhibits the gastrocnemius from contracting (via the principle of shortened active insufficiency). If the gastrocnemius is inhibited, the soleus can be palpated through the gastrocnemius (in addition to where the soleus is superficial laterally as well as medially). Note: Do not provide too much resistance to the client's plantarflexion, or the inhibition of the gastrocnemius will be overridden and it will contract, blocking the ability to palpate the soleus through it.

Palpation Key:
Gently resist foot plantarflexion with the knee joint flexed.

19

SOLEUS—PRONE—cont'd

TRIGGER POINTS

1. Trigger points (TrPs) in the soleus often result from or are perpetuated by an acute or chronic overuse of the muscle (e.g., walking/running uphill), prolonged position of shortening of the muscle (e.g., wearing high heels, sleeping with the feet in plantarflexion, driving with the foot plantarflexed on the gas pedal), trauma, and chilling of the muscle.

2. TrPs in the soleus may produce restricted ankle joint dorsiflexion, pain when walking (especially uphill or upstairs), entrapment of the tibial nerve and associated vessels, heel pain upon weight bearing, and foot/ankle edema.

3. The referral patterns of soleus TrPs must be distinguished from the referral patterns of TrPs in the gastrocnemius, plantaris, tibialis posterior, flexor digitorum longus, hamstrings, gluteus minimus, quadratus plantae, and abductor hallucis.

4. TrPs in the soleus are often incorrectly assessed as posterior compartment syndrome, posterior shin splints, growing pains, Achilles tendinitis, Baker's cyst, deep vein thrombosis, S1 nerve compression, intermittent claudication, plantar fasciitis, or heel spur.

5. Associated TrPs often occur in the gastrocnemius, tibialis posterior, flexor digitorum longus, flexor hallucis longus, and gluteus minimus.

Figure 19-39 Posterior views of common soleus TrPs and their corresponding referral zones.

STRETCHING THE SOLEUS

Figure 19-40 A stretch of the right soleus. With the knee joint flexed, the client leans forward with the leg, causing ankle joint dorsiflexion. It is important that the heel stays on the ground. Note: If the knee joint is extended, this becomes more of a gastrocnemius stretch.

19

POPLITEUS—PRONE

❏ ATTACHMENTS:
o Lateral surface of the lateral condyle of the femur *to the* medial side of the proximal posterior tibia (Figure 19-41)

❏ ACTIONS:
o Medially rotates and flexes the leg at the knee joint

Starting position (Figure 19-42):
o Client prone with the leg flexed 90 degrees at the knee joint
o Therapist standing to the side of the client
o Palpating fingers curled around the posterior side of the medial border of the proximal tibia
o If resistance will be given, support hand placed on the distal leg (just proximal to the ankle joint)

Palpation steps:
1. With your palpating fingers curled around and pressing against the tibia, ask the client to medially rotate the leg at the knee joint and feel for the contraction of the popliteus. Resistance with the support hand can be given if desired (Figure 19-43).
2. Once the tibial attachment of the popliteus has been felt, try to continue palpating the popliteus through the gastrocnemius toward its proximal attachment while the client is alternately contracting and relaxing it by medially rotating the leg at the knee joint.
3. Once the popliteus has been located, have the client relax it and palpate to assess its baseline tone.

Figure 19-41 Posterior view of the right popliteus. The soleus and cut distal tendon of semimembranosus have been ghosted in.

Figure 19-42 Starting position for prone palpation of the right popliteus.

Figure 19-43 Palpation of the tibial attachment of the popliteus as the client medially rotates the leg against resistance.

POPLITEUS—PRONE—cont'd

Palpation Notes:

1. Many people have trouble isolating and performing medial rotation of the leg at the knee joint. To assist the client in doing this, before the actual palpation is done, move the client's leg into medial rotation so that the client can sense what this motion feels like; then ask the client to perform the motion once to practice it. This will help the client perform this joint action more easily when the palpation procedure is actually done. It is easier for the client to perform medial rotation of the leg at the knee joint when in the seated position (Figure 19-44).

2. Most of the belly of the popliteus is located deep to the gastrocnemius. As you palpate the belly of the popliteus through the gastrocnemius, it can be helpful to close your eyes to prevent visual sensations from distracting you, and press very lightly with your palpating fingers, feeling for the subtle contraction of the popliteus when the client medially rotates the leg at the knee joint, either with or without resistance. Continue palpating the popliteus toward its proximal attachment on the femur. At a certain point, its proximal attachment enters the joint cavity of the knee and is no longer palpable.

3. The proximal attachment of the popliteus on the lateral femoral condyle can be palpated. Palpate on the lateral surface of the lateral femoral condyle (just posterior to the lateral [fibular] collateral ligament) and resist the client from medially rotating the leg at the knee joint; feel for the tensing of the distal tendon of the popliteus (Figure 19-45).

Figure 19-44 The advantage to palpating the popliteus with the client seated is that it is easier for the client to isolate medial rotation of the leg at the knee joint if the foot is flat on the floor. Palpate the popliteus with the client seated following the same steps used when the client is prone.

Alternate Palpation Position—Seated

Figure 19-45 Palpation of the proximal attachment of the popliteus on the lateral femoral condyle.

TRIGGER POINTS

1. Trigger points (TrPs) in the popliteus often result from or are perpetuated by an acute or chronic overuse of the muscle (e.g., running or skiing downhill, planting and cutting on a semiflexed knee joint), excessive foot subtalar joint pronation, wearing high-heeled shoes, and a torn posterior cruciate ligament.

2. TrPs in the popliteus may produce posterior knee pain when crouching or walking/running downhill or downstairs, or decreased lateral rotation or extension of the leg at the knee joint.

3. The referral patterns of popliteus TrPs must be distinguished from the referral patterns of TrPs in the gastrocnemius, soleus, plantaris, hamstrings, and gluteus minimus.

4. TrPs in the popliteus are often incorrectly assessed as Baker's cyst, instability of the knee joint, popliteus tendinitis/tenosynovitis, meniscal tear, or torn plantaris muscle.

5. Associated TrPs often occur in the gastrocnemius.

Figure 19-46 Posteromedial view showing a common popliteus TrP and its corresponding referral zone.

19

POPLITEUS—PRONE—cont'd

STRETCHING THE POPLITEUS

Palpation Key:
Curl your fingers around to the medial side of the proximal tibia.

Figure 19-47 A stretch of the right popliteus. The client holds the thigh fixed with his hands and then laterally rotates the leg at the knee joint. The knee joint is flexed approximately 45 degrees from full extension.

19

TIBIALIS POSTERIOR, FLEXOR DIGITORUM LONGUS, AND FLEXOR HALLUCIS LONGUS—PRONE

19-4

"Tom, Dick, and Harry Muscles"
(Tibialis Posterior = Tom; Flexor Digitorum
Longus = Dick; Flexor Hallucis Longus = Harry)

❑ ATTACHMENTS:

o Tibialis posterior (TP): proximal ⅔ of the posterior tibia and fibula *to the* plantar surface of the foot (metatarsals two to four and all tarsal except the talus)
o Flexor digitorum longus (FDL): Middle ⅓ of the posterior tibia *to the* plantar surfaces of the distal phalanges of toes two to five
o Flexor hallucis longus (FHL): Distal ⅔ of the posterior fibula *to the* plantar surface of the distal phalanx of the big toe

❑ ACTIONS:

o TP:
　o Inverts the foot at the tarsal joints; plantarflexes the foot at the ankle joint
o FDL:
　o Flexes toes two to five at the metatarsophalangeal (MTP) and interphalangeal (IP) joints
　o Inverts the foot at the tarsal joints; plantarflexes the foot at the ankle joint
o FHL:
　o Flexes the big toe at the MTP and IP joints
　o Inverts the foot at the tarsal joints; plantarflexes the foot at the ankle joint

Starting position (Figure 19-49, A):

o Client prone with a roll under the ankles
o Therapist standing or seated on the other side of the client
o Palpating fingers placed just posterior and distal to the medial malleolus of the tibia, but not until after its tendon has been visualized
o If resistance is needed, support hand placed on the foot

Palpation steps:

o Note: All three Tom, Dick, and Harry muscles are superficial and palpable in the distal medial leg; of the three, the FDL has the most exposure. The tendons of the TP and FDL are usually palpable and sometimes visible just posterior and distal to the medial malleolus of the tibia (Figure 19-49, B).

Tibialis Posterior (TP):

1. Ask the client to plantarflex the foot at the ankle joint and invert the foot at the tarsal joints, and look for the distal tendon of the tibialis posterior (TP) in the distal medial leg immediately posterior to the shaft of the distal tibia and immediately posterior and distal to the medial malleolus of the tibia. Resistance may be added with your support hand if needed to bring out the tendon (Figure 19-50, A).

Tibialis posterior

Flexor digitorum longus

Flexor hallucis longus

A   B

Figure 19-48 Posterior views of the right Tom, Dick, and Harry muscles. **A**, Tibialis posterior (Tom). **B**, Flexor digitorum longus (Dick) and flexor hallucis longus (Harry). Tibialis posterior has been ghosted in.

2. Once located, palpate the distal tendon of the TP by strumming perpendicularly across it as the client alternately contracts and relaxes the muscle. Palpate proximally and distally as far as possible. Note: The TP tendon is the closest of the three to the medial malleolus (Figure 19-50, B).
3. The belly of the TP is located very deep in the posterior compartment of the leg. To palpate its belly, press gently over it in the midline of the posterior leg, ask the client to invert the foot, and feel for its contraction (Figure 19-50, C).
4. Once the TP muscle has been located, have the client relax it and palpate to assess its baseline tone.

19

TIBIALIS POSTERIOR, FLEXOR DIGITORUM LONGUS, AND FLEXOR HALLUCIS LONGUS—PRONE—cont'd

Figure 19-49 A, Starting position for prone palpation of the Tom, Dick, and Harry group. First try to visualize the tendons. **B**, All three Tom, Dick, and Harry muscles' distal tendons near the medial malleolus. The gastrocnemius and soleus have been ghosted in. Tom = tibialis posterior (TP); Dick = flexor digitorum longus (FDL); Harry = flexor hallucis longus (FHL).

Figure 19-50 Palpation of the tibialis posterior (TP) as the client plantarflexes and inverts the foot against resistance. **A**, Visualization of the distal tendon near the medial malleolus and navicular tuberosity. **B**, Strumming across the distal tendon. **C**, Palpation proximally of the belly deep to the gastrocnemius and soleus. Note: The gastrocnemius and soleus have been ghosted in all three figures.

TIBIALIS POSTERIOR, FLEXOR DIGITORUM LONGUS, AND FLEXOR HALLUCIS LONGUS—PRONE—cont'd

Flexor Digitorum Longus (FDL):

5. Part of the belly of the flexor digitorum longus (FDL) is superficial in the distal medial leg between the soleus and the shaft of the tibia. Ask the client to flex toes two to five and feel for the contraction of the FDL (Figure 19-51, A). Resistance may be added with the fingers of your support hand if needed.

6. Once the FDL has been found, strum perpendicular to its fibers and follow it proximally and distally as far as possible as the client contracts and relaxes the muscle.

7. At the level of the medial malleolus, the distal tendon of the FDL is usually palpable and sometimes visible posterior and distal to the medial malleolus. It is located slightly farther from the medial malleolus than the distal tendon of the tibialis posterior (TP) (Figure 19-51, B).

8. Within the plantar foot, the distal tendons of the FDL are fairly superficial and can usually be palpated if the client alternately contracts and relaxes the FDL by flexing toes two to five at the metatarsophalangeal and interphalangeal joints (Note: Some clients have a difficult time isolating flexion of toes two to five from flexion of the big toe.) (Figure 19-51, C). However, precisely discerning the location of these tendons and their borders relative to adjacent musculature and soft tissue is sometimes difficult. Try to follow these tendons to the toes.

9. The belly of the FDL is located deep in the posterior compartment of the leg. To palpate its belly, press gently over it in the posterior medial leg, ask the client to flex toes two to five, and feel for its contraction (Figure 19-51, D).

10. Once the FDL muscle has been located, have the client relax it and palpate to assess its baseline tone.

Figure 19-51 Palpation of the flexor digitorum longus (FDL) as the client flexes toes two to five against resistance. **A**, Palpation of the belly in the distal medial leg. **B**, Palpation of the distal tendon near the medial malleolus. **C**, Palpation of the distal tendons in the plantar foot. **D**, Palpation proximally of the belly deep in the posterior leg. Note: The gastrocnemius and soleus have been ghosted in **A**, **B**, and **D**.

19

TIBIALIS POSTERIOR, FLEXOR DIGITORUM LONGUS, AND FLEXOR HALLUCIS LONGUS—PRONE—cont'd

Flexor Hallucis Longus (FHL):

11. A small part of the distal belly of the flexor hallucis longus (FHL) is superficial in the distal medial leg between the flexor digitorum longus (FDL) and the calcaneal tendon. Ask the client to flex the big toe and feel for the contraction of the FHL (Figure 19-52, A). Resistance may be added with fingers of your support hand if needed.
12. Once the FHL has been found, strum perpendicular to its fibers and try to follow it as far distally as possible. At the level of the medial malleolus, its distal tendon runs quite deep and is difficult to palpate.
13. Within the plantar foot, the distal tendon of the FHL is fairly superficial and can usually be palpated if the client

alternately contracts and relaxes the FHL by flexing the big toe at the metatarsophalangeal and interphalangeal joints. (Note: Some clients have a difficult time isolating flexion of the big toe from flexion of the other toes.) However, precisely discerning the location of its tendon and its borders relative to adjacent musculature and soft tissue is sometimes difficult. Try to follow its tendon to the big toe (Figure 19-52, B).
14. The belly of the FHL is located deep in the posterior compartment of the leg. To palpate its belly, press gently over it in the posterior lateral leg, ask the client to flex the big toe, and feel for its contraction (Figure 19-52, C).
15. Once the FHL muscle has been located, have the client relax it and palpate to assess its baseline tone.

Figure 19-52 Palpation of the flexor hallucis longus (FHL) as the client flexes the big toe against resistance. **A**, Palpation of the belly in the distal medial leg. **B**, Palpation of the distal tendon in the plantar foot. **C**, Palpation proximally of the belly deep in the posterior leg. Note: The gastrocnemius and soleus have been ghosted in **A** and **C**.

TIBIALIS POSTERIOR, FLEXOR DIGITORUM LONGUS, AND FLEXOR HALLUCIS LONGUS—PRONE—cont'd

Palpation Notes:

1. The "Tom, Dick, and Harry muscles" are so named because they all cross from the leg into the foot posterior and then distal to the medial malleolus of the tibia, with the TP closest to the medial malleolus, then the flexor digitorum longus (FDL), and then the flexor hallucis longus (FHL) farthest. Because they all cross the ankle joint posteriorly and the subtalar joint medially, they all plantarflex the foot at the ankle joint and invert the foot at the subtalar joint.

2. When first palpating the Tom, Dick, and Harry muscles, look for the tendons of the TP and the FDL before placing the palpating hand on the client; otherwise your palpating hand will obstruct your view and visual identification.

3. When palpating for the TP, if you ask the client to extend all five toes, it will inhibit and relax the FDL and FHL from contracting, making it easier to palpate and discern the TP.

4. Do not use plantarflexion and/or inversion of the foot when palpating the FDL and FHL, because these actions will make all three Tom, Dick, and Harry muscles contract, making it difficult to discern the separate muscles.

5. The majority of fibers of the distal attachment of the TP attach into the navicular tuberosity; this attachment site can be palpated in the medial foot (Figure 19-50, B). To do this, once the distal tendon of TP is located near the medial malleolus, continue strumming it perpendicularly as the client contracts and relaxes the muscle until you reach the navicular tuberosity. The rest of the attachments of the TP distal tendon in the plantar surface of the foot are very deep and extremely difficult to palpate and discern from adjacent tissue.

6. When palpating the bellies of the Tom, Dick, and Harry muscles in the deep posterior compartment of the leg, it can be helpful to close your eyes (to eliminate distracting visual stimuli) and press very gently into the tissues, feeling for the vibration of the muscle's contraction when the client engages the muscle as described in the Palpation Steps for each muscle. Note that in the posterior leg, the FDL belly is medial, the FHL belly is lateral, and the TP belly is in the middle.

7. A small part of the FHL can often be palpated in the lateral leg (see Figure 19-3). Palpate between the soleus posteriorly and the fibularis longus and brevis muscles anteriorly, while asking the client to flex the big toe against resistance. It is important that the client does not also plantarflex the foot at the ankle joint, because this will cause the soleus and fibularis longus/brevis muscles to also contract.

Alternate Palpation Position—Side Lying or Supine
The Tom, Dick, and Harry muscles can also be palpated with the client side lying or supine. If the client is side lying, the hip and knee joints of the lower extremity that is away from the table must be flexed to allow access to the medial side of the leg.

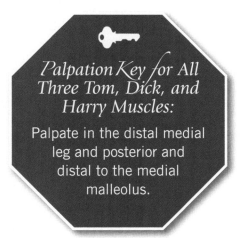

Palpation Key for All Three Tom, Dick, and Harry Muscles:

Palpate in the distal medial leg and posterior and distal to the medial malleolus.

TIBIALIS POSTERIOR, FLEXOR DIGITORUM LONGUS, AND FLEXOR HALLUCIS LONGUS—PRONE—cont'd

TRIGGER POINTS

1. Trigger points (TrPs) in the tibialis posterior (TP), flexor digitorum longus (FDL), and flexor hallucis longus (FHL) often result from or are perpetuated by an acute or chronic overuse of the muscle (e.g., walking on soft sand), walking/running on uneven (slanted side to side) ground, excessive foot subtalar joint pronation, wearing high-heeled shoes, and Morton's foot.
2. TrPs in the TP, FDL, and FHL may produce foot pain (plantar surface of the foot, especially the ball of the foot or the toes) when walking or running, spasm of the associated muscle, excessive foot subtalar joint pronation, and decreased extension range of motion of the associated toes.
3. The referral patterns of TP, FDL, and FHL TrPs must be distinguished from the referral patterns of TrPs in the other muscles of the deep posterior compartment; the gastrocnemius, soleus, and gluteus minimus (for TP); the adductor hallucis, plantar interossei, dorsal interossei pedis, and flexor digitorum brevis (for FDL and FHL); the abductor digiti minimi pedis (for FDL); and flexor hallucis brevis (for FHL).
4. TrPs in the TP, FDL, and FHL are often incorrectly assessed as shin splints, deep posterior compartment syndrome, tarsal tunnel syndrome, or tenosynovitis of the associated muscle's tendon.
5. Associated TrPs often occur in the other muscles of the deep posterior compartment; the fibularis longus, fibularis brevis, and fibularis tertius (for TP); the extensor digitorum longus, extensor digitorum brevis, and flexor digitorum brevis (for FDL); and the extensor hallucis longus, extensor hallucis brevis, and flexor hallucis brevis (for FHL).

Figure 19-53 A to C, Posterior views showing common TrPs and their corresponding referral zones for the tibialis posterior, flexor digitorum longus, and flexor hallucis longus muscles, respectively.

Figure 19-54 Stretches of the right Tom, Dick, and Harry group. **A,** Stretch of the right tibialis posterior. The client uses a towel to dorsiflex and evert the foot. **B,** Stretch of the right flexor digitorum longus. With the foot in neutral position or dorsiflexed, the client uses his hand to pull the toes (two to five) into extension. **C,** Stretch of the right flexor hallucis longus. With the foot in neutral position or dorsiflexed, the client uses his hand to pull the big toe into extension. Note: Eversion of the foot can be added to enhance the stretch of either the flexor digitorum longus or flexor hallucis longus.

Anterior Compartment Muscles: Client Supine with the Knee Joint Extended:

1. **Tibialis anterior:** Resist the client from dorsiflexing and inverting the foot, and look and feel for the tensing of the distal tendon of the tibialis anterior anteriorly and proximally on the dorsum of the foot. Continue palpating the tibialis anterior proximally along the lateral border of the tibia to its proximal attachment by strumming perpendicular to it.

2. **Extensor digitorum longus (EDL):** Resist the client from extending toes two to five and look and feel for the muscle's tendons on the dorsal surface of the foot. Continue palpating the EDL proximally to its proximal attachment by strumming perpendicular to it. Note: Proximally, the EDL is located between the tibialis anterior and the fibularis longus. Use eversion of the foot to engage and discern the EDL from the tibialis anterior; use dorsiflexion to engage and discern the EDL from the fibularis longus.

3. **Fibularis tertius:** Palpate just lateral to the tendon of the EDL that goes to the little toe, and ask the client to dorsiflex and/or evert the foot. Look and feel for the tendon of the fibularis tertius. Once located, follow the fibularis tertius proximally into the distal leg. Note: The fibularis tertius is often absent.

4. **Extensor hallucis longus (EHL):** Ask the client to extend the big toe against resistance and look and feel for the distal tendon of the EHL on the medial side of the dorsum of the foot. Follow the EHL proximally by strumming perpendicular to it. When it is deep to the tibialis anterior and the EDL, press gently and feel for its contraction as the client extends the big toe.

Lateral Compartment Muscles: Client Side Lying:

5. **Fibularis longus:** Ask the client to evert the foot against resistance, and feel for the contraction of the fibularis longus in the proximal lateral leg, just distal to the head of the fibula. Once located, continue palpating it distally to the lateral malleolus by strumming perpendicular. Note: The fibularis longus is located between the EDL and the soleus. Use plantarflexion of the foot to engage and discern the fibularis longus from the EDL; use eversion to engage and discern the fibularis longus from the soleus.

6. **Fibularis brevis:** Locate the tendon of the fibularis longus in the distal half of the leg. Then palpate on either side of it and feel for the fibularis brevis as the client everts the foot (resistance may be added). The distal tendon of the fibularis brevis can often be visualized and palpated between the lateral malleolus and the fifth metatarsal.

Superficial Posterior Compartment Muscles: Client Prone:

7. **Gastrocnemius:** With the client prone with the knee joints extended, ask the client to plantarflex the foot against resistance and feel for the contraction of the gastrocnemius in the proximal posterior leg. Palpate both the medial and lateral heads and then palpate to the attachment on the calcaneus.

8. **Plantaris:** Press gently into the center of the popliteal fossa as the client plantarflexes the foot (resistance can be added). Gradually move laterally until you feel the presence of muscle tissue that contracts with plantarflexion of the foot. You are now on the plantaris. Strum across it perpendicularly. It is usually not possible to discern the border between the plantaris and the lateral head of the gastrocnemius.

9. **Soleus:** With the client prone with the knee joint flexed to approximately 90 degrees, ask the client to plantarflex the foot (if resistance is given, offer only gentle resistance) and feel for the contraction of the soleus through the gastrocnemius in the proximal posterior leg. Continue palpating the soleus distally to the calcaneal attachment. Note: The soleus is superficial and palpable in the lateral leg between the gastrocnemius and the fibularis longus, and superficial and palpable proximally in the medial leg between the gastrocnemius and the tibia (and flexor digitorum longus).

Deep Posterior Compartment Muscles: Client Prone:

For the popliteus palpation, you are standing to the same side of the client; for the rest of the palpations, you are seated or standing on the opposite side of the client.

10. **Popliteus:** With the client prone and the knee joint flexed to approximately 90 degrees, find the tibial tuberosity. Then curl your fingers around the tibia and palpate against the posterior surface of the medial border of the tibia, feeling for the contraction of the popliteus as the client actively medially rotates the leg at the knee joint (resistance can be added if needed). Once located, try to follow the popliteus deep to the gastrocnemius toward its femoral attachment as the client alternately contracts and relaxes the muscle.

11. **Tibialis posterior:** The distal tendon of the tibialis posterior is superficial in the distal medial leg directly posterior to the tibia. Ask the client to plantarflex and invert the foot and feel for the tendon of the tibialis posterior to tense. Continue palpating the tendon to the navicular tuberosity by strumming perpendicularly across it. The tendon of the tibialis posterior is often visible and palpable directly posterior and then distal to the medial malleolus of the tibia. Palpate its belly proximally by pressing gently into

19

the center of the posterior leg as the client plantarflexes and inverts the foot.

12. **Flexor digitorum longus (FDL):** Part of the FDL is superficial in the distal medial leg between the shaft of the tibia and the soleus. Ask the client to flex toes two to five (against resistance if needed) and feel for the contraction of the FDL. Continue palpating it distally as far as possible by strumming perpendicularly across it. Its tendon may be visible and palpable running posterior and then distal to the medial malleolus; its tendons may also be palpable in the plantar foot as the client contracts the muscle. Palpate its belly proximally by pressing gently into the medial posterior leg as the client flexes toes two to five.

13. **Flexor hallucis longus (FHL):** A small part of the FHL is superficial in the distal medial leg between the FDL and the soleus. Ask the client to flex the big toe (against resistance if necessary) and feel for the contraction of the FHL. Continue palpating it as far distally as possible. It is usually not possible to palpate its distal tendon as it passes posteriorly and then distally to the medial malleolus; however, its distal tendon may be palpated in the plantar foot as the client contracts the muscle. Palpate its belly proximally by pressing gently into the lateral posterior leg as the client flexes the big toe.

Chapter 20

Tour #11—Palpation of the Intrinsic Muscles of the Foot

Overview

This chapter is a palpation tour of the intrinsic muscles of the foot. The tour begins with the dorsal muscles and then addresses the plantar muscles. Palpation of the muscles on the dorsum of the foot is shown in the supine position; palpation of the plantar muscles is shown in the prone position. Alternate palpation positions are also described. The major muscles or muscle groups of the region are each given a separate layout. There are also a few detours to other muscles of the region. Many intrinsic muscles of the foot are relatively easy to palpate and discern. However, one difficult aspect to intrinsic foot musculature palpation is that clients are often unable to isolate the joint action necessary for isolated contraction of the target muscle. Trigger point (TrP) information and stretching is given for each of the muscles covered in this chapter. The chapter closes with an advanced *Whirlwind Tour* that explains the sequential palpation of all of the muscles of the chapter.

Chapter Outline

Chapter Objectives

After completing this chapter, the student should be able to perform the following for each of the muscles covered in this chapter:

1. State the attachments.
2. State the actions.
3. Describe the starting position for palpation.
4. Describe and explain the purpose of each of the palpation steps.
5. Palpate each muscle.
6. State the "Palpation Key."
7. Describe alternate palpation positions.
8. State the locations of the most common TrP(s).
9. Describe the TrP referral zones.
10. State the most common factors that create and/or perpetuate TrPs.
11. State the symptoms most commonly caused by TrPs.
12. Describe and perform a stretch.

Go to http://evolve.elsevier.com/Muscolino/palpation for video demonstrations of the muscle palpations presented in this chapter.

Figure 20-1 Plantar views of the muscles of the right foot. **A**, Superficial view, including the fascia. **B**, Superficial muscular view.

Figure 20-1, cont'd C, Intermediate view. **D**, Deep view.

Extensor hallucis longus

Tibialis anterior

Fibularis longus and brevis

Extensor digitorum longus and fibularis tertius

Superior extensor retinaculum

Lateral malleolus of fibula

Inferior extensor retinaculum

Inferior fibular retinaculum

Fibularis longus tendon

Fibularis brevis tendon

Extensor hallucis brevis

Base of 5th metatarsal

Extensor digitorum brevis

Abductor digiti minimi pedis

Abductor hallucis

Dorsal interossei pedis

Dorsal digital expansion of 2nd toe

20

Figure 20-2 Dorsal view of the muscles of the right foot.

Figure 20-3 Lateral and medial views of the muscles of the right foot. **A**, Lateral view. **B**, Medial view.

EXTENSOR DIGITORUM BREVIS (EDB) AND EXTENSOR HALLUCIS BREVIS (EHB)—SUPINE

❏ ATTACHMENTS:

o Proximally, both the extensor digitorum brevis (EDB) and extensor hallucis brevis (EHB) attach to the dorsal surface of the calcaneus.
o Distally, the EDB attaches to the lateral side of the distal tendons of the extensor digitorum longus of toes two through four.
o Distally, the EHB attaches to the dorsal surface of the base of the proximal phalanx of the big toe (toe one).

❏ ACTIONS:

o The EDB extends toes two to four at the metatarsophalangeal (MTP) and proximal and distal interphalangeal joints.
o The EHB extends the big toe at the MTP joint.

Starting position (Figure 20-5):

o Client supine
o Therapist is seated to the side of the client
o After the common belly of the extensor digitorum brevis (EDB) and extensor hallucis brevis (EHB) is visualized, palpating fingers placed on the belly of these muscles on the proximal dorsolateral surface of the foot (approximately 1 inch [2.5 cm] distal to the lateral malleolus of the fibula)
o Fingers of the support hand placed on the proximal phalanges of toes two to four

Palpation steps:

1. Resist the client from extending toes two to four at the metatarsophalangeal joints by placing fingers of the support hand on the proximal phalanges of toes two to four, and look for the contraction of the belly of the EDB. After visualizing the contracted belly of the EDB, palpate it (Note: If the EDB cannot be visualized, then palpate for it on the proximal dorsolateral foot) (Figure 20-6, A).
2. To palpate the EHB, follow the same procedure used for the EDB except that the support hand is placed on the proximal phalanx of the big toe to provide resistance to extension of the big toe (Figure 20-6, B).
3. Asking the client to alternately contract and relax the EDB or the EHB against resistance, try to follow the EDB distally toward toes two to four and the EHB toward the big

Extensor digitorum brevis

Extensor hallucis brevis

Figure 20-4 Dorsal view of the extensors digitorum and hallucis brevis.

toe by strumming perpendicularly to the tendon(s) (Palpation Note #3).
4. Once the EDB and/or EHB have been located, have the client relax them and palpate to assess their baseline tone.

Figure 20-5 Starting position for supine palpation of the right extensors digitorum and hallucis brevis.

EXTENSOR DIGITORUM BREVIS (EDB) AND EXTENSOR HALLUCIS BREVIS (EHB)—SUPINE—cont'd

A   B

Figure 20-6 Palpation of the right extensor digitorum brevis (EDB) and extensor hallucis brevis (EHB). **A**, Palpation of the EDB as the client extends toes two to four against resistance. The EHB has been ghosted in. **B**, Palpation of the EHB as the client extends the big toe against resistance. The EDB has been ghosted in.

Palpation Notes:

1. Structurally, the EDB and EHB are actually one muscle. They are functionally divided into two separate muscles based on their distal attachments. The fibers that attach distally to toes two to four are named the EDB, and the fibers that attach distally to the big toe are named the EHB.
2. Within the common belly of these two muscles, the fibers of the EDB are on the lateral side and the fibers of the EHB are on the medial side.
3. The distal aspects of the EDB and EHB can be difficult to palpate and discern because they are located deep to the distal tendons of the extensor digitorum longus, whose tendons will (also) tense with extension of the proximal phalanges of toes two to four.

4. To discern the EDB from the EHB, it is necessary for the client to be able to isolate extension of the big toe from the other toes. Many people are unable to do this. It does not help to hold down whichever toe(s) you want the client to not move because even though the toe(s) might not move, the belly of the muscle that we want to be relaxed will be isometrically contracted, making it more difficult to discern these two muscles from each other. In other words, if you are palpating the EDB and you want the EHB to stay relaxed, but the client cannot extend toes two to four without also extending the big toe at the same time, it does not help to restrain the big toe by holding it down, because the belly of the EHB will isometrically contract against the resistance of your finger.

20

Alternate Position—Seated
Both the EDB and EHB can also be easily accessed with the client seated.

YOU ARE HERE ★

EXTENSOR DIGITORUM BREVIS (EDB) AND EXTENSOR HALLUCIS BREVIS (EHB)—SUPINE—cont'd

TRIGGER POINTS

1. Trigger points (TrPs) in the extensor digitorum brevis (EDB) and extensor hallucis brevis (EHB) often result from or are perpetuated by acute or chronic overuse of the muscles, sustained postures that cause the muscles to lengthen (e.g., sleeping supine with tight sheets that hold the toes in flexion), sustained postures that allow the muscles to shorten (e.g., wearing high-heeled shoes), wearing shoes with an inflexible sole (not allowing motion of the metatarsophalangeal [MTP] joints), wearing shoes that are too tight (or laced too tightly), trauma, or stress fractures of the metatarsals.
2. TrPs in the EDB and EHB may produce decreased flexion of the toes at the MTP joints, cramps in the foot, or an antalgic gait.
3. The referral patterns of EDB and EHB TrPs must be distinguished from the referral patterns of TrPs in the extensor digitorum longus, fibularis tertius, tibialis anterior, plantar and dorsal interossei pedis, and lumbricals pedis.
4. TrPs in the EDB and EHB may be incorrectly assessed as a metatarsal stress fracture or entrapment of a digital nerve between adjacent metatarsals.
5. Associated TrPs often occur in the extensor digitorum longus or extensor hallucis longus.
6. Note: The EDB and EHB share the same TrP pain referral pattern.

Figure 20-7 Anterolateral (dorsolateral) view showing common TrPs and their corresponding referral zone for the extensors digitorum and hallucis brevis.

STRETCHING THE EDB AND EHB

A

B

Figure 20-8 Stretches of the right extensor digitorum brevis (EDB) and extensor hallucis brevis (EHB). **A,** Stretch of the EDB in which the proximal, middle, and distal phalanges of toes two to four are flexed. **B,** Stretch of the EHB in which the proximal phalanx of the big toe is flexed.

Palpation Key:
Look for the bulge of the EDB and EHB laterally on the dorsum of the foot.

DORSAL INTEROSSEI PEDIS (DIP)—SUPINE

There are four dorsal interossei pedis muscles, numbered one to four from medial to lateral, respectively.

❏ ATTACHMENTS:

o Proximally, each dorsal interosseus pedis (DIP) attaches to both sides of the adjacent metatarsals.
o Distally, each one attaches to one side of the proximal phalanx of a toe (the side away from the center of the second toe), and to the tendon of the extensor digitorum longus to that toe.

❏ ACTIONS:

o Abduct and flex toes two to four at the metatarsophalan-geal (MTP) joints
o Extend toes two to four at the proximal and distal inter-phalangeal joints

Starting position (Figure 20-10, A):

o Client supine
o Therapist is seated to the side of the client
o Palpating fingers placed on the dorsal side of the foot between the fourth and fifth metatarsal bones
o Fingers of support hand placed on the lateral side of the proximal phalanx of the fourth toe

Palpation steps:

1. Fourth dorsal interosseus pedis (DIP): Ask the client to abduct the fourth toe against your resistance and feel for the contraction of the fourth DIP between the fourth and fifth metatarsals (Figure 20-10, A).
2. Palpate the fourth DIP proximally and distally while the client alternately contracts against your resistance and relaxes the muscle.
3. Third DIP: Repeat this procedure for the third DIP by pal-pating on the dorsal surface of the foot between the third and fourth metatarsals and resisting the client from abducting the third toe (Figure 20-10, B).
4. Second DIP: Repeat this procedure for the second DIP by palpating on the dorsal surface of the foot between the second and third metatarsals and resisting the client from performing fibular abduction of the second toe (Figure 20-10, C).
5. First DIP: Repeat this procedure for the first DIP by palpating on the dorsal surface of the foot between the first and second metatarsals and resisting the client from performing tibial abduction of the second toe (Figure 20-10, D).
6. Once each DIP has been located, have the client relax it and palpate to assess its baseline tone.

Extensor digitorum longus tendons and dorsal digital expansion

Figure 20-9 Dorsal view of the right dorsal interossei pedis.

20

DORSAL INTEROSSEI PEDIS (DIP)—SUPINE—cont'd

Figure 20-10 Palpation of the dorsal interossei pedis (DIP). **A**, Palpation of the fourth DIP as the client abducts the fourth toe against resistance. **B**, Palpation of the third DIP as the client abducts the third toe against resistance. **C**, Palpation of the second DIP as the client does fibular abduction of the second toe against resistance. **D**, Palpation of the first DIP as the client does tibial abduction of the second toe against resistance.

Palpation Notes:
1. The second toe abducts in both directions. Fibular abduction is moving it laterally (i.e., toward the fibula); tibial abduction is moving it medially (i.e., toward the tibia).
2. Many clients cannot isolate abduction of the toes, especially fibular versus tibial abduction of the second toe. If a client cannot isolate a motion to engage one of the dorsal interossei pedis (DIP) for palpation, then simply palpate the muscle in a relaxed state by its location.
3. Keep in mind that the extensor muscles of the toes (longus and brevis) lie superficial to the DIP. For this reason, it is important that the client does not attempt to extend the toes, or these extensor muscles will contract, making palpation and discernment of the DIP extremely difficult.

Alternate Position—Seated
The DIP can also be easily accessed with the client seated.

Palpation Key:
Palpate between the metatarsals on the dorsum of the foot.

DORSAL INTEROSSEI PEDIS (DIP)—SUPINE—cont'd

TRIGGER POINTS

1. Trigger points (TrPs) in the dorsal interossei pedis (DIP) often result from or are perpetuated by acute or chronic overuse of the muscle (e.g., walking in soft sand), sustained postures that cause the muscles to lengthen (e.g., wearing high-heeled shoes), wearing ill-fitting shoes (that are either too tight or laced too tightly, or have a pointed toe), wearing shoes with an inflexible sole (not allowing motion of the metatarsophalangeal [MTP] joints), immobilization due to a cast, excessive pronation of the foot (requiring greater stabilization by the intrinsic foot muscles), structural deformities of the foot, trauma, or stress fractures of the metatarsals.

2. TrPs in the DIP tend to produce pain in a vertical pattern along the dorsal and plantar sides of the ray (metatarsal and phalanges) to which the DIP attaches distally (Figure 20-11 shows the typical patterns for the first and fourth DIP muscles). DIP TrPs also tend to produce tender and sore feet (especially when weight bearing), pain when walking, decreased or painful adduction or extension of toes two to five at the MTP joints, cramps in the foot, or an antalgic gait. Furthermore, TrPs in the first DIP may produce tingling in the big toe.

3. The referral patterns of DIP TrPs must be distinguished from the referral patterns of TrPs in the flexor digitorum brevis, abductor digiti minimi pedis, adductor hallucis, plantar interossei, lumbricals pedis, extensor digitorum longus, and flexor digitorum longus.

4. TrPs in the DIP are often incorrectly assessed as plantar fasciitis, metatarsal stress fracture, entrapment of a digital nerve between adjacent metatarsals, or tarsal joint dysfunction.

5. Associated TrPs often occur in the plantar interossei and lumbricals pedis.

6. Note: The plantar interossei and lumbricals pedis share the same TrP pain referral patterns as the DIP.

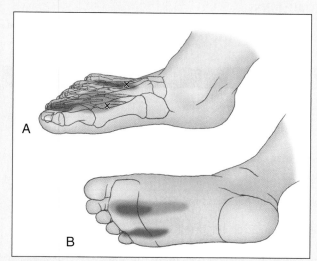

Figure 20-11 Views of common TrPs of the first and fourth dorsal interossei pedis (DIP) muscles and their corresponding referral zones. **A,** Medial view showing common TrPs and their corresponding referral zones. **B,** Medial-plantar view that shows the remainder of the referral zones. Note: TrPs commonly occur in all four DIP muscles.

STRETCHING THE DORSAL INTEROSSEI PEDIS (DIP)

Figure 20-12 Stretches of the four dorsal interossei pedis (DIP) muscles in which each toe is moved at the metatarsophalangeal joint. **A,** Stretch of the first DIP by moving the second toe into fibular abduction. **B,** Stretch of the second DIP by moving the second toe into tibial abduction. **C,** Stretch of the third DIP by moving the third toe into adduction. **D,** Stretch of the fourth DIP by moving the fourth toe into adduction.

20

ABDUCTOR HALLUCIS (AbH) AND FLEXOR HALLUCIS BREVIS (FHB)—PRONE

Abductor Hallucis (AbH):

❑ ATTACHMENTS:
o Tuberosity of the calcaneus *to the* medial plantar side of the base of the proximal phalanx of the big toe

❑ ACTIONS:
o Abducts and flexes the big toe at the metatarsophalangeal (MTP) joint

Flexor Hallucis Brevis (FHB):

❑ ATTACHMENTS:
o Cuboid and third cuneiform *to the* medial and lateral sides of the plantar surface of the base of the proximal phalanx of the big toe

❑ ACTIONS:
o Flexes the big toe at the MTP joint

Starting position (Figure 20-15):
o Client prone
o Therapist seated at the end of the table
o Palpating fingers placed on the medial side of the foot, close to the plantar surface

Palpation steps:
1. Begin by palpating the abductor hallucis, which is superficial and easily palpable.
2. Ask the client to abduct the big toe at the metatarsophalangeal (MTP) joint and feel for the contraction of the abductor hallucis. If desired, resistance can be given with the support hand on the medial side of the proximal phalanx of the big toe (Figure 20-16).
3. Once located, palpate it proximally and distally toward its attachments by strumming perpendicular to its fibers.
4. Once the abductor hallucis has been located, have the client relax it and palpate to assess its baseline tone.
5. To now palpate the flexor hallucis brevis, which is also superficial and easily palpable, move your palpating fingers over the first metatarsal bone on the plantar side of the foot.
6. Ask the client to flex the big toe at the MTP joint and feel for the contraction of the flexor hallucis brevis. If desired, resistance can be given with the support hand on the plantar surface of the proximal phalanx of the big toe (Figure 20-17).
7. Once located, palpate it distally to the proximal phalanx of the big toe by strumming perpendicular to its fibers. Then palpate it proximally as far as possible.
8. Once the flexor hallucis brevis has been located, have the client relax it and palpate to assess its baseline tone.

Figure 20-13 Plantar view of the right abductor hallucis.

Figure 20-14 Plantar view of the right flexor hallucis brevis.

20

ABDUCTOR HALLUCIS (AbH) AND FLEXOR HALLUCIS BREVIS (FHB)—PRONE—cont'd

Figure 20-15 Starting position for prone palpation of the right abductor hallucis.

Figure 20-17 Palpation of the right flexor hallucis brevis as the client flexes the big toe against resistance.

Figure 20-16 Palpation of the right abductor hallucis as the client abducts the big toe against resistance.

Abductor Hallucis Palpation Notes:

1. Abduction of the big toe at the MTP joint is a medial motion.
2. The entire abductor hallucis can usually be palpated and discerned.
3. Many clients are unable to isolate big toe abduction. If this occurs, place a finger of your support hand against the medial side of the proximal phalanx of the big toe and ask the client to press against it. Having the pressure of the resistance finger often helps the client create this motion.
4. If the client is still unable to perform abduction of the big toe against pressure (as in Palpation Note #3), then try resisting the client from flexing the proximal phalanx of the big toe at the MTP joint, feeling for the abductor hallucis to contract on the medial side of the foot. Have the client keep the interphalangeal joint of the big toe extended; otherwise flexion of the proximal phalanx of the big toe will be carried out by the flexor hallucis longus and the abductor hallucis will not contract. Note: The flexor hallucis brevis (FHB) will also contract with flexion of the big toe at the MTP joint, so be sure that you are not palpating too far onto the plantar surface of the foot.
5. Another method to discern the abductor hallucis from the FHB is to ask the client to abduct and extend the big toe at the MTP joint. Extension will reciprocally inhibit and relax the FHB.

20

ABDUCTOR HALLUCIS (AbH) AND FLEXOR HALLUCIS BREVIS (FHB)—PRONE—cont'd

Flexor Hallucis Brevis Palpation Notes:

1. Even though the FHB is in the second plantar layer of the foot, the vast majority of it is fairly easily palpable. The most challenging aspect to palpate is the proximal attachment at the cuboid and third cuneiform. If the client is able to isolate flexion of the big toe without also flexing the other toes, even this proximal attachment can usually be well palpated and discerned from the more superficial flexor digitorum brevis. However, many clients cannot isolate this motion.

2. It does not help to stop toes two to five from flexing with the fingers of your support hand, because even though these other toes might not move, the belly of the flexor digitorum brevis that we want to be relaxed will still contract (isometri-

cally), making it more difficult to palpate the proximal attachment of the FHB through it.

3. Directly superficial to the FHB is the distal tendon of the flexor hallucis longus. Given that both these muscles contract with flexion of the big toe, it can be difficult to discern them from each other.

4. To discern the FHB from the more superficial distal tendon of the flexor hallucis longus, try to have the client isolate flexion of the big toe at the MTP joint while keeping the interphalangeal joint of the big toe extended. This will tend to engage the FHB more than the flexor hallucis longus. However, many clients are unable to do this.

Alternate Position—Supine

Both the abductor hallucis and flexor hallucis brevis can also be easily palpated with the client supine.

TRIGGER POINTS

1. Trigger points (TrPs) in the abductor hallucis (AbH) and flexor hallucis brevis (FHB) often result from or are perpetuated by acute or chronic overuse of the muscle (e.g., walking in soft sand), sustained postures that cause the muscles to lengthen (e.g., wearing high-heeled shoes), wearing ill-fitting shoes (that are either too tight or laced too tightly, or have a pointed toe), wearing shoes with an inflexible sole (not allowing motion of the metatarsophalangeal [MTP] joint), immobilization due to a cast, excessive pronation of the foot (requiring greater stabilization by the intrinsic foot muscles), structural deformities of the foot, trauma, or stress fractures of the metatarsals.

2. TrPs in the AbH and FHB tend to produce tender and sore feet (especially when weight bearing), pain when walking, decreased or painful adduction (AbH) or extension (FHB or AbH) of the big toe at the MTP joint, cramps in the foot, or an antalgic gait. Furthermore, the AbH may produce entrapment of the posterior tibial nerve and/or its two branches, the medial and lateral plantar nerves (resulting in sensory symptoms on the plantar surface of the foot and/or weakness of the intrinsic muscles of the sole of the foot).

3. The referral patterns of AbH TrPs must be distinguished from the referral patterns of TrPs in the plantar interossei, dorsal interossei pedis, and lumbricals pedis between the first and second toes, quadratus plantae, and medial head of the gastrocnemius. The referral patterns of FHB TrPs must be distinguished from the referral patterns of TrPs in the flexor hallucis longus, adductor hallucis, tibialis anterior, and extensor hallucis longus.

4. TrPs in the AbH are often incorrectly assessed as calcaneal (Achilles) tendinitis or tarsal joint dysfunction. TrPs in the FHB are often incorrectly assessed as gout, plantar fasciitis, metatarsal stress fracture, or tarsal joint dysfunction.

5. Associated TrPs for the AbH often occur in the FHB and flexor digitorum brevis. Associated TrPs for the FHB often occur in the AbH, quadratus plantae, and flexor digitorum longus.

Figure 20-18 A, Medial-plantar view showing common abductor hallucis TrPs and their corresponding referral zone. **B** and **C**, Plantar and medial views, respectively, of common flexor hallucis brevis TrPs and their corresponding referral zones.

ABDUCTOR HALLUCIS (AbH) AND FLEXOR HALLUCIS BREVIS (FHB)—PRONE—cont'd

STRETCHING THE AbH AND FHB

A

B

Palpation Keys:

Abductor hallucis: Palpate on the medial side of the foot, strumming up and down. Flexor hallucis brevis: Palpate over the plantar surface of the first metatarsal while flexing the big toe.

Figure 20-19 Stretches of the abductor hallucis and flexor hallucis brevis muscles at the metatarsophalangeal joint. **A**, Stretch of the abductor hallucis in which the big toe is adducted and extended. **B**, Stretch of the flexor hallucis brevis in which the big toe is extended.

20

ABDUCTOR HALLUCIS (AbH) AND FLEXOR HALLUCIS BREVIS (FHB)—PRONE—cont'd

DETOUR

Adductor Hallucis: The adductor hallucis has two heads, an oblique head and a transverse head, and attaches from metatarsals two to four, the tendon of the fibularis longus, and the plantar metatarsophalangeal ligaments to the proximal phalanx of the big toe. Its actions are adduction and flexion of the big toe at the metatarsophalangeal joint. It is deep to the plantar fascia and the flexor digitorum brevis. Given its depth and the difficulty that most clients have isolating adduction of the big toe, this muscle can be challenging to palpate and discern. When palpating this muscle, palpate over the heads of the metatarsals of the second, third, and fourth toes while resisting the client from adducting the big toe and feel for the contraction of the transverse head. Try to palpate the oblique head in a similar manner.

Trigger Points:
1. Trigger points (TrPs) in the adductor hallucis usually result from the same factors that create or perpetuate TrPs in the abductor hallucis and flexor hallucis brevis.
2. TrPs in the adductor hallucis often produce sore feet that cause pain when weight bearing and walking, antalgic gait, cramps, decreased abduction or extension of the big toe, or numbness in its TrP referral area.
3. The referral patterns of adductor hallucis TrPs must be distinguished from the referral patterns of TrPs in the flexor digitorum brevis, flexor and abductor digiti minimi pedis, flexor hallucis brevis, plantar and dorsal interossei pedis, lumbricals pedis, flexor digitorum longus, and flexor hallucis longus.
4. TrPs in the adductor hallucis are often incorrectly assessed as plantar fasciitis, metatarsal stress fracture, or tarsal joint dysfunction.
5. Associated TrPs often occur in the flexor hallucis brevis and abductor hallucis.

Figure 20-20 Views of the right adductor hallucis. **A,** Plantar view of the adductor hallucis.
B, Plantar view showing common adductor hallucis TrPs and their corresponding referral zone.
C, Stretch of the adductor hallucis in which the big toe is abducted away from the second toe and also slightly extended.

20

ABDUCTOR DIGITI MINIMI PEDIS (ADMP) AND FLEXOR DIGITI MINIMI PEDIS (FDMP)—PRONE

Abductor Digiti Minimi Pedis:

❏ **ATTACHMENTS:**

o Tuberosity of the calcaneus *to the* lateral plantar side of the proximal phalanx of the little toe

❏ **ACTIONS:**

o Abducts and flexes the little toe at the metatarsophalangeal (MTP) joint

Flexor Digiti Minimi Pedis:

❏ **ATTACHMENTS:**

o The plantar surface of the base of the fifth metatarsal and the tendon of the fibularis longus *to the* plantar surface of the base of the proximal phalanx of the little toe

❏ **ACTIONS:**

o Flexes the little toe at the MTP joint

Starting position (Figure 20-23):

o Client prone
o Therapist seated at the end of the table
o Palpating fingers placed on the lateral side of the distal foot, close to the plantar surface

Palpation steps:

1. Begin by palpating the abductor digiti minimi pedis, which is superficial and easily palpable.
2. Ask the client to abduct the little toe at the metatarsophalangeal (MTP) joint and feel for the contraction of the abductor digiti minimi pedis (ADMP). If desired, resistance can be given by placing fingers of the support hand on the lateral side of the proximal phalanx of the little toe (Figure 20-24).
3. Once located, palpate it proximally and distally toward its attachments by strumming perpendicular to its fibers.
4. Once the ADMP has been located, have the client relax it and palpate to assess its baseline tone.
5. To now palpate the flexor digiti minimi pedis, which is also superficial and easily palpable, move your palpating fingers over the fifth metatarsal bone on the plantar side of the foot.
6. Ask the client to flex the little toe at the metatarsophalangeal (MTP) joint and feel for the contraction of the flexor digiti minimi pedis (FDMP). If desired, resistance can be given with the support hand on the plantar surface of the proximal phalanx of the little toe (Figure 20-25).
7. Once located, palpate it distally to the proximal phalanx of the little toe by strumming perpendicular to its fibers. Then palpate it proximally as far as possible.
8. Once the FDMP has been located, have the client relax it and palpate to assess its baseline tone.

Figure 20-21 Plantar view of the right abductor digiti minimi pedis.

Fibularis longus tendon

Figure 20-22 Plantar view of the right flexor digiti minimi pedis.

20

ABDUCTOR DIGITI MINIMI PEDIS (ADMP) AND FLEXOR DIGITI MINIMI PEDIS (FDMP)—PRONE—cont'd

Figure 20-23 Starting position for prone palpation of the right abductor digiti minimi pedis.

Figure 20-25 Palpation of the right flexor digiti minimi pedis as the client flexes the little toe against resistance.

Figure 20-24 Palpation of the right abductor digiti minimi pedis as the client abducts the little toe against resistance.

Abductor Digiti Minimi Pedis (ADMP) Palpation Notes:

1. The ADMP is superficial and easily palpable.
2. Abduction of the little toe at the MTP joint is a lateral motion.
3. Although all of the ADMP can usually be palpated and discerned, it is easiest to palpate it in the distal half of the foot.
4. Many clients are unable to isolate the motion of abduction of the little toe. If this occurs, place a finger of your support hand against the lateral side of the proximal phalanx of the little toe and ask the client to press against it. Having the pressure of the resistance finger often helps the client create this motion.
5. To discern the border of the ADMP from the flexor digiti minimi pedis, make sure that the client is not flexing the little toe as abduction is done. If necessary, the client can be asked to abduct and extend the little toe at the MTP joint. Extension will reciprocally inhibit and relax the flexor digiti minimi pedis.

20

ABDUCTOR DIGITI MINIMI PEDIS (ADMP) AND FLEXOR DIGITI MINIMI PEDIS (FDMP)—PRONE—cont'd

Flexor Digiti Minimi Pedis Palpation Notes:

1. The flexor digitorum brevis and the tendon of the flexor digitorum longus to the little toe lie superficial to the FDMP. For this reason, it can be difficult to discern the FDMP from these other muscles because they also contract when the little toe flexes.
2. To discern the FDMP from the more superficial flexors digitorum brevis and longus, try to have the client isolate flexion of the little toe at the MTP joint while keeping the interphalangeal joints of the little toe extended. This will tend to engage the FDMP more than the flexors digitorum brevis and longus. Unfortunately, most clients are unable to do this.

Alternate Position—Supine

Both the abductor and flexor digiti minimi pedis can also be easily accessed with the client supine.

Palpation Key:

Abductor digiti minimi pedis: Palpate on the lateral side of the foot, strumming up and down.
Flexor digiti minimi pedis: Palpate over the plantar surface of the fifth metatarsal while flexing the little toe.

TRIGGER POINTS

1. Trigger points (TrPs) in the abductor digiti minimi pedis (ADMP) and flexor digiti minimi pedis (FDMP) often result from or are perpetuated by acute or chronic overuse of the muscle (e.g., walking in soft sand), sustained postures that cause the muscles to lengthen (e.g., wearing high-heeled shoes), wearing ill-fitting shoes (that are either too tight or laced too tightly, or have a pointed toe), wearing shoes with an inflexible sole (not allowing motion of the metatarsophalangeal [MTP] joint), immobilization due to a cast, excessive pronation of the foot (requiring greater stabilization by the intrinsic foot muscles), structural deformities of the foot, trauma, or stress fractures of the metatarsals.
2. TrPs in the ADMP and FDMP tend to produce tender and sore feet (especially when weight bearing), pain when walking, decreased or painful adduction (ADMP) or extension (FDMP or ADMP) of the little toe at the MTP joint, cramps in the foot, or an antalgic gait.
3. The referral patterns of ADMP and FDMP TrPs must be distinguished from the referral patterns of TrPs in the flexor digitorum brevis, plantar interossei, dorsal interossei pedis, and lumbricals pedis between the fourth and fifth toes, adductor hallucis, and flexor digitorum longus.
4. TrPs in the ADMP and FDMP are often incorrectly assessed as plantar fasciitis, metatarsal stress fracture, or tarsal joint dysfunction.
5. Associated TrPs often occur in the flexor digitorum brevis.
6. Note: The ADMP and FDMP share the same TrP pain referral pattern.

Figure 20-26 Plantar view showing common TrPs and their corresponding referral zone in the abductor and flexor digiti minimi pedis muscles.

ABDUCTOR DIGITI MINIMI PEDIS (ADMP) AND FLEXOR DIGITI MINIMI PEDIS (FDMP)—PRONE—cont'd

STRETCHING THE ABDUCTOR DIGITI MINIMI PEDIS AND FLEXOR DIGITI MINIMI PEDIS

Figure 20-27 Stretches of the abductor and flexor digiti minimi pedis muscles at the metatarsophalangeal joint. **A**, Stretch of the abductor digiti minimi pedis in which the little toe is adducted and extended. **B**, Stretch of the flexor digiti minimi pedis in which the little toe is extended.

A

B

20

ABDUCTOR DIGITI MINIMI PEDIS (ADMP) AND FLEXOR DIGITI MINIMI PEDIS (FDMP)—PRONE—cont'd

DETOUR ▶

Lumbricals Pedis: There are four lumbricals pedis muscles, numbered one to four from medial to lateral. Even though they are located in the second plantar layer of the foot, they are fairly accessible to palpation. They attach from the distal tendons of the flexor digitorum longus to the distal tendons of the extensor digitorum longus (Figure 20-28, A). They flex toes two to five at the metatarsophalangeal (MTP) joints and extend them at the interphalangeal (IP) joints. To palpate these muscles, palpate between the metatarsal bones. If the client is able to flex toes two to five at the MTP joints while keeping them extended at the IP joints, ask the client to do this and feel for their contraction. To stretch the lumbricals pedis, move toes two to five into extension at the MTP joints and flexion at the IP joints (Figure 20-28, B).

Plantar Interossei: There are three plantar interossei (PI) muscles, numbered one to three from medial to lateral. The plantar interossei attach from metatarsals three to five to the medial side of the proximal phalanges of toes three to five (Figure 20-28, C) and are located deep to the lumbricals pedis; parts of them are also deep to the flexor digitorum brevis as well as the plantar fascia. Their main action is to adduct toes three to five at the MTP joints; however, many clients are unable to isolate their action of toe adduction. Given their depth and the difficulty of isolating their action, the plantar

interossei are usually difficult to palpate and discern from adjacent soft tissues. To stretch them, move toes three to five into abduction (away from the second toe) at the MTP joints (Figure 20-28, D).

Trigger Points:
1. Trigger points (TrPs) in the lumbricals pedis and plantar interossei usually result from the same factors that create or perpetuate TrPs in the abductor and flexor digiti minimi pedis muscles, and they produce approximately the same symptoms.
2. As with many intrinsic foot muscles of the plantar side, TrPs in the lumbricals pedis and plantar interossei tend to produce tender and sore feet (especially when weight bearing), pain when walking, decreased or painful extension of the affected toe at the MTP joint, cramps in the foot, or an antalgic gait.
3. Lumbricals pedis and plantar interossei TrP referral patterns are the same as for the dorsal interossei pedis (see page 497), and their TrPs are often incorrectly assessed as plantar fasciitis, metatarsal stress fracture, tarsal joint dysfunction, or entrapment of a digital nerve between adjacent metatarsals.
4. Associated TrPs often occur in the flexor digitorum brevis, flexor hallucis brevis, and flexor digiti minimi pedis.

Flexor digitorum longus tendon

Quadratus plantae

PI#3
PI#2
PI#1

A   B   C   D

20

Figure 20-28 Views of the right lumbricals pedis and plantar interossei muscles. **A,** Plantar view of the lumbricals pedis; the quadratus plantae is ghosted in. **B,** Stretch of the lumbricals pedis. Toes two to five are extended at the metatarsophalangeal (MTP) joints and flexed at the interphalangeal joints. **C,** Plantar view of the plantar interossei; the dorsal interossei pedis are ghosted in. **D,** Stretch of the plantar interossei. Toes three to five are abducted at the MTP joints.

FLEXOR DIGITORUM BREVIS—PRONE

❑ **ATTACHMENTS:**

o Tuberosity of the calcaneus *to the* plantar surface of the middle phalanges of toes two to five

❑ **ACTIONS:**

o Flexes toes two to five at the metatarsophalangeal (MTP) and proximal interphalangeal joints

Starting position (Figure 20-30):

o Client prone
o Therapist seated at the end of the table
o Palpating fingers placed on the midline of the plantar surface of the proximal foot.
o If resistance is necessary, place fingers of the support hand on the plantar surface of the proximal or middle phalanges of toes two to five

Palpation steps:

1. Ask the client to flex toes two to five at the metatarsophalangeal (MTP) joints and feel for the contraction of the flexor digitorum brevis. If desired, resistance can be given with the support hand (Figure 20-31).
2. Once located, palpate it proximally to the calcaneus by strumming perpendicular to its fibers. Then palpate it distally as far as possible.
3. Once the flexor digitorum brevis has been located, have the client relax it and palpate to assess its baseline tone.

Figure 20-29 Plantar view of the right flexor digitorum brevis.

Figure 20-30 Starting position for prone palpation of the right flexor digitorum brevis.

Figure 20-31 Palpation of the right flexor digitorum brevis as the client flexes toes two to five against resistance.

FLEXOR DIGITORUM BREVIS—PRONE—cont'd

Palpation Notes:

1. Even though the flexor digitorum brevis is deep to the plantar fascia, the contraction of its belly can usually be fairly easily palpated.

2. Directly deep to the flexor digitorum brevis are the distal tendons of the flexor digitorum longus. Given that both these muscles contract with flexion of toes two to five, it can be difficult to discern them from each other. This is especially true in the distal end of the foot where the tendons of the flexor digitorum brevis directly overlie the tendons of the flexor digitorum longus.

3. To discern the flexor digitorum brevis from the deeper distal tendons of the flexor digitorum longus, try to have the client isolate flexion of the toes at the metatarsophalangeal joints while keeping the interphalangeal joints extended. This will tend to engage the flexor digitorum brevis more than the flexor digitorum longus. Unfortunately, many clients are unable to isolate this action.

4. The quadratus plantae muscle is located directly deep to the flexor digitorum brevis in the proximal foot and also flexes toes two to five. Therefore these two muscles can be difficult to discern from each other.

Alternate Position—Supine

The flexor digitorum brevis can also be fairly easily palpated with the client supine.

Palpation Key:
Palpate in the center of the proximal plantar foot while flexing the toes.

TRIGGER POINTS

1. Trigger points (TrPs) in the flexor digitorum brevis (FDB) often result from or are perpetuated by acute or chronic overuse of the muscle (e.g., walking in soft sand), sustained postures that cause the muscles to lengthen (e.g., wearing high-heeled shoes), wearing ill-fitting shoes (that are either too tight or laced too tightly, or have a pointed toe), wearing shoes with an inflexible sole (not allowing motion of the metatarsophalangeal [MTP] joints), immobilization due to a cast, excessive pronation of the foot (requiring greater stabilization by the intrinsic foot muscles), structural deformities of the foot, trauma, or stress fractures of the metatarsals.

2. TrPs in the FDB tend to produce tender and sore feet (especially when weight bearing), pain when walking, decreased or painful extension of toes two to five at the MTP joints, plantar fasciitis, cramps in the foot, or an antalgic gait.

3. The referral pattern of FDB TrPs must be distinguished from the referral patterns of TrPs in the adductor hallucis, flexor digitorum longus, flexor hallucis longus, abductor digiti minimi pedis, flexor hallucis brevis, and plantar interossei, dorsal interossei pedis, and lumbricals pedis.

4. TrPs in the FDB are often incorrectly assessed as plantar fasciitis, metatarsal stress fracture, or tarsal joint dysfunction.

5. Associated TrPs often occur in the flexor digitorum longus, flexor hallucis brevis, and flexor digiti minimi pedis.

Figure 20-32 Plantar view showing common flexor digitorum brevis TrPs and their corresponding referral zone.

YOU ARE HERE

FLEXOR DIGITORUM BREVIS—PRONE—cont'd

STRETCHING THE FLEXOR DIGITORUM BREVIS

Figure 20-33 A stretch of the flexor digitorum brevis in which the proximal and middle phalanges of toes two to five are extended at the metatarsophalangeal and proximal interphalangeal joints.

DETOUR

Quadratus Plantae: The quadratus plantae attaches from the calcaneus to the distal tendon of the flexor digitorum longus. To palpate this muscle, palpate on the midline of the plantar surface of the proximal foot and ask the client to flex toes two to five. Because the quadratus plantae lies immediately deep to the flexor digitorum brevis, and both these muscles flex toes two to five, it can be very difficult to palpate and discern the quadratus plantae from the flexor digitorum brevis.

Trigger Points:

1. Trigger points (TrPs) in the quadratus plantae usually result from the same factors that create or perpetuate TrPs in the flexor digitorum brevis. (However, their referral zones are quite different.)
2. The referral pattern for quadratus plantae TrPs must be distinguished from the referral patterns of TrPs in the soleus and abductor hallucis.
3. Associated TrPs often occur in the flexor digitorum brevis and flexor digitorum longus.

Flexor digitorum longus tendon

A

B

Figure 20-34 Views of the right quadratus plantae. **A,** Planter view of the quadratus plantae. **B,** Medial-plantar view showing a common quadratus plantae TrP and its corresponding referral zone.

20

Intrinsic Muscles of the Foot

Client Supine:

For the palpations of the following intrinsic muscles of the foot on the dorsal side, the client is supine with a roll under the knees and you are seated to the side of the client.

1. **Extensor digitorum brevis (EDB) and extensor hallucis brevis (EHB):** Visualize, locate, and palpate the belly of the EDB and EHB just distal to the lateral malleolus on the dorsal foot. Feel for its contraction as the client extends toes two to four at the metatarsophalangeal (MTP) and interphalangeal (IP) joints and the big toe at the MTP joint. The EDB fibers are located more laterally within the common belly, and the EHB fibers are located more medially within the common belly. Once the contraction is felt, continue palpating each of the tendons distally to its attachment on a toe by strumming perpendicular to it as the client alternately contracts and relaxes the muscle. Resistance can be added if needed.

2. **Dorsal interossei pedis (DIP):** Palpate between the metatarsals on the dorsal foot. To confirm that you are on a DIP muscle, ask the client to abduct the toe to which that muscle is attached. The fourth DIP between metatarsals four and five abducts the fourth toe; the third DIP between metatarsals three and four abducts the third toe; the second DIP between metatarsals two and three does fibular abduction of the second toe; and the first DIP between metatarsals one and two does tibial abduction of the second toe. Palpate proximally and distally as far as possible. Resistance can be added if needed.

Client Prone:

For the palpations of the following intrinsic muscles of the foot on the plantar side, the client is prone with a bolster under the ankles and you are seated at the end of the table.

3. **Abductor hallucis (AbH):** Palpate on the medial side of the foot, close to the plantar surface, and feel for the contraction of the belly of the AbH as the client abducts the big toe at the MTP joint. Once located, palpate proximally and distally as far as possible by strumming perpendicular to its fibers. Resistance can be added if needed.

4. **Abductor digiti minimi pedis (ADMP):** Palpate on the lateral side of the foot, close to the plantar surface, and feel for the contraction of the belly of the ADMP as the client abducts the little toe at the MTP joint. Once located, palpate proximally and distally as far as possible by strumming perpendicular to its fibers. Resistance can be added if needed.

5. **Flexor digitorum brevis (FDB):** Palpate on the midline of the plantar surface of the proximal foot and feel for the contraction of the belly of the FDB as the client flexes toes two to five at the MTP and proximal interphalangeal (PIP) joints. Once located, palpate proximally to the calcaneus and distally as far as possible by strumming perpendicular to the fibers. Resistance can be added if needed. Detour: The quadratus plantae may be palpated in the midline of the proximal plantar foot as the client flexes toes two to five. However, it is deep to the FDB and difficult to discern from this muscle.

6. **Flexor hallucis brevis (FHB):** Palpate over the first metatarsal on the plantar side of the foot and feel for the contraction of the FHB as the client flexes the big toe at the MTP joint. Once located, palpate as far proximally and distally as possible by strumming perpendicular to its fibers. Resistance can be added if needed.

7. **Flexor digiti minimi pedis (FDMP):** Palpate over the fifth metatarsal on the plantar side of the foot and feel for the contraction of the FDMP as the client flexes the little toe at the MTP joint. Once located, palpate proximally and distally as far as possible by strumming perpendicular to its fibers. Resistance can be added if needed. Detour(s): (1) The lumbricals pedis can be palpated between the metatarsals in the plantar foot. If the client is able, ask the client to flex toes two to five at the MTP joints while keeping them extended at the IP joints. (2) The plantar interossei are extremely difficult to palpate and discern. To attempt to palpate them, ask the client to adduct toes three to five as you palpate between metatarsals two to five in the plantar foot.

20

INDEX

Page numbers followed by *f* indicate figure; *t*, tables; *b*, boxes.